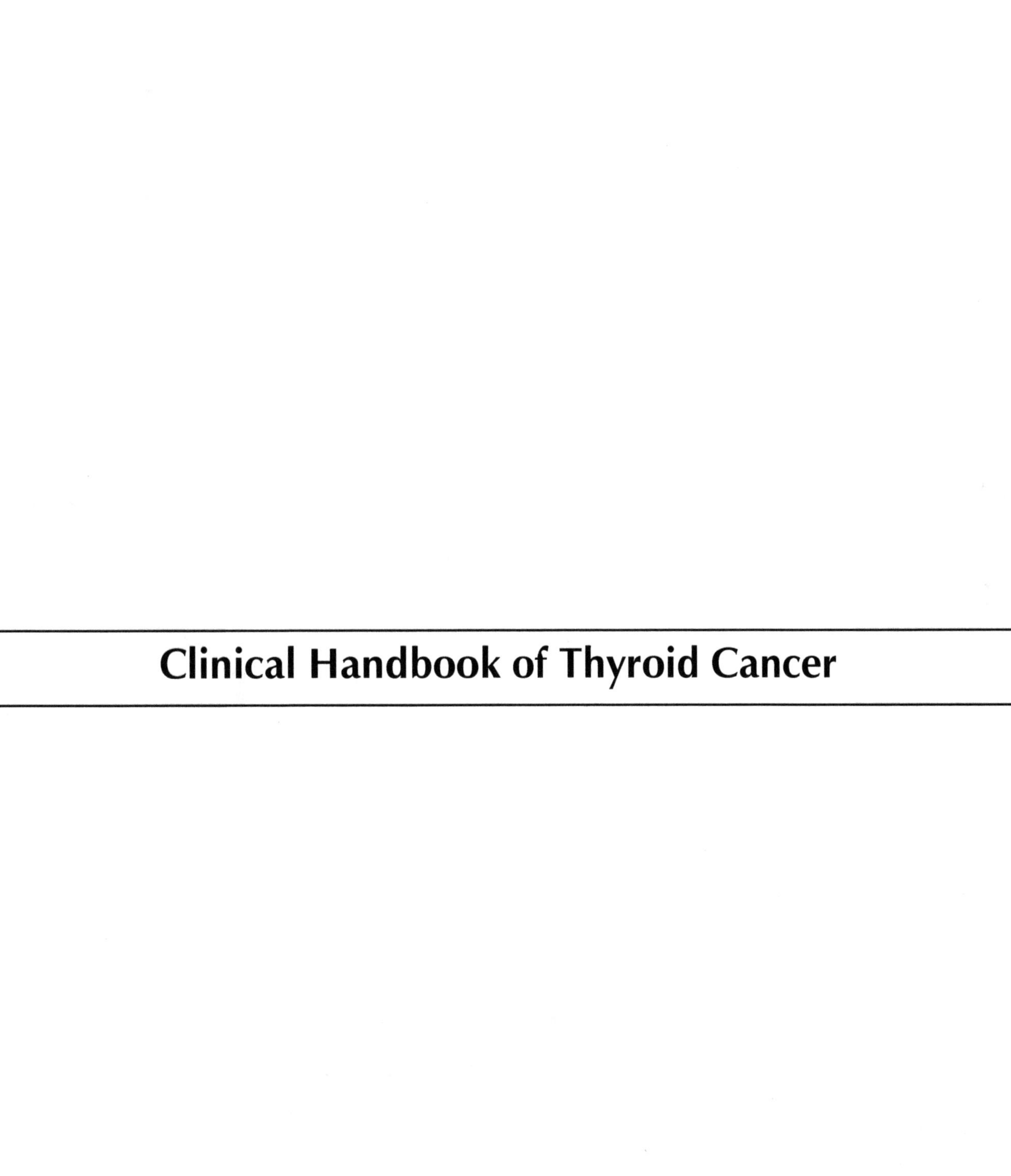

Clinical Handbook of Thyroid Cancer

Clinical Handbook of Thyroid Cancer

Editor: Nell Bingham

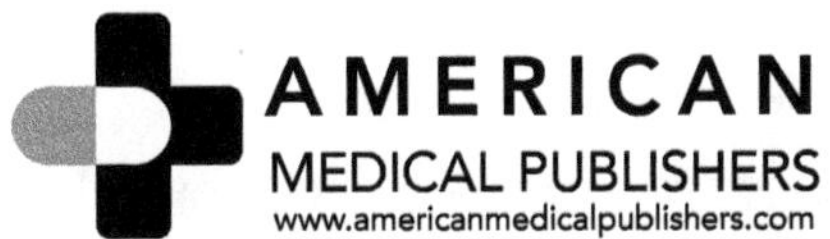

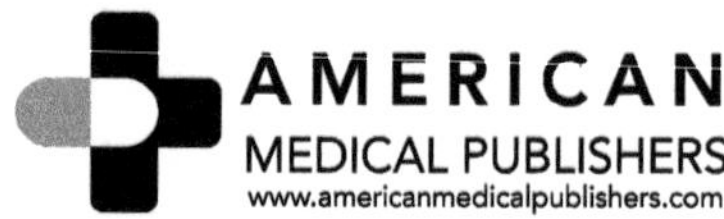

Cataloging-in-Publication Data

Clinical handbook of thyroid cancer / edited by Nell Bingham.
p. cm.
Includes bibliographical references and index.
ISBN 978-1-63927-636-3
1. Thyroid gland--Cancer. 2. Thyroid gland--Cancer--Diagnosis.
3. Thyroid gland--Cancer--Treatment. I. Bingham, Nell.
RC280.T6 C55 2023
616.994 44--dc23

American Medical Publishers,
41 Flatbush Avenue,
1st Floor, New York,
NY 11217, USA

ISBN 978-1-63927-636-3 (Hardback)

Contents

Preface

Every book is a source of knowledge and this one is no exception. The idea that led to the conceptualization of this book was the fact that the world is advancing rapidly; which makes it crucial to document the progress in every field. I am aware that a lot of data is already available, yet, there is a lot more to learn. Hence, I accepted the responsibility of editing this book and contributing my knowledge to the community.

Thyroid cancer refers to a type of cancer which grows from the tissues of the thyroid gland. It is a condition in which cells develop unusually and can spread to other parts of the body. A protrusion or swelling in the neck are its common symptoms. There are several risk factors of thyroid cancer, including a family history, radiation exposure at a young age and having an enlarged thyroid. There are four major types of thyroid cancer, namely, medullary thyroid cancer, papillary thyroid cancer, anaplastic thyroid cancer and follicular thyroid cancer. Fine needle aspiration and ultrasound are frequently used for its diagnosis. There are several treatment options available for thyroid cancer, such as chemotherapy, targeted therapy, surgery, and thyroid hormone and radiation therapy. Surgery can include the removal of all or a part of the thyroid gland. This book provides comprehensive insights on thyroid cancer. It is appropriate for students seeking detailed information in this area as well as for experts.

While editing this book, I had multiple visions for it. Then I finally narrowed down to make every chapter a sole standing text explaining a particular topic, so that they can be used independently. However, the umbrella subject sinews them into a common theme. This makes the book a unique platform of knowledge.

I would like to give the major credit of this book to the experts from every corner of the world, who took the time to share their expertise with us. Also, I owe the completion of this book to the never-ending support of my family, who supported me throughout the project.

Editor

1

Differentiated Thyroid Cancer—Treatment: State of the Art

Benedikt Schmidbauer †, Karin Menhart †, Dirk Hellwig and Jirka Grosse *

Department of Nuclear Medicine, University of Regensburg, 93053 Regensburg, Germany; benedikt.schmidbauer@ukr.de (B.S.); karin.menhart@ukr.de (K.M.); dirk.hellwig@ukr.de (D.H.)

* Correspondence: jirka.grosse@ukr.de

† These authors contributed equally to this work.

Abstract: Differentiated thyroid cancer (DTC) is a rare malignant disease, although its incidence has increased over the last few decades. It derives from follicular thyroid cells. Generally speaking, the prognosis is excellent. If treatment according to the current guidelines is given, cases of recurrence or persistence are rare. DTC requires special expertise by the treating physician. In recent years, new therapeutic options for these patients have become available. For this article we performed a systematic literature review with special focus on the guidelines of the American Thyroid Association, the European Association of Nuclear Medicine, and the German Society of Nuclear Medicine. For DTC, surgery and radioiodine therapy followed by levothyroxine substitution remain the established therapeutic procedures. Even metastasized tumors can be cured this way. However, in rare cases of radioiodine-refractory tumors, additional options are to be discussed. These include strict suppression of thyroid-stimulating hormone (also known as thyrotropin, TSH) and external local radiotherapy. Systemic cytostatic chemotherapy does not play a significant role. Recently, multikinase or tyrosine kinase inhibitors have been approved for the treatment of radioiodine-refractory DTC. Although a benefit for overall survival has not been shown yet, these new drugs can slow down tumor progression. However, they are frequently associated with severe side effects and should be reserved for patients with threatening symptoms only.

Keywords: differentiated thyroid cancer; radioiodine therapy; targeted therapy; tyrosine kinase inhibitors

---

1. Introduction

Patients with differentiated thyroid carcinoma have an excellent prognosis. The multimodal therapeutic approach is risk-adapted to achieve optimal treatment of differentiated thyroid cancer (DTC) and to minimize treatment-related morbidity. The treatment includes surgery (near-/total thyroidectomy) usually followed by remnant ablation using radioiodine according to the guidelines of the American Thyroid Association (ATA) and European Association of Nuclear Medicine (EANM) as well as a risk-stratified follow-up including hormone substitution.

However, in patients with primary or secondary radioiodine-refractory thyroid carcinoma the prognosis becomes significantly poorer. External beam irradiation may be used for locoregional control. Receptor tyrosine kinase inhibitors (TKIs) have shown clinical effectiveness in iodine-refractory DTC.

In this review, we present the current state of treatment of DTC.

2. Epidemiology and Classification

DTC is a rare disease with mostly excellent prognosis. The appearance of DTC depends on age, sex, family history, radiation exposure and many other factors [1]. DTC occurs in 7–15% of patients with thyroid surgery. In the year 2014, approximately 63,000 new cases of DTC were diagnosed in the

US [2] compared to 2009 with only 31,200 new cases. In Germany there are about 6000 new cases of DTC per year. The growing incidence of thyroid cancer and the tumor shift to diagnosis of smaller tumors is due to the increased usage of diagnostic methods, such as ultrasound of the neck [3].

Differentiated thyroid cancer includes papillary and follicular cancer that derive from thyrocytes and express the sodium iodine symporter. DTC represents the majority (90%) of all types of thyroid cancer [4]. One study predicts that papillary thyroid cancer will become the third most expensive cancer in women, with costs of US$ 19–21 billion in the US in 2019 [5].

Worldwide, there are many clinical practice guidelines for diagnosis, therapy and follow-up of DTC. The European Thyroid Association (ETA) published new guidelines for the management of DTC in 2013 [6]. The Society for Nuclear Medicine and Molecular Imaging and European Association of Nuclear Medicine published their most recent guidelines for radioiodine therapy of differentiated thyroid cancer in 2012 and 2008, respectively [7,8]. The Japanese Association of Endocrine Surgeons and the Japanese Society of Thyroid Surgeons recently reviewed their guidelines in 2014 [9]. The new ATA guidelines for management of differentiated thyroid cancer for adults were published in 2015 [10]. The updated ATA guidelines for management of DTC for children were also published in 2015 [11].

The risk classification of DTC using multiple staging systems is based on a combination of the size of the primary tumor, specific histology, extrathyroidal spread of the tumor and the age at diagnosis. It helps to predict the risk of local recurrence and developing metastases and the mortality in patients with DTC. The TNM classification depends on the size of primary tumor, the number and localization of metastatic lymph nodes and number of distant metastases (Table 1) [12]. The American Joint Committee on Cancer (AJCC) uses the combination of TNM Classification and an age of more than 55 years at diagnosis as risk factor [13]. The differentiation of lymphatic invasion and angioinvasion is of high importance, because angioinvasion is associated with an intermediate risk of recurrence. A common risk-stratification of DTC is based on the TNM classification (see also Section 4.2) [14]:

- high-risk group: pT3, pT4, each N1, all M1;
- low-risk group: pT1b, pT2, cN0/pN0, cM0;
- very low risk-group: pT1a, cN0/pN0, cM0.

Table 1. TNM Classification of thyroid cancer, 8th edition (modified from [12]).

TX	Primary Tumor Cannot be Assessed
T0	No evidence of primary tumor
T1	Tumor size maximum 2 cm, limited to the thyroid
T1a	Tumor size maximum 1 cm, limited to the thyroid
T1b	Tumor size >1 cm up to a maximum of 2 cm, limited to the thyroid
T2	Tumor size >2 cm up to 4 cm, limited to the thyroid
T3	Tumor size >4 cm, limited to the thyroid, or any tumor with macroscopic extrathyroidal extension (*Musculus sternohyoideus, Musculus sternothyreoideus, Musculus omohyoideus*)
T3a	Tumor size >4 cm, limited to the thyroid
T3b	Any tumor with macroscopic extrathyroidal extension (*M. sternohyoideus, M. sternothyreoideus, M. omohyoideus*)
T4a	Any tumor size with extrathyroidal extension beyond the thyroid capsule and invasion of subcutaneous soft tissue, larynx, trachea, esophagus and/or recurrent laryngeal nerve
T4b	Any tumor size with invasion of prevertebral fascia, mediastinal vessels or carotid artery
NX	Regional lymph nodes cannot be assessed
N0	No regional lymph node metastases
N1	Regional lymph node metastases
N1a	Lymph node metastases unilateral in level VI or upper mediastinum
N1b	Metastases in other unilateral, bilateral or contralateral cervical lymph nodes (level I, II, III, IV and V) or retropharyngeal
M0	No distant metastases
M1	Distant metastases

The American Thyroid Association defines in their current guideline a stratification based on the risk of structural disease recurrence [10]:

- high-risk group: gross extrathyreoidal extension, incomplete tumor resection, distant metastases, or lymph node >3 cm;
- intermediate-risk: aggressive histology, minor extrathyreoidal extension, vascular invasion, or >5 involved lymph nodes (0.2–3 cm);
- low-risk: intrathyreoidal DTC, ≤5 lymph nodes micrometastases (<0.2 cm).

In the last few years new molecular and genetic biomarkers, such as BRAF (V600E), phosphatidylinositol 4,5-bisphosphate 3-kinase catalytic subunit α (PIK3CA), tumor protein p53 (TP53), RAC-α serine/threonine-protein kinase 1 (AKT1) and telomerase reverse transcriptase (TERT) became more important for the management of diagnosis, therapy and observing of DTC. The role of RAS is discussed controversally. Table 2 shows the impact of the two well-evaluated molecular markers BRAF and TERT [15]. Some of these alterations might be interesting molecular targets for new therapies.

Table 2. Mutations of BRAF and TERTp in follicular-derived thyroid carcinoma and clinicopathological impact (modified from [15]).

Mutation	Histology	Clinicopathological Associations
BRAF	papillary thyroid carcinoma (PTC)	recurrence, multifocality, extrathyreoidal extension, lymph nodes metastasis, advanced stage, absence of capsule, vascular invasion, more aggressive histological subtype
BRAF	micro PTC	multifocality, extrathyreoidal extension, advanced stage, lymph node metastasis
BRAF	thyroid carcinoma derived from follicular cells	no association
TERT	papillary thyroid carcinoma	more advanced stage by tall cell variant, higher tumor size, vascular invasion, older age, poor outcome, lymph node and distant metastasis
TERT	thyroid carcinoma derived from follicular cells	more aggressive histologic variants, concomitant presence of mutated RAS/BRAF, age > 45, higher tumor size, vascular invasion, persistent or recurrent disease, lymph node metastasis

2.1. *Papillary Thyroid Cancer*

Papillary thyroid carcinoma (PTC) is the most common form of DTC. Histologically it is a tumor of follicular cells of the thyroid gland with characteristic nuclear signs. There are more than 10 histological variants of papillary thyroid cancer documented, can be seen in Table 3 [16,17]. Due to this microscopic diversity, different risk stratifications are needed.

The tall cell variant is one of the tumor entities with unfavorable outcome. This type of thyroid cancer is presented in tall columnar cells and occurs in older age showing a higher rate of lymph node metastases. In nearly 80% of these tumors the BRAF (V600E) mutation is found [18]. A new aggressive variant of papillary thyroid carcinoma, which is characterized by cells with hobnail appearance and apically placed nuclei, was described recently. The BRAF (V600E) mutation is found frequently and associated with distant metastases [19]. In children and adults affected by the Chernobyl incident the solid variant of PTC appears predominantly. Mortality within the first 10 years after initial diagnosis and treatment is low (<1%) [20,21]. It is very important to recognize that there are histological differences compared to poorly differentiated carcinomas, because of the very different therapy strategy. In poorly differentiated thyroid cancer the capability to take up (radio) iodine is clearly reduced (e.g., decreased expression of sodium iodine symporter) and therefore not sufficient to achieve a significant therapeutic effect. Another form of PTC is the diffuse sclerosing variant. It is characterized by a higher incidence of lymph node and distant metastases. Nevertheless, overall mortality appears low. The encapsulated follicular variant of papillary carcinoma very rarely shows capsular or vascular invasion. Histologically it is characterized by follicular growth, typical nuclear features of papillary carcinoma and total tumor encapsulation. RAS mutations can be detected frequently. The non-encapsulated follicular variant of papillary cancer shows BRAF (V600E) mutations quite often [22,23]. This tumor is associated with lymph node metastases in about 25–30% and low rates of distant metastases.

Table 3. WHO classification of papillary and follicular carcinoma of the thyroid (modified from [17]).

Histology	Histological Variants
Papillary carcinoma	Classic (usual) Clear cell variant Columnar cell variant Cribriform-morular variant Diffuse sclerosing variant Follicular variant Macrofollicular variant Microcarcinoma (occult, latent, small, microtumor) Oncocytic or oxyphilic variant (follicular/nonfollicular variant) Solid variant Tall cell variant Warthin-like variant
Follicular carcinoma	Clear cell variant Oncocytic (Hürthle cell) variant Mucinous variant With signet-ring cells

PTC presents distant metastases mainly in bones or lungs.

Papillary microcarcinoma is a PTC < 1 cm corresponding to the classification of the World Health Organization (WHO) which is often found incidentally. In some autopsy studies the papillary microcarcinoma was found in 6–35% of the thyroids by incident [10]. Papillary microcarcinoma may also exhibit RET proto-oncogene (RET)/PTC-rearrangements or BRAF (V600E) mutations.

2.2. Follicular Thyroid Cancer

Follicular thyroid carcinoma (FTC) is a malignant tumor, histologically derived from follicular thyroid cells, showing transcapsular or vascular invasion and missing the typical nuclear signs of papillary carcinoma. In the traditional classification of FTC there are two groups: minimally invasive and widely invasive [24–26]. The widely invasive FTC shows an extensive vascular invasion, often also associated with extrathyroidal growth.

Oncocytic follicular carcinoma is a special form of FTC with some microscopic differences compared to conventional FTC. One of them is the accumulation of innumerable mitochondria. Due to its histological differences, oncocytic carcinoma shows some different biological behavior with a higher ability to metastasize to lymph nodes and a possibly higher rate of recurrence and tumor-related mortality [27–29].

2.3. Familial Tumor Syndromes

Some of the histopathological variants of DTC are associated with familial tumor syndromes. For example, the cribriform-morular form of papillary thyroid cancer is frequently seen in patients with a germline mutation in adenomatous polyposis coli gene [30,31]. About 40% of patients with this special histological form of papillary thyroid carcinoma show simultaneously a familial adenomatous polyposis (FAP) [32]. Due to this high rate of association of cribriform-morular PTC and FAP it is very important to complete the diagnostic work-up with colonoscopy and genetic counseling.

Another type of FTC is associated with the germline mutation of the phosphatase and tensin homolog (PTEN) gene [33–35]. The follicular variant of thyroid carcinoma is in this case very characteristic and should be known by pathologists. The syndrome is associated with a high risk of appearance of other tumors, such as colon hamartomas or breast and endometrium tumors. Genetic counseling is recommended.

3. Diagnostic Approach to Thyroid Nodules

The prevalence of sonographically-detected thyroid nodules in the U.S. is described between 19% and 35% [36]. Toxic adenomas are found in up to 4 percent of the population. In Europe the incidence of thyroid nodules is higher in some areas. In Germany, a country with relative iodine deficiency, nodules are found in 33% of the population.

Risk factors for malignancy are exposure to ionizing radiation through radiotherapy or fallout especially in younger years, familial thyroid carcinoma, or syndromes that are associated with thyroid cancer like PTEN, Cowdens disease or multiple endocrine neoplasia type 2 (MEN2). Warning signs in clinical examination are rapid nodule growth, fixation in the surrounding tissue, vocal cord paralysis, possibly accompanied by hoarseness.

The diagnostic cornerstone of thyroid nodules remains the ultrasound examination. It should be performed in any case of known or suspected thyroid nodules or cervical lymphadenopathy to assess if further diagnostic is needed. Sonographic patterns suspicious of malignancy are microcalcifications, irregular margins, solid consistency, hypoechogenity, extrathyroidal extension (ETE) and a tall shape rather than a wide one. Intranodulary vascularization does not seem to have a clear correlation with malignancy [10].

Roughly one third of thyroid nodules are larger than 1 cm and eligible for scintigraphy [37]. The guidelines of the German Society of Nuclear Medicine recommend a scintigraphic examination of every thyroid nodule >1 cm. By routinely performing a Tc-99m thyroid scan autonomous adenomas that have not yet an impact on thyroid-stimulating hormone (TSH) level can be detected without subjecting the patient to the risks and stress of fine-needle aspiration (FNA). This applies especially to groups at increased risk for complications like patients that are treated with coagulation inhibitors. The diagnostic algorithm for evaluation of thyroid nodules according to the German guidelines that was recently published by Feldkamp et al. is shown in Figure 1 [38].

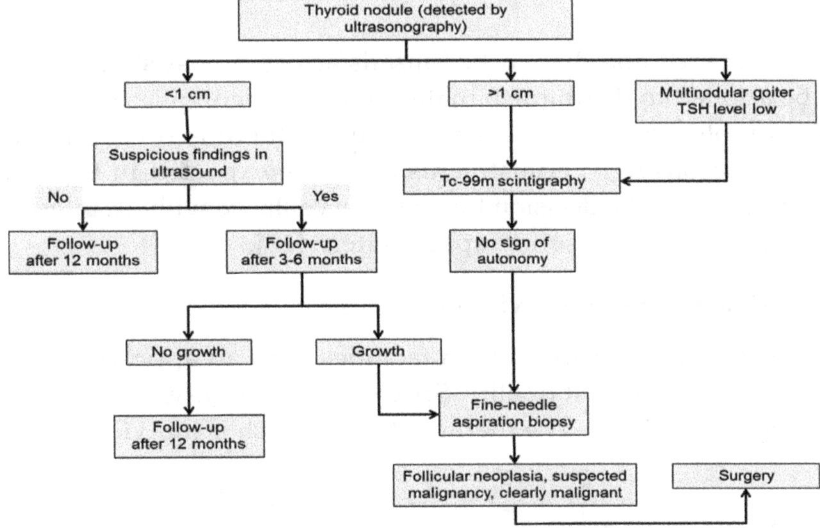

Figure 1. Diagnostic algorithm for the evaluation of thyroid nodules (modified from [38]). TSH: thyroid-stimulating hormone.

The ATA guidelines recommend measurement of the TSH level if a thyroid nodule is found. A radionuclide scan (Tc-99m, preferable I-123) should be performed only if TSH level is subnormal [10]. Nevertheless, the American guidelines cannot be applied to the rest of the world without adjustment for differences in the patient populations. Except for clearly benign cysts, for every lesion of a certain size ultrasound guided fine-needle aspiration biopsy (FNA) is recommended (Table 4) [10]. Furthermore, the measurement of serum calcitonin is recommended when new thyroid nodules are detected time to rule out medullary thyroid cancer that derives from c-cells and is not added to group of DTC.

Table 4. Sonographic patterns and risk of malignancy (modified from [10]).

Ultrasound Features	Estimated Risk of Malignancy	Sonographic Pattern	FNA Size Cutoff
Solid hypoechogenic nodule or solid hypoechogenic component of a partially cystic nodule with one or more of the following features: irregular margins, microcalcification, taller rather than wide shape, rim calcifications with small extrusive soft tissue component, evidence of extrathyroidal extension (ETE)	>70–90%	Highly suspicious	>1 cm
Solid hypoechogenic nodule with smooth margins without microcalcification, taller rather than wide shape or signs of ETE	10–20%	Intermediate suspicion	>1 cm
Isoechogenic solid nodule or partally cystic nodule with eccentric solid areas without microcalcification, taller rather than wide shape or signs of ETE	5–10%	Low suspicion	>1.5 cm
Spongiform or partially cystic nodule without any of the sonographic features described above	<3%	Very low suspicion	>2 cm, alternative: observation without fine needle aspiration (FNA)
Purely cystic nodules without solid components	<1%	Benign	No biopsy

Cytological analysis is performed according to the Bethesda System for Reporting Thyroid Cytopathology. The findings are graded into six categories:

I: nondiagnostic/unsatisfactory;
II: benign;
III: atypia of undetermined significance/follicular lesion of undetermined significance;
IV: follicular neoplasm/suspicious for follicular neoplasm;
V: suspicious for malignancy;
VI: malignant.

If the FNA biopsy is graded non-diagnostic/unsatisfactory, biopsy should be repeated. Numerous molecular tests can be applied to distinguish malignant from benign lesions, such as BRAF (V600E), PIK3CA and TERT promoter, AKT1, and TP53, although there is no explicit recommendation in the current guidelines. Accordingly, adjustments are to be expected in the future [15]. For more non-diagnostic biopsies in a row, the decision for close surveillance without intervention or for surgery should be made in dependence of the sonographic pattern [10].

4. Therapy of Differentiated Thyroid Carcinoma

DTC should be treated interdisciplinary in facilities with an appropriate expertise in order to ensure an optimal long-term treatment quality. Specialists in surgery, endocrinology, pathology and nuclear medicine should be available. The therapeutic approach is individualized and risk-adapted.

4.1. Surgery

For widely invasive follicular thyroid carcinomas and FTC with vascular infiltration, thyreoidectomy is recommended. Lymph node dissection is recommended if lymph node metastases can be detected pre- or intraoperatively by sonographic examination and/or palpation. The solitary minimally invasive FTC without vascular invasion does not require a second surgical intervention as completion, if the tumor has been completely removed (R0). Thyreoidectomy and lymph node dissection of the central compartment are recommended for prognostically unfavorable variants.

For all papillary thyroid carcinomas >1 cm and/or for all metastasized or macroscopically invasive PTC irrespective of size, thyreoidectomy is recommended [10,39]. If lymph node metastases have been detected sonographically or intraoperatively, lymph node dissection in the affected compartment should be done to reduce the risk of (local) recurrence. On the other hand, the diagnostic or therapeutic extirpation of only single lymph nodes as a part of the primary intervention is not recommended. Although at present the importance of central lymph dissection with prophylactic intention is still unclear, the high probability of lymph node metastases is a substantial argument to expand the surgical procedure. Furthermore, it is difficult to exclude lymph node metastases pre- or intraoperatively. After all, the increased risk of a local recurrence associated with an increased morbidity due to the surgical intervention in the situation of relapse should be mentioned. On the other hand, the main arguments against a prophylactic dissection are the lack of evidence regarding a better outcome of the patients and the remarkably higher complication rate due to the more extensive intervention (e.g., vocal cord paralysis, parathyreoprival tetany). Specifically, papillary thyroid microcarcinoma that is found incidentally does not require a further surgical treatment.

After all, accurate histopathological examination of the specimen after (hemi)thyroidectomy and lymphadenectomy (if done) is regarded as the gold standard and is indispensable for the management and further diagnostic and therapeutic approach.

4.2. *Adjuvant Radioiodine Therapy*

Radioiodine therapy (RIT) has been established for more than 60 years. The benefit was demonstrated in DTC patients with a high risk for recurrence. In patients with very low-risk DTC a positive effect of a RIT on tumor-free and overall survival has not been proven by prospective clinical trials.

RIT is defined as the systemic administration of I-131 (radioiodine as sodium iodide or potassium iodide) to irradiate thyroid remnants as well as non-resectable or incompletely resected DTC.

Adjuvant ablative RIT of thyroid remnants or tumor tissue is the optimal precondition for the follow-up including determination of serum thyroglobulin (Tg) and I-131 whole-body scans. The rationale that underlies this approach is to detect a local recurrence or distant metastases in an early and potentially curable stage to minimize mortality. However, regional or distant metastases frequently are only detectable by rising Tg levels after a successful remnant-ablation. It was shown that an ablative RIT decreases the rate of recurrence and mortality over a follow-up period of more than 10 years [40–43]. RIT is indicated in high-risk DTC (pT3, pT4, each N1, every M1), in low-risk DTC (pT1b, pT2, cN0, pN0, M0) and in small papillary thyroid carcinoma (very low-risk DTC), if there are risk factors (see Section 4.7) [44,45]. Furthermore, RIT can be used for the treatment of radioiodine-positive tumor residues, lymph node and distant metastases with curative or palliative intention. In the case of tumor activity shown by an increasing serum level of thyroglobulin without a macroscopically detectable tumor using morphological and functional imaging RIT can be carried out after carefully weighing risks and benefits [14].

To ensure a high uptake of radioiodine (I-131) in remnant tissue, (suspected) tumor, or metastases, an elevated serum level of TSH is required (>30 mU/L). This level is believed to increase the expression of the sodium iodine symporter (NIS) in benign and malignant follicular cells of the thyroid [46]. According to the guidelines of the ATA and EANM [8,10] this TSH level can be reached by waiting not less than 3 weeks after thyroidectomy or after a withdrawal (4–5 weeks) of levothyroxine (LT4). The subsequent period of hypothyroidism decreases the quality of life significantly in many patients. The physical and psychological symptoms of hypothyroidism include gain of weight, impaired renal function, cardiovascular abnormalities, dyslipidemia (exacerbation), constipation, dry skin, hoarseness, fatigue, sleep disturbance, impaired ability to concentrate and depression [47].

Alternatively, recombinant TSH (rhTSH) can be administered intramuscularly (2 times 0.9 mg rhTSH) to avoid inconvenience and morbidity due to the lack of thyroid hormone. This drug is approved for radioiodine ablation (without known distant metastases) of T1–4 tumors, diagnostic whole-body scan and preparation for testing of serum Tg in adults [48–51].

Absolute contraindications of RIT are pregnancy and breastfeeding. Relative contraindications include depression of the bone marrow (especially if the administration of high activities of I-131 is planned), a restriction of salivary gland function, pulmonary function restriction (if a high accumulation of I-131 in lung metastases is possible) and symptomatic metastases of the central nervous system, because local edema and inflammation caused by RIT and hypothyroidism can lead to severe compression effects [8].

The activity of I-131 for remnant ablation is still discussed controversially. The HiLo study (Great Britain) and the ESTIMABL study (France) both compared ablative RIT with 1.1 GBq I-131 versus administration of 3.7 GBq (100 mCi) I-131 after thyroid hormone withdrawal or stimulation with rhTSH in patients with low-risk carcinoma [52,53]. Both studies showed that RIT with only 1.1 GBq (30 mCi) I-131 is not inferior compared to the higher activity in regard to the success of ablation. However, the definition of "success of ablation" used in both studies is not accepted by all departments and associations. Several authors report that the rate of a second RIT increases when low therapy activities were used initially [54,55].

In the ESTIMABL study the diagnostic I-131-whole-body scan 8 months after I-131 ablation was limited to patients with elevated Tg antibodies and disturbed Tg recovery. Even in this subgroup this concept was not consistently implemented. Based on an observation study, iodine-accumulating metastases are possible with a measurable Tg level of up to 1 ng/mL [56]. Due to the open question of the "optimal" activity for remnant ablation, the German Society of Nuclear Medicine for example recommends a single administration of 1 to 3.7 GBq (about 30–100 mCi) I-131 [14]. Preablation scanning with Tc-99m pertechnetate on the day of ablation (as used in the HiLo trial [52]) can give very useful information in clinical decision making. In low-risk DTC patients with a large remnant (multiple foci or one large focus) ablation with 3.7 GBq (30 mCi) may be prefered.

Although RIT is generally well tolerated, the procedure has some potential short- and long-term side effects [8]. Short-term risks/side effects are: thyroiditis due to irradiation, swelling of the tumor or metastases (including compression symptoms), gastritis and nausea, sialadenitis and abnormalities of taste and smell, bone marrow depression, and hypospermia.

Long-term risks and side effects include permanent bone marrow depression, second primary malignancy after RIT with a high cumulative activity (leukemia and solid tumors) [57], chronic sialadenitis (including abnormalities of taste and smell, xerostomia,) and pulmonary fibrosis (in patients with diffuse iodine-avid pulmonary metastases). Due to the risk of chronic hypospermia or azoospermia, sperm banking should be considered if high cumulative activities are expected [58]. These risks have to be weighed against the expected benefits of the RIT.

4.3. Metastatic Differentiated Thyroid Carcinoma

Distant metastases occur in patients with differentiated thyroid carcinoma with a prevalence of up to 10%. In particular, they affect lung and bone [59]. If a sufficient uptake of I-131 in metastases is measurable, different therapeutic approaches are to be weighed regarding risk and benefit.

If locoregional lymph node metastases are detectable, surgery should be performed. I-131 is used for iodine-avid metastases for treatment control after surgery or as an alternative therapy if no surgery is possible/planned (e.g., additional detection of distant metastases requiring RIT, previously performed radiotherapy, previous lymph node dissection).

In the case of micronodulary metastases of the lung RIT is carried out as a treatment with curative intent. Macronodulary pulmonary metastases should also be treated with I-131 in a curative intention but a complete remission is unlikely. Alternatively, (or in combination) the resectability can be evaluated.

The complete surgical resection of isolated bone metastases leads to an improved outcome. A combination of different therapeutic approaches like percutaneous radiotherapy, RIT and local interventional therapy could be helpful if symptomatic metastases of the bone cannot be (completely) resected. The same strategy is applied to brain metastases [14].

For the treatment of metastases, standard activities of 4–11 GBq (about 100–300 mCi) I-131 are given depending on individual patient characteristics like age, renal function, bone marrow depression and tumor load.

4.4. Thyroid Hormone Treatment

After thyroidectomy, life-long thyroid hormone therapy is required, usually as monotherapy with levothyroxine (LT4). Since TSH is able to promote the growth of remaining DTC cells, the dosage of LT4 should initially be high enough to achieve a suppression of thyrotropin. The thyroid function should be checked after 6 to 8 weeks. Depending on the result the dosage should be adjusted. An elevated level of triiodothyronine has to be avoided.

A long-term suppression of TSH to values <0.1 mU/L is currently only recommended for high-risk patients and patients with persistent disease indefinitely in the absence of specific contraindications [10]. In these cases, a better prognosis was demonstrated for the suppression of thyrotropin. No evidence-based data are available for optimal duration of TSH suppression.

According to the guidelines of the ATA, serum TSH should be maintained between 0.1 and 0.5 mU/L in patients with high-risk disease but excellent or intermediate response to therapy for up to 5 years and also in patients with a biochemical incomplete response taking into account the initial ATA risk classification published by Haugen et al. [10]. This recommendation is rated as weak with low-quality evidence. If the response to therapy is excellent biochemically and clinically in patients with a low risk for recurrence and there is no evidence of disease in the course of time, the serum level of TSH may be kept in a range of 0.5–2.0 mU/L, because there is no data showing a benefit of TSH suppression for low-risk patients.

Individual patient-related factors such as osteoporosis or osteopenia and cardiac co-morbidities like atrial fibrillation should always be taken into account during thyroid hormone therapy and weighed against the risk of recurrence. Especially in elderly patients >60 years, the use of TSH suppressive therapy should be carefully considered since the risk of such complications is significantly increased [60].

4.5. Follow-Up

Although the cumulative relapse rate is up to 30%, the life expectancy of DTC patients (pT1-3, pN0-1, M0) is not significantly different from the general population after therapy according to the current guidelines. Lifelong follow-up examinations should be carried out because relapses can occur even after decades and may be cured again. Initial checks should be carried out every six months (e.g., for the first 5 years after diagnosis). If there are no pathological findings later on, annual examinations are adequate [61]. The follow-up examination is based on the medical interview, clinical examination, cervical sonography, determination of TSH, triiodothyronine, levothyroxine, and thyroglobulin including Tg antibodies. In the case of postoperative hypoparathyroidism, the substitution therapy (cholecalciferol, calcium) should be checked and adapted (if necessary) to minimize the risk of osteoporosis.

A diagnostic whole-body scan is obligatory 6–12 months after initial RIT, a second scan is only needed in the case of relapse [10,62].

The criteria for a disease-free stage 6–12 months after primary therapy of DTC with total thyroidectomy $\pm$ radioiodine therapy are no clinical signs of DTC, no pathological uptake in the I-131 whole-body scan (only after remnant ablation) and a serum Tg below the detection limit (under suppression and after TSH stimulation, with absence of Tg antibodies) [10,62,63]. Under these conditions patients have a very low probability of relapse. If there are signs of relapse (e.g., elevated/rising serum levels of Tg) and no radioiodine-accumulating tumor tissue is detectable, clinical diagnostics should include the search for non-radioiodine-avid tumor tissue using F-18-fluorodeoxy-glucose positron emission tomography (FDG-PET) combined with computed tomography ideally under TSH-stimulation.

4.6. Tyrosine Kinase Inhibitors

For poorly differentiated thyroid carcinoma without relevant iodine metabolism and therefore very low radioiodine uptake, RIT is not a therapeutic option. Radioiodine resistance is currently defined as lesions without iodine uptake under TSH stimulation, progression in size in the year following RIT or persistent metastases after a cumulative dose of 22 GBq (600 mCi) I-131 of radioiodine. In these cases, complimentary diagnostic using FDG-PET/computed tomography (CT) is essential. FDG uptake is typically increased in poorly differentiated lesions that can be overlooked on radioiodine scans. Prognosis for radioiodine resistant thyroid cancer with distant metastases is very poor, with an estimated median survival time of about 2.5 to 3.5 years [64,65].

Chemotherapy comes at high toxicity with disappointing response rates [66]. For these patients a strict LT4 regime with TSH suppression is the best way to go. On showing rapid progression under such a regime, therapy options were few until recently.

Tyrosine kinase inhibitors like vandetanib, sorafenib and lenvatinib are a relatively new approach to systemic therapy in these cases. Tyrosine kinase receptors, the target structure of TKI, are trans-membrane proteins that mediate cell survival and proliferation [67]. If mutated, they can cause uncontrolled cell proliferation, dedifferentiation and apoptosis reduction. A large part of DTC show at least one mutation of RAF, RET or paired box gene 8 (PAX8)/peroxisome proliferator-activated receptor gamma (PPARγ) which makes them targets for TKI therapy. Furthermore, TKIs block receptors of the vascular endothelial growth factor (VEGF), fibroblast growth factor receptors and platelet-derived growth factor and thus inhibit tumor angiogenesis and lymphangiogenesis and cause hypoxia in malignant tissue [68]. TKIs, already approved for the treatment of irresectable liver cancer and renal carcinoma, promise to be an effective new tool for the treatment of poorly differentiated thyroid carcinoma (PDTC) [66].

A recent review on the use of sorafenib, sunitinib and lenvatinib showed a benefit for progression-free survival of up to five months [69]. While initially showing partial response or at least disease stabilization after sorafenib, the first TKI approved for thyroid cancer, patients almost always develop resistance over the course of the following one to two years. Switching to another TKI is possible at this point [70]. A study using lenvatinib was able to indicate prolonged progression-free survival regardless of BRAF or RAS mutation status, suggesting a diminished role of these pathways [71]. However, a benefit in overall survival could not be found.

Therapy with kinase inhibitors may be accompanied by severe side effects. Induced hypertension is one of the most common; the underlying pathophysiology is yet unclear. Vasoconstriction following reduced nitric oxide production via inhibition of the VEGF-PI3K pathway is discussed. A reduction of peripheral arterioles due to antiangiogenic effects resulting in increased peripheral resistance and an activation of the endothelin-1-system causing vasoconstriction have also been suggested [72]. Other side effects may include diarrhea, fatigue, hepatotoxicity, skin changes, nausea, increased LT4 dosage requirement, changes in taste and weight loss and associated with a severe decrease of quality of life [69].

Keeping this in mind kinase inhibitors can certainly not be considered as a standard regime or an alternative to TSH-suppression. For patients with radioiodine-refractory DTC they can be a useful complementation to standard therapy.

While undergoing TKI therapy patients can display somewhat inconclusive lab results. Normally a reliable parameter, thyroglobulin levels can fluctuate under TKI treatment. These changes do not necessarily represent the actual course of the disease as it is monitored in anatomical imaging. Sufficient therapeutic monitoring not only by relying on lab tests but also on CT or PET/CT diagnosis to determine a morphologic or metabolic response is essential [73].

Considering the extensive side effects, this therapy should be reserved for patients with rapid tumor progression and severe to life threatening symptoms. In these cases, the decision for TKI therapy should be made in a interdisciplinary manner, carefully weighed against local strategies like radiotherapy and local surgery [74]. TKI treatment should only be performed by a team of physicians experienced with side effects management.

The European guidelines for treating differentiated thyroid carcinoma are from 2008. Kinase inhibitors are therefore not considered there [8] and a unanimous European recommendation is still awaited.

4.7. Papillary Microcarcinoma

Because of the excellent prognosis of papillary microcarcinoma (PTMC), a hemithyroidectomy without RIT is regarded as sufficient therapy, if there is no sign of local invasion, lymph node and/or distant metastases. The substitution of LT4 should keep the serum level of TSH in a euthyroid metabolic state.

In a meta-analysis, PTMC showed a prevalence of distant metastases of 0.4%, a probability of locoregional relapse of 2.5% but also a prevalence of micrometastases in locoregional lymph nodes of 12–50% [45]. The risk of lymphogenic micrometastases increases with increasing tumor diameter [75]. Using single photon emission computed tomography (SPECT) combined with CT, other studies showed a prevalence of lymph node metastases up to 57% [76,77]. The relapse-free survival in patients with PTMC after 5 years was 78.6% without RIT compared to 95.0% in patients that have had a remnant ablation with RIT [78]. The recommendation for a RIT in PTMC is based on the extent of resection and the individual risk profile. Risk factors are multifocality, infiltration of the thyroid gland, histological variants of papillary thyroid carcinoma, low degree of differentiation, tumor diameter 6–10 mm, molecular markers like BRAF-V600E mutation, infiltrative tumor growth, surrounding desmoplastic fibrosis and previous percutaneous irradiation of the neck [14]. In patients with a residual thyroid gland (e.g., after lobectomy) an ablative RIT is not indicated.

5. Summary and Conclusion

Differentiated thyroid cancer is a rare tumor entity but shows a strongly increasing incidence over the last decades. It derives from the follicular epithelium of the thyroid and shows basic biological characteristics of healthy thyroid tissue. The expression of the sodium iodide symporter is the key feature for specific iodine uptake. Patients with DTC have an excellent prognosis.

The therapeutic approach including surgery and remnant ablation with radioiodine should be risk-adapted to achieve an optimal treatment and to minimize treatment-related morbidity. Overtreatment should be avoided.

With regard to so-called low-risk carcinoma defined by the ATA there are controversial therapeutic approaches. The guidelines of the ATA recommend a lobectomy under certain conditions. Following the guidelines of the EANM a thyreodectomy with RIT should be performed (except PTC pT1a). However, long-term studies are currently not available. These studies are certainly necessary (against the background of the slow growth of the well-differentiated thyroid carcinoma) to decide which approach is appropriate. A risk-stratified follow-up is required since recurrences can occur over years. Furthermore, thyroid hormone substitution must be controlled.

The life span of most DTC patients does not differ from general population when appropriate treatment is given. The prognosis becomes poorer in patients with radioiodine refractory thyroid carcinoma. TKI have shown clinical effectiveness in iodine-refractory DTC with regard to progression free survival. A positive effect on overall survival could not be shown yet and has to be evaluated in further studies. However, therapy should be carried out in centers with special expertise.

In the current guidelines of the ATA and EANM there is no evidence-based treatment concept (or strong recommendation) for every situation. There are still open questions:

- The value of RIT under the condition of increasing serum level of Tg without a detectable correlatation in the morphological or functional imaging (i.e. iodine-negative whole-body scan);
- The benefit of a remnant ablation in patients with papillary microcarcinoma (very low risk of relapse, lymph node metastasis possible);
- Optimal activities of I-131 for safe and effective radioiodine ablation;
- The role of rhTSH as preparation for RIT to treat incomplete or non-resectable local recurrence or metastases;
- The role of a short LT4 withdrawal to reduce blood levels of iodine before RIT or diagnostic whole-body scan.

An analysis by the Cancer Genome Atlas Research Network identifies previously unknown genetic alterations and molecular subtypes of PTC. These alterations may lead to a more accurate diagnosis of tumors and potentially more targeted treatment [79]. Although in the current guidelines no explicit recommendation concerning the determination of molecular markers in the cyto-/histopathological specimen is made, further adjustments are to be expected in the future.

Author Contributions: The manuscript was written by Benedikt Schmidbauer, Karin Menhart and Jirka Grosse, the systematic literature research and corrections were done by Dirk Hellwig and Jirka Grosse, Jirka Grosse concieved the manuscript.

Abbreviations

AKT1	RAC-α serine/threonine-protein kinase 1
ATA	American Thyroid Association
CT	computed tomography
DTC	differentiated thyroid carcinoma
EANM	European Association of Nuclear Medicine
ETE	extrathyroidal extension
ETA	European Thyroid Association
FAP	familial adenomatous polyposis
FNA	fine-needle aspiration biopsy
FTC	follicular thyroid carcinoma
FDG-PET	F-18-fluorodeoxy-glucose positron emission tomography
LT4	levothyroxine
MEN2	multiple endocrine neoplasia type 2
PAX8	paired box gene 8
PDTC	poorly differentiated thyroid carcinoma
PIK3CA	phosphatidylinositol 4,5-bisphosphate 3-kinase catalytic subunit α
PPARγ	peroxisome proliferator-activated receptor gamma
PTC	papillary thyroid carcinoma
PTEN	phosphatase and tensin homolog
PTMC	papillary microcarcinoma
RET	RET proto-oncogene
rhTSH	recombinant thyrotropin
RIT	radioiodine therapy
SPECT	single photon emission computed tomography
TERT	telomerase reverse transcriptase
Tg	serum thyroglobulin
TKI	receptor tyrosine kinase inhibitors
TP53	tumor protein p53
TSH	thyroid-stimulating hormone (also known as thyrotropin)
VEGF	vascular endothelial growth factor
WHO	World Health Organization

References

1. Hegedüs, L. Clinical practice. The thyroid nodule. *N. Engl. J. Med.* **2004**, *351*, 1764–1771. [CrossRef] [PubMed]
2. Siegel, R.; Ma, J.; Zou, Z.; Jemal, A. Cancer statistics, 2014. *CA Cancer J. Clin.* **2014**, *64*, 9–29. [CrossRef] [PubMed]
3. Leenhardt, L.; Bernier, M.O.; Boin-Pineau, M.H.; Conte Devolx, B.; Maréchaud, R.; Niccoli-Sire, P.; Nocaudie, M.; Orgiazzi, J.; Schlumberger, M.; Wémeau, J.L.; et al. Advances in diagnostic practices affect thyroid cancer incidence in France. *Eur. J. Endocrinol.* **2004**, *150*, 133–139. [CrossRef] [PubMed]
4. Sherman, S.I. Thyroid carcinoma. *Lancet* **2003**, *361*, 501–511. [CrossRef]
5. Aschebrook-Kilfoy, B.; Schechter, R.B.; Shih, Y.C.; Kaplan, E.L.; Chiu, B.C.; Angelos, P.; Grogan, R.H. The clinical and economic burden of a sustained increase in thyroid cancer incidence. *Cancer Epidemiol. Biomark. Prev.* **2013**, *22*, 1252–1259. [CrossRef] [PubMed]
6. Leenhardt, L.; Erdogan, M.F.; Hegedus, L.; Mandel, S.J.; Paschke, R.; Rago, T.; Russ, G. 2013 European thyroid association guidelines for cervical ultrasound scan and ultrasound-guided techniques in the postoperative management of patients with thyroid cancer. *Eur. Thyroid J.* **2013**, *2*, 147–159. [CrossRef] [PubMed]
7. Silberstein, E.B.; Alavi, A.; Balon, H.R.; Clarke, S.E.; Divgi, C.; Gelfand, M.J.; Goldsmith, S.J.; Jadvar, H.; Marcus, C.S.; Martin, W.H.; et al. The SNMMI practice guideline for therapy of thyroid disease with 131I 3.0. *J. Nucl. Med.* **2012**, *53*, 1633–1651. [CrossRef] [PubMed]
8. Luster, M.; Clarke, S.E.; Dietlein, M.; Lassmann, M.; Lind, P.; Oyen, W.J.; Tennvall, J.; Bombardieri, E.; European Association of Nuclear Medicine (EANM). Guidelines for radioiodine therapy of differentiated thyroid cancer. *Eur. J. Nucl. Med. Mol. Imaging* **2008**, *35*, 1941–1959. [CrossRef] [PubMed]
9. Takami, H.; Ito, Y.; Okamoto, T.; Onoda, N.; Noguchi, H.; Yoshida, A. Revisiting the guidelines issued by the Japanese Society of Thyroid Surgeons and Japan Association of Endocrine Surgeons: A gradual move towards consensus between Japanese and western practice in the management of thyroid carcinoma. *World J. Surg.* **2014**, *38*, 2002–2010. [CrossRef] [PubMed]
10. Haugen, B.R.; Alexander, E.K.; Bible, K.C.; Doherty, G.M.; Mandel, S.J.; Nikiforov, Y.E.; Pacini, F.; Randolph, G.W.; Sawka, A.M.; Schlumberger, M.; et al. 2015 American Thyroid Association Management Guidelines for Adult Patients with Thyroid Nodules and Differentiated Thyroid Cancer: The American Thyroid Association Guidelines Task Force on Thyroid Nodules and Differentiated Thyroid Cancer. *Thyroid* **2016**, *26*, 1–133. [CrossRef] [PubMed]
11. Francis, G.L.; Waguespack, S.G.; Bauer, A.J.; Angelos, P.; Benvenga, S.; Cerutti, J.M.; Dinauer, C.A.; Hamilton, J.; Hay, I.D.; Luster, M.; et al. Management guidelines for children with thyroid nodules and differentiated thyroid cancer. *Thyroid* **2015**, *25*, 716–759. [CrossRef] [PubMed]
12. Brierley, J.D.; Gospodarowicz, M.K.; Wittekind, C. *TNM Classification of Malignant Tumours*, 8th ed.; John Wiley & Sons: Weinheim, Germany, 2017; pp. 69–71.
13. Armin, M.B.; Edge, S.; Greene, F.; Byrd, D.R.; Brookland, R.K.; Washington, M.K.; Gershenwald, J.E.; Compton, C.C.; Hess, K.R.; Sullivan, D.C.; et al. *AJCC Cancer Staging Manual*, 8th ed.; Springer: New York, NY, USA, 2017; pp. 1–19.
14. Dietlein, M.; Eschner, W.; Grünwald, F.; Lassmann, M.; Verburg, F.A.; Luster, M. Procedure guidelines for radioiodine therapy of differentiated thyroid cancer. Version 4. *Nuklearmedizin* **2016**, *55*, 77–89. [CrossRef] [PubMed]
15. Penna, G.C.; Vaisman, F.; Vaisman, M.; Sobrinho-Simões, M.; Soares, P. Molecular Markers Involved in Tumorigenesis of Thyroid Carcinoma: Focus on Aggressive Histotypes. *Cytogenet. Genome Res.* **2016**, *150*, 194–207. [CrossRef] [PubMed]
16. Nikiforov, Y.E.; Ohori, N.P. Papillary Carcinoma. In *Diagnostic Pathology and Molecular Genetics of the Thyroid*, 1st ed.; Nikiforov, Y.E., Biddinger, P.W., Thompson, L.D.R., Eds.; Lippincott: Philadelphia, PA, USA, 2012; pp. 183–262.
17. Seethala, R.R.; Asa, S.L.; Carty, S.E.; Hodak, S.P.; McHugh, J.B.; Richardson, M.S.; Shah, J.; Thompson, L.D.R.; Nikiforov, Y.E. For the Members of the Cancer Committee, College of American Pathologists. Protocol for the Examination of Specimens From Patients With Carcinomas of the Thyroid Gland, Based on AJCC/UICC TNM, 7th edition. Version: Thyroid 3.2.0.0. Available online: http://www.cap.org/ShowProperty?nodePath=/UCMCon/Contribution%20Folders/WebContent/pdf/cp-thyroid-16protocol-3200.pdf (accessed on 2 June 2017).

18. Nikiforova, M.N.; Kimura, E.T.; Gandhi, M.; Biddinger, P.W.; Knauf, J.A.; Basolo, F.; Zhu, Z.; Giannini, R.; Salvatore, G.; Fusco, A.; et al. BRAF mutations in thyroid tumors are restricted to papillary carcinomas and anaplastic or poorly differentiated carcinomas arising from papillary carcinomas. *J. Clin. Endocrinol. Metab.* **2003**, *88*, 5399–5404. [CrossRef] [PubMed]
19. Asioli, S.; Erickson, L.A.; Sebo, T.J.; Zhang, J.; Jin, L.; Thompson, G.B.; Lloyd, R.V. Papillary thyroid carcinoma with prominent hobnail features: A new aggressive variant of moderately differentiated papillary carcinoma. A clinicopathologic, immunohistochemical, and molecular study of eight cases. *Am. J. Surg. Pathol.* **2010**, *34*, 44–52. [CrossRef] [PubMed]
20. Cardis, E.; Howe, G.; Ron, E.; Bebeshko, V.; Bogdanova, T.; Bouville, A.; Carr, Z.; Chumak, V.; Davis, S.; Demidchik, Y.; et al. Cancer consequences of the Chernobyl accident: 20 years on. *J. Radiol. Prot.* **2006**, *26*, 127–140. [CrossRef] [PubMed]
21. Nikiforov, Y.E. Radiation-induced thyroid cancer: What we have learned from Chernobyl. *Endocr. Pathol.* **2006**, *17*, 307–317. [CrossRef] [PubMed]
22. Howitt, B.E.; Jia, Y.; Sholl, L.M.; Barletta, J.A. Molecular alterations in partially-encapsulated or well-circumscribed follicular variant of papillary thyroid carcinoma. *Thyroid* **2013**, *23*, 1256–1262. [CrossRef] [PubMed]
23. Liu, J.; Singh, B.; Tallini, G.; Carlson, D.L.; Katabi, N.; Shaha, A.; Tuttle, R.M.; Ghossein, R.A. Follicular variant of papillary thyroid carcinoma: A clinicopathologic study of a problematic entity. *Cancer* **2006**, *107*, 1255–1264. [CrossRef] [PubMed]
24. Brennan, M.D.; Bergstralh, E.J.; van Heerden, J.A.; McConahey, W.M. Follicular thyroid cancer treated at the Mayo Clinic, 1946 through 1970: Initial manifestations, pathologic findings, therapy, and outcome. *Mayo Clin. Proc.* **1991**, *66*, 11–22. [CrossRef]
25. Collini, P.; Sampietro, G.; Pilotti, S. Extensive vascular invasion is a marker of risk of relapse in encapsulated non-Hürthle cell follicular carcinoma of the thyroid gland: A clinicopathological study of 18 consecutive cases from a single institution with a 11-year median follow-up. *Histopathology* **2004**, *44*, 35–39. [CrossRef] [PubMed]
26. Lang, W.; Choritz, H.; Hundeshagen, H. Risk factors in follicular thyroid carcinomas. A retrospective follow-up study covering a 14-year period with emphasis on morphological findings. *Am. J. Surg. Pathol.* **1986**, *10*, 246–255. [CrossRef] [PubMed]
27. Hundahl, S.A.; Fleming, I.D.; Fremgen, A.M.; Menck, H.R. A National Cancer Data Base report on 53,856 cases of thyroid carcinoma treated in the U.S., 1985–1995. *Cancer* **1998**, *83*, 2638–2648. [CrossRef]
28. Haigh, P.I.; Urbach, D.R. The treatment and prognosis of Hürthle cell follicular thyroid carcinoma compared with its non-Hürthle cell counterpart. *Surgery* **2005**, *138*, 1152–1157. [CrossRef] [PubMed]
29. Shaha, A.R.; Loree, T.R.; Shah, J.P. Prognostic factors and risk group analysis in follicular carcinoma of the thyroid. *Surgery* **1995**, *118*, 1131–1136. [CrossRef]
30. Cetta, F.; Montalto, G.; Gori, M.; Curia, M.C.; Cama, A.; Olschwang, S. Germline mutations of the APC gene in patients with familial adenomatous polyposis-associated thyroid carcinoma: Results from a European cooperative study. *J. Clin. Endocrinol. Metab.* **2000**, *85*, 286–292. [PubMed]
31. Harach, H.R.; Williams, G.T.; Williams, E.D. Familial adenomatous polyposis associated thyroid carcinoma: A distinct type of follicular cell neoplasm. *Histopathology* **1994**, *25*, 549–561. [CrossRef] [PubMed]
32. Ito, Y.; Miyauchi, A.; Ishikawa, H.; Hirokawa, M.; Kudo, T.; Tomoda, C.; Miya, A. Our experience of treatment of cribriform morular variant of papillary thyroid carcinoma; difference in clinicopathological features of FAP-associated and sporadic patients. *Endocr. J.* **2011**, *58*, 685–689. [CrossRef] [PubMed]
33. Hollander, M.C.; Blumenthal, G.M.; Dennis, P.A. PTEN loss in the continuum of common cancers, rare syndromes and mouse models. *Nat. Rev. Cancer* **2011**, *11*, 289–301. [CrossRef] [PubMed]
34. Laury, A.R.; Bongiovanni, M.; Tille, J.C.; Kozakewich, H.; Nosé, V. Thyroid pathology in PTEN-hamartoma tumor syndrome: Characteristic findings of a distinct entity. *Thyroid* **2011**, *21*, 135–144. [CrossRef] [PubMed]
35. Nosé, V. Familial thyroid cancer: A review. *Mod. Pathol.* **2011**, *24*, S19–S33. [CrossRef] [PubMed]
36. Dean, D.S.; Gharib, H. Epidemiology of thyroid nodules. *Best Pract. Res. Clin. Endocrinol. Metab.* **2008**, *22*, 901–911. [CrossRef] [PubMed]
37. Vanderpump, M.P. The epidemiology of thyroid disease. *Br. Med. Bull.* **2011**, *99*, 39–51. [CrossRef] [PubMed]
38. Feldkamp, J.; Führer, D.; Luster, M.; Musholt, T.J.; Spitzweg, C.; Schott, M. Fine Needle Aspiration in the Investigation of Thyroid Nodules. *Dtsch. Arztebl. Int.* **2016**, *113*, 353–359. [PubMed]

39. Dralle, H.; Musholt, T.J.; Schabram, J.; Steinmüller, T.; Frilling, A.; Simon, D.; Goretzki, P.E.; Niederle, B.; Scheuba, C.; Clerici, T.; et al. German Association of Endocrine Surgeons practice guideline for the surgical management of malignant thyroid tumors. *Langenbecks Arch. Surg.* **2013**, *398*, 347–375. [CrossRef] [PubMed]
40. Mazzaferri, E.L.; Jhiang, S.M. Long-term impact of initial surgical and medical therapy on papillary and follicular thyroid cancer. *Am. J. Med.* **1994**, *97*, 418–428. [CrossRef]
41. Samaan, N.A.; Schultz, P.N.; Hickey, R.C.; Goepfert, H.; Haynie, T.P.; Johnston, D.A.; Ordonez, N.G. The results of various modalities of treatment of well differentiated thyroid carcinomas: A retrospective review of 1599 patients. *J. Clin. Endocrinol. Metab.* **1992**, *75*, 714–720. [PubMed]
42. Sawka, A.M.; Thephamongkhol, K.; Brouwers, M.; Thabane, L.; Browman, G.; Gerstein, H.C. Clinical review 170: A systematic review and metaanalysis of the effectiveness of radioactive iodine remnant ablation for well-differentiated thyroid cancer. *J. Clin. Endocrinol. Metab.* **2004**, *89*, 3668–3676. [CrossRef] [PubMed]
43. Sawka, A.M.; Brierley, J.D.; Tsang, R.W.; Thabane, L.; Rotstein, L.; Gafni, A.; Straus, S.; Goldstein, D.P. An updated systematic review and commentary examining the effectiveness of radioactive iodine remnant ablation in well-differentiated thyroid cancer. *Endocrinol. Metab. Clin. N. Am.* **2008**, *37*, 457–480. [CrossRef] [PubMed]
44. Mehanna, H.; Al-Maqbili, T.; Carter, B.; Martin, E.; Campain, N.; Watkinson, J.; McCabe, C.; Boelaert, K.; Franklyn, J.A. Differences in the recurrence and mortality outcomes rates of incidental and nonincidental papillary thyroid microcarcinoma: A systematic review and meta-analysis of 21,329 person-years of follow-up. *J. Clin. Endocrinol. Metab.* **2014**, *99*, 2834–2843. [CrossRef] [PubMed]
45. Perros, P.; Boelaert, K.; Colley, S.; Evans, C.; Evans, R.M.; Gerrard, B.G.; Gilbert, J.; Harrison, B.; Johnson, S.J.; Giles, T.E.; et al. British Thyroid Association. Guidelines for the management of thyroid cancer. *Clin. Endocrinol.* **2014**, *81*, 1–122. [CrossRef] [PubMed]
46. Cooper, D.S.; Doherty, G.M.; Haugen, B.R.; Kloos, R.T.; Lee, S.L.; Mandel, S.J.; Mazzaferri, E.L.; McIver, B.; Sherman, S.I.; Tuttle, R.M.; et al. Management guidelines for patients with thyroid nodules and differentiated thyroid cancer. *Thyroid* **2006**, *16*, 109–142. [CrossRef] [PubMed]
47. Luster, M.; Felbinger, R.; Dietlein, M.; Reiners, C. Thyroid hormone withdrawal in patients with differentiated thyroid carcinoma: A one hundred thirty-patient pilot survey on consequences of hypothyroidism and a pharmacoeconomic comparison to recombinant thyrotropin administration. *Thyroid* **2005**, *15*, 1147–1155. [CrossRef] [PubMed]
48. Pacini, F.; Ladenson, P.W.; Schlumberger, M.; Driedger, A.; Luster, M.; Kloos, R.T.; Sherman, S.; Haugen, B.; Corone, C.; Molinaro, E.; et al. Radioiodine ablation of thyroid remnants after preparation with recombinant human thyrotropin in differentiated thyroid carcinoma: Results of an international, randomized, controlled study. *J. Clin. Endocrinol. Metab.* **2006**, *91*, 926–932. [CrossRef] [PubMed]
49. Ladenson, P.W.; Braverman, L.E.; Mazzaferri, E.L.; Brucker-Davis, F.; Cooper, D.S.; Garber, J.R.; Wondisford, F.E.; Davies, T.F.; DeGroot, L.J.; Daniels, G.H.; et al. Comparison of administration of recombinant human thyrotropin with withdrawal of thyroid hormone for radioactive iodine scanning in patients with thyroid carcinoma. *N. Engl. J. Med.* **1997**, *337*, 888–896. [CrossRef] [PubMed]
50. Luster, M. Acta Oncologica Lecture. Present status of the use of recombinant human TSH in thyroid cancer management. *Acta Oncol.* **2006**, *45*, 1018–1030. [CrossRef] [PubMed]
51. Schlumberger, M.; Ricard, M.; De Pouvourville, G.; Pacini, F. How the availability of recombinant human TSH has changed the management of patients who have thyroid cancer. *Nat. Clin. Pract. Endocrinol. Metab.* **2007**, *3*, 641–650. [CrossRef] [PubMed]
52. Mallick, U.; Harmer, C.; Yap, B.; Wadsley, J.; Clarke, S.; Moss, L.; Nicol, A.; Clark, P.M.; Farnell, K.; McCready, R.; et al. Ablation with low-dose radioiodine and thyrotropin alfa in thyroid cancer. *N. Engl. J. Med.* **2012**, *366*, 1674–1685. [CrossRef] [PubMed]
53. Schlumberger, M.; Catargi, B.; Borget, I.; Deandreis, D.; Zerdoud, S.; Bridji, B.; Bardet, S.; Leenhardt, L.; Bastie, D.; Schvartz, C.; et al. Strategies of radioiodine ablation in patients with low-risk thyroid cancer. *N. Engl. J. Med.* **2012**, *366*, 1663–1673. [CrossRef] [PubMed]
54. Kukulska, A.; Krajewska, J.; Gawkowska-Suwińska, M.; Puch, Z.; Paliczka-Cieslik, E.; Roskosz, J.; Handkiewicz-Junak, D.; Jarzab, M.; Gubała, E.; Jarzab, B. Radioiodine thyroid remnant ablation in patients with differentiated thyroid carcinoma (DTC): Prospective comparison of long-term outcomes of treatment with 30, 60 and 100 mCi. *Thyroid Res.* **2010**, *3*, 9. [CrossRef] [PubMed]

55. Fallahi, B.; Beiki, D.; Takavar, A.; Fard-Esfahani, A.; Gilani, K.A.; Saghari, M.; Eftekhari, M. Low versus high radioiodine dose in postoperative ablation of residual thyroid tissue in patients with differentiated thyroid carcinoma: A large randomized clinical trial. *Nucl. Med. Commun.* **2012**, *33*, 275–282. [CrossRef] [PubMed]
56. Robbins, R.J.; Chon, J.T.; Fleisher, M.; Larson, S.M.; Tuttle, R.M. Is the serum thyroglobulin response to recombinant human thyrotropin sufficient, by itself, to monitor for residual thyroid carcinoma? *J. Clin. Endocrinol. Metab.* **2002**, *87*, 3242–3247. [CrossRef] [PubMed]
57. Rubino, C.; de Vathaire, F.; Dottorini, M.E.; Hall, P.; Schvartz, C.; Couette, J.E.; Dondon, M.G.; Abbas, M.T.; Langlois, C.; Schlumberger, M. Second primary malignancies in thyroid cancer patients. *Br. J. Cancer* **2003**, *89*, 1638–1644. [CrossRef] [PubMed]
58. Wichers, M.; Benz, E.; Palmedo, H.; Biersack, H.J.; Grünwald, F.; Klingmüller, D. Testicular function after radioiodine therapy for thyroid carcinoma. *Eur. J. Nucl. Med.* **2000**, *27*, 503–507. [CrossRef] [PubMed]
59. Benbassat, C.A.; Mechlis-Frish, S.; Hirsch, D. Clinicopathological characteristics and long-term outcome in patients with distant metastases from differentiated thyroid cancer. *World J. Surg.* **2006**, *30*, 1088–1095. [CrossRef] [PubMed]
60. Abonowara, A.; Quraishi, A.; Sapp, J.L.; Alqambar, M.H.; Saric, A.; O'Connell, C.M.; Rajaraman, M.M.; Hart, R.D.; Imran, S.A. Prevalence of atrial fibrillation in patients taking TSH suppression therapy for management of thyroid cancer. *Clin. Investig. Med.* **2012**, *35*, E152–E156. [CrossRef] [PubMed]
61. Tiedje, V.; Schmid, K.W.; Weber, F.; Bockisch, A.; Führer, D. Differentiated thyroid cancer. *Internist* **2015**, *56*, 153–166. [CrossRef] [PubMed]
62. Pacini, F.; Schlumberger, M.; Dralle, H.; Elisei, R.; Smit, J.W.; Wiersinga, W.; European Thyroid Cancer Taskforce. European consensus for the management of patients with differentiated thyroid carcinoma of the follicular epithelium. *Eur. J. Endocrinol.* **2006**, *154*, 787–803. [CrossRef] [PubMed]
63. Tuttle, R.M.; Tala, H.; Shah, J.; Leboeuf, R.; Ghossein, R.; Gonen, M.; Brokhin, M.; Omry, G.; Fagin, J.A.; Shaha, A. Estimating risk of recurrence in differentiated thyroid cancer after total thyroidectomy and radioactive iodine remnant ablation: Using response to therapy variables to modify the initial risk estimates predicted by the new American Thyroid Association staging system. *Thyroid* **2010**, *20*, 1341–1349. [PubMed]
64. Durante, C.; Haddy, N.; Baudin, E.; Leboulleux, S.; Hartl, D.; Travagli, J.P.; Caillou, B.; Ricard, M.; Lumbroso, J.D.; De Vathaire, F.; et al. Long-term outcome of 444 patients with distant metastases from papillary and follicular thyroid carcinoma: Benefits and limits of radioiodine therapy. *J. Clin. Endocrinol. Metab.* **2006**, *91*, 2892–2899. [CrossRef] [PubMed]
65. Robbins, R.J.; Wan, Q.; Grewal, R.K.; Reibke, R.; Gonen, M.; Strauss, H.W.; Tuttle, R.M.; Drucker, W.; Larson, S.M. Real-time prognosis for metastatic thyroid carcinoma based on 2-[18F]fluoro-2-deoxy-D-glucose-positron emission tomography scanning. *J. Clin. Endocrinol. Metab.* **2006**, *91*, 498–505. [CrossRef] [PubMed]
66. Sherman, S.I. Early clinical studies of novel therapies for thyroid cancers. *Endocrinol. Metab. Clin. N. Am.* **2008**, *37*, 511–524. [CrossRef] [PubMed]
67. Fassnacht, M.; Kreissl, M.C.; Weismann, D.; Allolio, B. New targets and therapeutic approaches for endocrine malignancies. *Pharmacol. Ther.* **2009**, *123*, 117–141. [CrossRef] [PubMed]
68. Lorusso, L.; Pieruzzi, L.; Biagini, A.; Sabini, E.; Valerio, L.; Giani, C.; Passannanti, P.; Pontillo-Contillo, B.; Battaglia, V.; Mazzeo, S.; et al. Lenvatinib and other tyrosine kinase inhibitors for the treatment of radioiodine refractory, advanced, and progressive thyroid cancer. *Onco Targets Ther.* **2016**, *9*, 6467–6477. [CrossRef] [PubMed]
69. Laursen, R.; Wehland, M.; Kopp, S.; Pietsch, J.; Infanger, M.; Grosse, J.; Grimm, D. Effects and Role of Multikinase Inhibitors in Thyroid Cancer. *Curr. Pharm. Des.* **2016**, *22*, 5915–5926. [CrossRef] [PubMed]
70. Pitoia, F.; Jerkovich, F. Selective use of sorafenib in the treatment of thyroid cancer. *Drug Des. Dev. Ther.* **2016**, *10*, 1119–1131. [CrossRef] [PubMed]
71. Schlumberger, M.; Tahara, M.; Wirth, L.J.; Robinson, B.; Brose, M.S.; Elisei, R.; Habra, M.A.; Newbold, K.; Shah, M.H.; Hoff, A.O.; et al. Lenvatinib versus placebo in radioiodine-refractory thyroid cancer. *N. Engl. J. Med.* **2015**, *372*, 621–630. [CrossRef] [PubMed]
72. Ancker, O.V.; Wehland, M.; Bauer, J.; Infanger, M.; Grimm, D. The Adverse Effect of Hypertension in the Treatment of Thyroid Cancer with Multi-Kinase Inhibitors. *Int. J. Mol. Sci.* **2017**, *18*, 625. [CrossRef] [PubMed]

73. Werner, R.A.; Lückerath, K.; Schmid, J.S.; Higuchi, T.; Kreissl, M.C.; Grelle, I.; Reiners, C.; Buck, A.K.; Lapa, C. Thyroglobulin fluctuations in patients with iodine-refractory differentiated thyroid carcinoma on lenvatinib treatment—initial experience. *Sci. Rep.* **2016**, *6*, 28081. [CrossRef] [PubMed]
74. Kreissl, M.C.; Fassnacht, M.; Mueller, S.P. Systemic treatment of advanced differentiated and medullary thyroid cancer. Overview and practical aspects. *Nuklearmedizin* **2015**, *54*, 88–93. [PubMed]
75. Machens, A.; Holzhausen, H.J.; Dralle, H. The prognostic value of primary tumor size in papillary and follicular thyroid carcinoma. *Cancer* **2005**, *103*, 2269–2273. [CrossRef] [PubMed]
76. Gallicchio, R.; Giacomobono, S.; Capacchione, D.; Nardelli, A.; Barbato, F.; Nappi, A.; Pellegrino, T.; Storto, G. Should patients with remnants from thyroid microcarcinoma really not be treated with iodine-131 ablation? *Endocrine* **2013**, *44*, 426–433. [CrossRef] [PubMed]
77. Avram, A.M.; Fig, L.M.; Frey, K.A.; Gross, M.D.; Wong, K.K. Preablation 131-I scans with SPECT/CT in postoperative thyroid cancer patients: What is the impact on staging? *J. Clin. Endocrinol. Metab.* **2013**, *98*, 1163–1171. [CrossRef] [PubMed]
78. Creach, K.M.; Siegel, B.A.; Nussenbaum, B.; Grigsby, P.W. Radioactive iodine therapy decreases recurrence in thyroid papillary microcarcinoma. *ISRN Endocrinol.* **2012**, *2012*, 816386. [CrossRef] [PubMed]
79. Cancer Genome Atlas Research Network. Integrated genomic characterization of papillary thyroid carcinoma. *Cell* **2014**, *159*, 676–690.

2

Genetic Mutations and Variants in the Susceptibility of Familial Non-Medullary Thyroid Cancer

Fabíola Yukiko Miasaki [1], Cesar Seigi Fuziwara [2], Gisah Amaral de Carvalho [1] and Edna Teruko Kimura [2,*]

1 Department of Endocrinology and Metabolism (SEMPR), Hospital de Clínicas, Federal University of Paraná, Curitiba 80030-110, Brazil; fymiasaki@gmail.com (F.Y.M.); carvalho.gisah@gmail.com (G.A.d.C.)

2 Department of Cell and Developmental Biology, Institute of Biomedical Sciences, University of São Paulo, São Paulo 05508-000, Brazil; cesar.fuziwara@usp.br

* Correspondence: etkimura@usp.br

Abstract: Thyroid cancer is the most frequent endocrine malignancy with the majority of cases derived from thyroid follicular cells and caused by sporadic mutations. However, when at least two or more first degree relatives present thyroid cancer, it is classified as familial non-medullary thyroid cancer (FNMTC) that may comprise 3–9% of all thyroid cancer. In this context, 5% of FNMTC are related to hereditary syndromes such as Cowden and Werner Syndromes, displaying specific genetic predisposition factors. On the other hand, the other 95% of cases are classified as non-syndromic FNMTC. Over the last 20 years, several candidate genes emerged in different studies of families worldwide. Nevertheless, the identification of a prevalent polymorphism or germinative mutation has not progressed in FNMTC. In this work, an overview of genetic alteration related to syndromic and non-syndromic FNMTC is presented.

Keywords: thyroid cancer; thyroid neoplasms; genetic predisposition to disease; genetic variants

---

1. Introduction

The most common type of thyroid cancer derives from thyroid follicular cells and is named as non-medullary thyroid cancer (NMTC) in order to be distinguished from the less frequent medullary thyroid cancer (MTC) that originates from the thyroid C-cells. The MTC occurs as sporadic and hereditary cancer, in contrast to the NMTC, which is mainly sporadic (Figure 1). The hereditary MTC can be a component of a syndrome or have a familial background. In this context, the NMTC can also be associated with syndromic conditions, such as in Cowden syndrome, Carney complex, Werner syndrome, and familial adenomatous polyposis but to a lesser extent than in MTC. Moreover, a high prevalence of NMTC in ataxia-telangiectasia, DICER1, and Pendred syndromes has been described [1,2].

Besides these well-known genetic syndromes, the characterization of the non-syndromic form of familial non-medullary thyroid cancer (FNMTC) remains to be consolidated. In 1953, Firminger and Skelton reported the first case of papillary thyroid cancer (PTC) in twins [3]. However, the concept of FNMTC and the genetic predisposition to PTC has emerged only in recent decades. Currently, it is accepted that FNMTC occurs when two or more first-degree relatives are diagnosed with NMTC cancer [4].

The initial FNMTC studies were performed by linkage analysis and described some specific loci, although they did not identify a precise gene associated with FMNTC [5–10]. Furthermore, despite the efforts of many groups in investigating FNMTC using Sanger sequencing, no conclusive information was found, suggesting genetic heterogeneity, multigenic inheritance, and multifactorial inheritance [11]. However, a new genomic perspective emerged with the application of Next Generation Sequencing

(NGS) technology that covered the entire genome. In this extent, some new insights into genetics of FNMTC have emerged by the recent genome-wide association studies (GWAS) in populations of PTC. The finding of several single nucleotide polymorphisms (SNPs), such as in *DIRC3*, *NIRG1*, *FOXE1*, *NKX2-1*, and *PCNXL2*, were observed in the European, Korean, and American populations [12]. Increasing evidence suggests that genetic predisposition factors play an essential role in carcinogenesis besides environmental factors [13]. In this review, we cover the genetic findings associated with FNMTC and in syndromes related to NMTC.

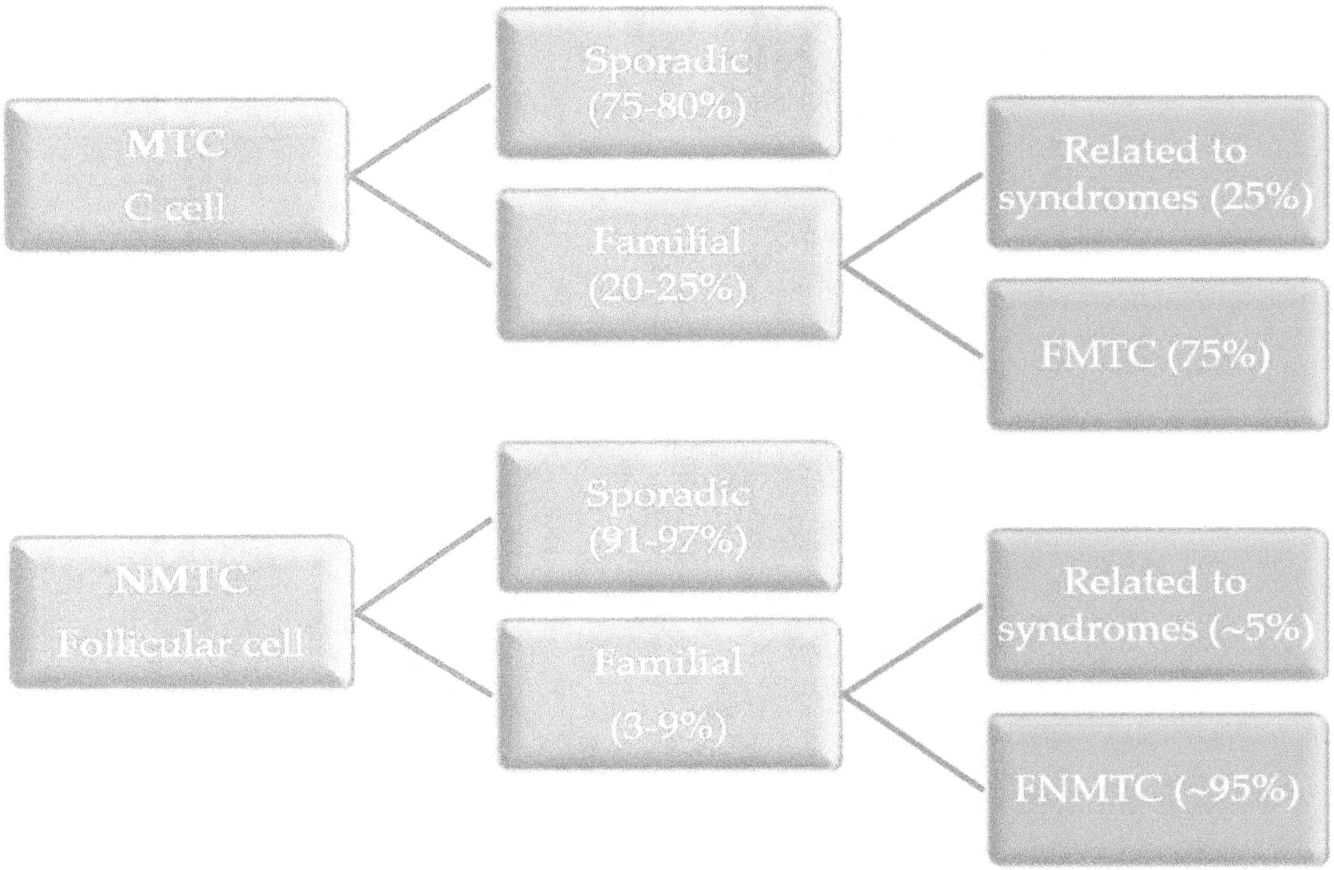

Figure 1. Incidence of sporadic and familial medullary thyroid cancer (MTC) and non-medullary thyroid cancer (NMTC).

2. Syndromic Causes of Non-Medullary Thyroid Cancer

Many syndromes associated with thyroid tumor predisposition have Mendelian patterns of inheritance, and they are related to mutations that may influence the mechanism of DNA repair, the microRNA processing, and maturation, the genome integrity maintenance, the cell signaling, or mitochondrial regulated cellular processes (Table 1) [13]. These syndromes are characterized by several other main malignancies and sometimes lack to present thyroid cancer. Some authors have suggested surveillance in syndromic FNMTC (see below). However, the guidelines, such as the 2015 American Thyroid Association's guideline, are precautious due to insufficient evidence in order to recommend the thyroid cancer screening [14].

Table 1. Genetic alterations in syndromes related to non-medullary thyroid cancer (NMTC).

Syndrome	Gene	Inheritance Pattern	Other Malignant Tumors	Prevalent Types of Thyroid Tumors	Benign Manifestations	Reference
Ataxia-telangiectasia syndrome *	*ATM*	AR *	Lymphocytic leukemia, lymphoma, stomach adenocarcinoma, medulloblastoma, glioma	FTC, PTC •	degenerative cerebellar atrophy, telangiectasias, immune defects	[15]
	ATM	AD	breast cancer, digestive tract cancer, lymphoma, leukemia			[15,16]
Carney complex	*PRKAR1A*	AD	-	Follicular hyperplasia, nodular hyperplasia, FA, cystic changes, PTC, FTC	Spotty skin pigmentation (lips, conjunctiva, vaginal, and penile mucosa), cutaneous and mucosal myxoma, cardiac myxoma, breast myxomatosis, primary pigmented nodular adrenocortical disease, GH-producing adenoma, large cell calcifying Sertoli cell tumors, psammomatous melanotic schwannomas	[17]
Cowden syndrome	*PTEN, SDHB-D, SEC23B, KLLN, PARP4, AKT1, PIK3CA, USF3, TTN, RASAL1*	AD	FTC, breast cancer, epithelial endometrial cancer, colon cancer, renal cell carcinoma melanoma	MNG, Hashimoto thyroiditis, FA, FTC, cPTC, FVPTC, C-cell hyperplasia	Macrocephaly	[18,19]
DICER1 syndrome	*DICER1*	AD	Pleuropulmonary blastoma, ovarian Sertoli-Leydig cell tumor, genitourinary and cerebral sarcomas	MNG, PTC, FA	MNG, cystic nephroma	[20,21]
Familial adenomatous polyposis	*APC*	AD	Digestive tract cancers, fibrosarcomas	CMVPTC, PTC	Intestinal polyps, osteomas, fibromas, desmoid tumors, dental abnormalities, leiomyomas, congenital hypertrophy of the retinal pigment epithelium	[22,23]
Li-Fraumeni syndrome	*TP53*	AD	Breast, brain, and adreno cortical cancers and sarcomas	cPTC, FVPTC		[13,24]
Werner syndrome	*WRN*	AR	Atypical melanoma, bone, or soft tissue sarcomas	FTC, PTC, ATC	Aging, bilateral cataract, type 2 diabetes mellitus, hypogonadism, meningioma	[2,25]

* Ataxia-telangiectasia syndrome occurs only in autosomal recessive pattern. However, heterozygotic carriers have an increased risk to cancer radio ionizing-induced. • An increased risk for thyroid cancer was observed in relatives of A-T patients, but the histological type was not specified in those epidemiological analysis. The above information is inferred from susceptibility thyroid cancer studies [26,27].

2.1. *Cowden Syndrome*

Cowden syndrome (OMIM #158350) is characterized by hamartomas in different parts of the body (gastrointestinal hamartomas, ganglioneuromas, trichilemmomas) associated with melanomas, breast, endometrial and thyroid cancer, macrocephaly, and, eventually, autism spectrum disorder and/or mental retardation [18,28]. One of the major diagnosis criteria is the presence of follicular thyroid carcinoma (FTC). However, if it is not detected, a biannual thyroid ultrasound is advocated in patients older than seven years [29].

Cowden syndrome is classically associated with mutations in the phosphatase and tensin homolog (*PTEN*) gene on chromosome 10q22–23, although variants in several other genes have been described in patients without *PTEN* mutations (*SDHB-D, SEC23B, KLLN, PARP4, AKT1, PIK3CA, USF3, TTN, MUTYH, RET, TSC2, BRCA1, BRCA2, ERCC2, HRAS,* and *RASAL1*) [19,30–32].

PTEN dephosphorylates PI (3,4,5) P3 (PIP3) and PI (3, 4) P2 to PI (4,5) P2 and PI (4) P, respectively. Thus, PIP3 and PI (3,4) P2 do not activate AKT serine/threonine kinase (AKT), and the phosphatidilinositol 3-kinase (PI3K)/AKT signaling pathway remains inhibited. PTEN mutation results in loss of function, leading to a high concentration of PI (3,4) P2 that activates AKT and enhances cell proliferation, cell migration, and reduces cell death [33,34]. In addition, mechanisms that regulate PTEN expression and compartmentalization are involved in tumorigenesis [35].

The first correlations between the PIK3-AKT pathway activation and thyroid cancer were observed in Cowden syndrome studies. Since Cowden syndrome mainly presents with FTC and PTEN activates the PIK3-AKT pathway, some authors have postulated that PIK3-AKT activation is required for FTC oncogenesis, and these preliminary findings were further corroborated [36,37].

Another intriguing fact was the association of RAS protein activator like 1 (*RASAL1*) with Cowden Syndrome. RASAL1 is a negative modulator of the RAS signaling pathway and suppresses both mitogen-activated protein kinase (MAPK) and PI3K pathways. However, *RASAL1* is frequently found methylated or mutated in sporadic follicular and anaplastic thyroid cancer [38].

In a large series of 155 patients with Cowden syndrome and thyroid cancer, 39 presented with *PTEN* germline mutations, while *RASAL1* germline alteration (*RASAL1*, c.982C>T, R328W) was observed in two patients without *PTEN* mutations [32]. In the same study, the authors also analyzed the germline database of The Cancer Genome Atlas (TCGA) and discovered that 0.6% of PTC patients harbored the deleterious germline *RASAL1* mutation [32].

2.2. *Carney Complex*

The Carney complex (OMIM #160980) is an autosomal dominant disorder in 70% of the cases, characterized by loss-of-function mutations in the *PRKAR1A* gene (17q22–24).

Under a normal condition of several endocrine related ligands, such as TSH, FSH, ACTH, GHRH, and MSH, when binding to the G-protein coupled receptor activates protein kinase A (PKA). *PRKAR1A* encodes the R1α subunit of PKA. Thus, when mutated, it increases cAMP-dependent PKA activity and drives tumorigenesis [17,39,40]. Therefore, thyrocytes, Sertoli cells, adrenocortical cells, somatotrophs, and melanocytes are directly affected by the *PRKAR1a* mutation. As a result, variable endocrine tumors are observed in the Carney complex disease, including primary pigmented nodular adrenocortical disease, pituitary adenomas, testicular tumors, ovarian lesions, and myxomas and lentiginosis syndromes [17]. Since thyroid cancer could also be part of this syndrome, annual long-term surveillance is recommended [17].

Evidence shows that PRKAR1A acts as a tumor suppressor gene in sporadic thyroid cancers [41]. However, the traditional thyroid cancer pathways (MAPK and PIK3-AKT pathways) are not involved in the Carney complex [42]. Instead, a recent in vitro study suggests that PKA activates AMP-activated kinase (AMPK) through serine/threonine kinase 11 (LKB1, also named SKT11) in Carney-related FTC without inhibiting mTOR activation [43].

2.3. *Werner Syndrome*

Werner syndrome is one of the progeroid syndromes (OMIM #27770) characterized by early aging, scleroderma-like skin changes, bilateral cataracts, and subcutaneous calcifications, premature arteriosclerosis, and diabetes mellitus. Different types of cancers are associated with this syndrome, such as meningiomas, myeloid disorders, soft tissue sarcomas, and thyroid carcinoma [1,44]. Their regular surveillance is recommended [45]. The Werner Syndrome's patients carry autosomal recessive WRN RecQ like helicase (*WRN*) gene mutations on 8p11.1–21.1. *WRN* gene encodes RecQ helicase that regulate DNA replication, recombination, repair, transcription, and telomerase maintenance. Dysregulation of this pathway triggers DNA instability, telomeric fusions of homologous chromosomes, and, ultimately, oncogenesis [13]. However, the precise mechanisms that contribute to genome instability in Werner syndrome remains unclear [46]. In a Japanese series, mutations in the N-terminal portion of *WRN* was correlated with PTC, while mutations in C-terminal with FTC [47]. The N-terminal portion of *WRN* contains exonuclease activity, whereas the central part contains the DNA-dependent ATPase, 3′–5′ helicase, and annealing activity [46]. Overall, these studies suggest specific effects in WRN activity depending on the site of mutation. Moreover, an in vitro study showed that mutations in *WRN*'s nuclease domain, helicase domain, or DNA binding domain aborted its canonical stimulatory effect on nonhomologous end-joining (c-NHEJ) pathway during DNA double-strand break (DSB) repair [46].

2.4. *Familial Adenomatous Polyposis*

The phenotype of familial adenomatous polyposis (FAP) (OMIM #175100) is characterized by numerous intestinal polyps, colon cancer, and other cancers that include thyroid cancer [2,22,48]. FAP is an autosomal dominant disorder caused by mutations in APC regulator of WNT signaling pathway (*APC*) gene on chromosome 5q21. The *APC* gene is a suppressor of the Wnt signaling pathway and regulates β-catenin activation by multiple mechanisms. In normal conditions, the Axin complex—formed by APC, glycogen synthase kinase 3 (GSK3), and casein kinase 1 (CK1)—phosphorylates the amino-terminal of the free β-catenin, permitting its recognition and further ubiquitination [49,50]. By this process of continuous degradation, β-catenin remains in the cytoplasm without reaching the promoter region of target genes in the nucleus. Thus, when the APC protein is mutated or truncated, β-catenin is released from its degradation and migrates to the nucleus, activating gene transcription of oncogenic pathways. Truncated APC protein also interferes with chromosome stability and cell migration [50].

In addition to the germline mutation, biallelic inactivation of the wild-type APC allele is frequently necessary for tumorigenesis, and the second-hit is commonly acquired by somatic mutation [51]. In the FAP-associated thyroid cancer, the concomitant presence of germline and distinct somatic mutation were observed in several Japanese families [48,52,53]. Most of FAP-associated thyroid cancers present the histological subtype called cribriform-morular variant of PTC (CMVPTC) [2,51]. An annual thyroid ultrasound is recommended to late teen years' patients [54,55].

2.5. *Ataxia-Telangiectasia Syndrome*

Ataxia-telangiectasia (A-T) syndrome (OMIM #208900) is an autosomal recessive disorder linked to the mutation of the ATM serine/threonine kinase (*ATM*) gene and characterized by degenerative cerebellar atrophy, telangiectasias, immune defects, and malignancy [56,57]. It is also well-known that relatives of patients with ataxia-telangiectasia have an increased cancer incidence [16].

ATM protein belongs to the PI-3 kinase-like protein kinases family. Besides TP53, BRCA1, and BRCA2, ATM is considered a genome's guardian and participates directly in the DNA damage response (DDR). For its activation, MRE11-RAD50-NBS1 (MRN) complex—A sensor of DSB (double strand-break)—induces several autophosphorylations and acetylations. Activated ATM then phosphorylates different proteins involved in the DSB (double-strand break) response [58].

For instance, ATM phosphorylates CHK2 and p53, which are both involved in senescence and apoptosis [58].

An increased incidence of thyroid cancer was observed in obligate *ATM* mutation carriers (RR adjusted = 2.6) [16]. Later, selective mutations in the *ATM* gene are related to thyroid cancer. *ATM* c.2119T>C p.S707P (rs4986761) heterozygotes were associated with an adjusted HR (hazard ratio for cancer) of 10 for thyroid/endocrine tumors, while no association was observed in *ATM* c.146C>G p.S49C (rs1800054) heterozygote carriers [56]. Nonetheless, recent population studies revealed that some ATM polymorphisms have a protective role, while other studies reported a damaging effect [59–62]. There are even controversial observations for the same polymorphism [26,27,59,60,63]. Despite these controversies, consistent *ATM* variants (*ATM* p.P1054R-rs1800057- and rs149711770) were recently described in families with FNMTC and other cancers (as kidney, lung, stomach, and prostate) [11]. Nonetheless, in A-T Syndrome´s patient, the only screening recommended is for breast cancer [15].

2.6. DICER 1 Syndrome and miRNA Processing

A non-toxic multinodular goiter (MNG) is frequently diagnosed in the adult population and studies correlate the presence of MNG and the development of differentiated thyroid cancer [14,64,65]. On the other hand, familial cases of MNG are a common characteristic associated with the DICER1 syndrome (OMIM #601200), which predisposes patients to thyroid cancer [66], and other types of tumors such as Sertoli-Leydig cell tumors of the ovary (SLCT) [20] and pleuropulmonary blastomas [21].

DICER is an endonuclease essential for the maturation of microRNAs (miRNAs), small non-coding RNAs with ~22 nt, that block mRNA translation post-transcriptionally by binding to the 3′-UTR (untranslated region) of target mRNAs, and tightly controlling cell signaling and cell biology [67]. A mutation in dicer1, ribonuclease III (*DICER1*) gene, especially those present in the ribonuclease domain, leads to DICER loss of function and downregulation of microRNA levels [20,68]. The correct control of miRNA expression is essential for the development of a functional thyroid gland [69]. Studies with transgenic mice with dysfunctional DICER lead to disturbance of thyroid architecture, cell proliferation and disarrangement of follicular structures, and loss of differentiation [70,71], indicating the influence of DICER loss in thyroid tumorigenesis.

A familial approach to investigate the risk of thyroid malignancy in DICER1 syndrome patients revealed a 16-fold higher risk of development of thyroid cancer when *DICER1* is mutated compared to non-mutated patients [66]. Thus, there is a suggestion to monitor the thyroid status by a thyroid ultrasound every two-three years in patients after the age of eight [29,72]. Enforced evidence of *DICER1* mutation with familial thyroid cancer was also shown in a study with six individuals of the same family harboring *DICER1* mutation (c.5441C>T, p.S1814L) and multiple cases of differentiated thyroid cancer and MNG [73].

The Cancer Genome Atlas (TCGA) database shows *DICER1* mutation in 0.8% of patients with PTC/PDTC (p.E1813G, p.D1810H, p.E1813K, p.R1906S, p.M1402T) [74–78]. A recent study revealed high prevalence of *DICER1* mutations in pediatric-adolescent poorly differentiated thyroid cancer (83%) at a hotspot in the metal-ion binding sites of the RNase IIIb domain of DICER1 (c.5113G>A, p.E1705K, c.5125G>A, p.D1709N (rs1595331264), c.5137G>A, p.1713Y, c.5437G>A, p.E1813K, c.5437G>C, p.E1813Q) [79]. Another study linked hotspot *DICER1* mutations to pediatric PTC (c.5125G>A p.D1709N, c.5428G>T p.D1801Y, c.5438A>G p.E1813G, c.5439G>C p.E1813D) with increased incidence in the patients that do not harbor MAPK classic alterations [80], suggesting a role for *DICER1* mutation detection in thyroid tumors. A recent study detected *DICER1* (c.5429A>T, p.D1810V, c.5437G>A, p.E1813K) and drosha ribonuclease III (*DROSHA*) mutation (c.2943C>T, p.S981S, c.3597C>T, p.Y1199Y (rs61748189)) in benign follicular adenoma, even though *DICER1* mutations were not detected in a follicular variant of PTC that harbored *HRAS* mutations [68]. On the other hand, a recent study associated MAPK alterations with germline mutations in *DICER1* [81]. Altogether, these studies suggest that *DICER1* haploinsufficiency is associated with thyroid tumorigenesis.

DROSHA is another endonuclease of miRNA processing machinery and acts together with DGCR8 to form the Microprocessor complex to excise the precursor miRNA out of the primary transcript in the nucleus [67]. Then, DICER acts in the next step in the cytoplasm and cleaves the precursor miRNA to form mature functional miRNAs. In a similar extent to *DICER1* mutations, *DGCR8* mutations were also detected in familial cases of MNG and are associated with schwannoma [82]. Altogether, these studies indicate the essential role of proper miRNA processing and expression for thyroid gland physiology.

2.7. Li-Fraumeni Syndrome

The Li-Fraumeni syndrome is caused by a heterozygous mutation in *TP53* and is typically characterized by soft tissue and bone sarcomas, breast cancers, central nervous system tumors, leukemia, and adrenal tumors. p53 interacts with a complex network and drives DNA repair, cell-cycle arrest, senescence, or apoptosis when it is phosphorylated by DNA damage response (DDR) kinases [13,83]. The PTC occurs in 10% of Li-Fraumeni syndrome patients, mainly when associated with *TP53* mutation p.R337H [24]. Therefore, imaging screening for thyroid malignancy in Li-Fraumeni families has been advocated [24].

3. Non-Syndromic FNMTC

Even if FNMTC comprises only 3–9% of all thyroid cancer, the first-degree relatives of NMTC have an 8-12-fold increased risk of developing the disease [84,85]. Non-syndromic FNMTC comprises 95% of all FNMTC and is defined by two or more first-degree relatives present with NMTC without associated syndromes. Moreover, the transmission pattern is not yet well defined, which seems to be autosomal dominant in most cases. Like sporadic NMTC, more than 85% are PTC, approximately 10% are FTC, and around 5% are anaplastic thyroid cancer. Furthermore, FNMTC is more aggressive, presents with nodal disease, and recurs more often. In addition, thyroid cancer tends to occur earlier in subsequent generations in FNMTC, called the anticipation phenomenon [2,86,87].

3.1. Linkage Analysis

From 1997 to 2006, the linkage analysis was the main method to study the familial condition. Using this approach, a positive logarithm of odds (LOD) would mean a high likelihood that locus cosegregates with the FNMTC trait, which is a linkage. In this way, several loci were associated with non-syndromic FNMTC (Table 2).

Table 2. Loci and genes associated with non-syndromic familial non-medullary thyroid cancer (FNMTC).

Loci/Gene	Localization	Characteristics	Reference
	Linkage analysis		
TCO	19p13.2	Oxyphilic PTC	[6]
NMTC1	2q21		[9]
PRN1	1q21	Papillary renal cancer	[8]
MNG1/*DICER1*	14q32	MNG	[7]
	Linkage analysis and NGS		
SRGAP1	12q14		[88]
	8p23.1–p22		[10]
	6q22		[89]
lncRNA inside TG	8q24	Melanoma in 1 family	[90]
Enhancer associated with POU2F1 and YY1	4q32		[91]
	Other methodology		
NKX2-1	14q13.3		[92]

3.1.1. TCO Locus (19p13.2)

The 'thyroid carcinoma, nonmedullary, with cell oxyphilia' (TCO) locus was identified in a French family with oxyphilic thyroid cancer in the short arm of chromosome 19 (19p13.2). This region includes several genes, such as *ICAM1* gene, which is overexpressed in thyroid cancer cells, and the JunB proto-oncogene, AP-1 transcription factor subunit (*JUNB*) [6]. However, some other genes in the locus, such as several zinc-finger-protein genes, were not yet identified. Moreover, the TCO locus does not seem to be involved in the majority of oxyphilic sporadic NMTC. An additional Tyrolean family with high LOD in the same locus was also described [93].

3.1.2. PRN1 Locus (1q21)

Papillary thyroid cancer is associated with papillary renal cancer. Linkage analysis identified this locus with the highest LOD of 3.58 in a family with three generations affected by PTC and papillary renal carcinoma. MET proto-oncogene, receptor tyrosine kinase (*MET*) mutations, frequently associated with familial papillary renal cancer, and mutations associated with other thyroid cancer syndromes were excluded [8]. However, this finding was limited to this family.

3.1.3. NMTC1 Locus (2q21)

This locus was described in a large Tasmanian family study [9], and when the authors further analyzed 17 families with FNMTC, they found an LOD heterogeneity of 4.17. At that time, it was hypothesized that multiple environmental and genetic causes could be involved in the pathogenesis of FNMTC [93].

3.1.4. q32 Locus (an Enhancer of Unknown Function)

A rare mutation in 4q32 was found in the linkage analysis and targeted deep sequencing in a large family with four individuals with benign thyroid disease, nine PTC patients, and one anaplastic thyroid cancer (ATC) patient. This nucleotide exchange in chr4:165491559 (GRCh37/hg19), named 4q32A>C, is in a highly conserved region. The chromatin immunoprecipitation (ChIP) assays showed that both POU2F1 and YY1 transcription factors related to specific thyroid genes and thyroid development bind to this region. As consequence of the allele's change, a decrease of both POUF2 and YY1 bindings were observed. Transcription factors' disruption has already been associated with cancer [91].

3.1.5. 6q22 Locus

The finding of 6q22 locus with LOD + 3.30 was observed in 38 families of FNMTC by linkage analysis and a genome-wide SNP array [89]. However, no further studies have confirmed this locus in additional families.

3.1.6. 8p23.1–p22 Locus

A locus associated with FNMTC in a huge Portuguese family was identified by linkage analysis, with a maximum parametric haplotype-based LOD score of 4.41. Among 17 candidate genes in the locus (*PPP1R3B, MIRN597, MIRN124A1, MSRA, C8orf74, SOX7, PINX1, MIRN598, C8orf15, C8orf16, MTMR9, C8orf13, NEIL2, CTSB, DUB3, DLC1, TUSC3*), no deleterious alteration was detected in the genes' coding region. [10].

3.1.7. 8q24 Locus, a lncRNA inside the Thyroglobulin (TG) Gene

Linkage analysis was also performed in a group of 26 families of PTC [90], which revealed a LOD of + 1.3 in a locus that harbors *TG* and *SLA* (Src like adaptor) genes. However, no polymorphism or mutation was found in the coding genes, suggesting that this alteration could be associated with a lncRNA related to the *TG* gene.

3.1.8. SRGAP1 (12q14 Locus)

The study of 38 families with FNMTC by genome-wide linkage analysis indicated a high peak in 12q14 in 55% (21 of 38), but with a modest OR = 1.21 (p = 0.0008). Nonetheless, it was observed six different germline mutations/variants in the *SRGAP1* gene (c.447A>C, p.Q149H, c.823G>A, p.A275T, c.1534G>A, p.V512I, rs74691643, c.1849C>T, p.R617C, rs114817817, c.2274T>C, p.S758S, rs789722, c.2624A>G, p.H875R, rs61754221). In vitro functional testing in thyroid cancer cells showed decreased GTPase activating protein (GAP) activity in two of these *SGARP1* polymorphisms (Q149H and R617C). The SRGAP1 could mediate tumorigenesis by interacting with CDC42 [88], which is a common signal transduction convergence point of many signaling pathways and can play a role in thyroid cancer cell migration via RAGE/Dia-1 signaling [94].

3.1.9. NKX2-1 (14q13.3 Locus)

The mutation in *NKX2-1* gene (c.1016 C>T, p. A339V) was described in two families associated with PTC and MNG [87]. Even though most patients had only MNG, the authors hypothesized that MNG could be the first step to malignancy [92,95–97].

3.1.10. MNG1 Locus (14q32)-DICER1

The MNG1 (OMIM # 138800) locus was revealed by linkage analysis in families with multinodular goiter and NMTC [7]. Furthermore, it was observed that MNG1 corresponded to *DICER1* gene, related to microRNA biogenesis (described in "Syndromic causes of non-medullary thyroid cancer" section).

3.2. Genome-Wide Linkage Analysis in the Population of PTC Patients

The sequencing of the genome by NGS) uncovered the genetic variation and the potential association with several pathologies, including cancer. In particular, the GWAS (genome-wide association study) revealed numerous SNPs in the genes related to thyroid physiology and tumorigenesis (Table 3) [12].

Table 3. Genes associated with genetic predisposition of sporadic papillary thyroid cancer.

Locus	Nearest Gene	Population	Reference
9q22.33	*FOXE1, PTCSC2*	Belarus, Iceland, Italy, Korea, Netherlands Poland, Spain, USA	[98–100]
14q13.3	*PTCSC3, NKX2-1, MBIP1*	Iceland, Italy, Korea, Netherlands, Poland, Spain, USA	[98,99]
2q35	*DIRC3*	Iceland, Italy, Korea, Netherlands, Poland, Spain, UK, USA	[99,101]
8p12	*NRG1*	Iceland, Korea, Netherlands, Spain, USA	[99,102]
1q42.2	*PCNXL2*	Iceland, Korea, Netherlands, Spain, USA	[102,103]
European Only			
3q26.2	*LRRC34*	Iceland, Netherlands, Spain, USA	[103]
5p15.33	*TERT*	Iceland, Netherlands, Spain, USA	[103]
5q22.1	*EPB41L4A*	Iceland, Netherlands, Spain, USA	[103]
10q24.33	*OBFC1*	Iceland, Netherlands, Spain, USA	[103]
15q22.33	*SMAD3*	Iceland, Netherlands, Spain, USA	[103]
Korean Only			
12q14.3	*MSRB3*	Korea	[102]
1p13.3	*VAV3*	Korea	[102]
4q21.1	*SEPT11*	Korea	[102]
3p14.2	*FHIT*	Korea	[102]
19p13.2	*INSR*	Korea	[102]
12q24.13	*SLC8B1*	Korea	[102]

3.2.1. *FOXE1/PTCSC2*

Located in 9q22.3 and close to the forkhead box E1 (*FOXE1*) gene, rs965513 conferred an increased risk for thyroid cancer and was named 'papillary thyroid carcinoma susceptibility candidate 2' (*PTCSC2*) gene. The carriers of rs965513 (homozygous of A allele present a 3.1-fold increased risk for thyroid cancer in large European series [98]. The same polymorphism rs965513 was observed in Japanese and Belarusian populations, but with an OR of 1.6-1.9 [104]. Similarly, a variant in the promoter region of the *FOXE1* gene (rs1867277) was identified as a risk factor for PTC (OR = 1.49) in a Spanish series and further confirmed in an Italian one [105]. Subsequently, new studies showed a tumor suppressor effect of FOXE1 and demonstrated that rs1867277 is involved in differential recruitment of USF1/ USF2 transcription factors, which interferes with FOXE1 expression [12,106]. Moreover, myosin heavy chain-9 (MYH9) can bind and suppress the shared promoter of *PTCSC2* and *FOXE1* genes bilaterally (that includes rs1867277 region), an effect that is abolished by PTCSC2 that sequesters MYH9 [107]. Therefore, MYH9, which is a lncRNA binding protein, can also play a role in PTC susceptibility.

A rare *FOXE1* variant (c.743C>G; p.A248G) was identified in one of 60 Portuguese FNMTC cases and one sporadic case. Besides, polymorphisms in *FOXE1* locus (rs965513 and rs1867277) were associated with increased familial and sporadic NMTC risk [104,108].

3.2.2. *NKX2-1*

A consistent finding in the 14q13.3 locus was rs944289. Located close to the NKX2-1 gene, this variant of uncertain significance (VUS) is in PTCSC3's promoter region and regulates the lncRNA PTCSC3 expression by affecting the binding site of C/EBPα and C/EBPβ (PTCSC3 activators) [98,99,109,110]. PTCSC3 downregulates S100A4, reducing cell motility and invasiveness. Thus, *PTCSC3* mutations could predispose to PTC through the S100A4 pathway [111]. Moreover, *NKX2-1* mutation (c.1016C>T, p.A339V) was observed in a family with multinodular goiter and papillary thyroid cancer [87], but this was not confirmed by another FNMTC study [112].

3.2.3. *NRG1*

NRG1 polymorphisms produced an association signal in GWAS for thyroid cancer. NRG1 is highly expressed in the thyroid and participates in cell growth pathways, mainly via erb-b2 receptor tyrosin kinase (ERBB)/MAPK [113]. However, NRG1 expression is detected in follicular adenomas, suggesting they are linked to thyroid tumorigenesis [12].

3.2.4. *DIRC3*

Polymorphisms in the *DIRC3* (disrupted in renal carcinoma 3) gene have also been found in thyroid cancer GWAS [12,102,103]. *DIRC3* codifies a lncRNA that was first associated with renal cancer, suggesting a tumor suppressor role [101]. *DIRC3* and *IGFBP5* (insulin-like growth factor binding protein 5) tumor suppressors are within the same topologically associated domain. Moreover, it was observed that *DIRC3* depletion induces an increased *SOX10* (SRY-box transcription factor 10) repression of *IGFBP5* in melanoma cell cultures, corroborating the tumor suppressor role of *DIRC3* [114].

In addition, the TT variant of rs966423 (*DIRC3*, g.217445617C>T) has been associated with worse PTC presentation and prognosis. An increased tumor size, staging, lymph node involvement, and overall mortality was observed in the TT-haplotype [115]. In a Chinese series, rs966423 was also correlated to tumor invasion and multifocality [1]. Nevertheless, no difference in these parameters was observed in a Polish series [116].

3.2.5. Polygenic Contribution

Recently, an increased risk for PTC was associated with a cumulative number of deleterious polymorphisms detected in the same patient. Ten different polymorphisms (rs12129938, rs11693806, rs6793295, rs73227498, rs2466076, rs1588635, rs7902587, rs368187, rs116909374, and rs2289261) related to the PTC development were analyzed, and the presence of each of these SNPs increased the risk to PTC. Nevertheless, if a patient harbors all 10 variants at the same time, the risk of developing thyroid cancer is 6.9-fold greater than those with no variants [117].

3.2.6. Telomere Abnormalities

A decade ago, three independent groups observed that relative telomere length (RTL) is shorter in patients with FNMTC [118–120]. As telomerase controls the telomere length, one of these groups investigated *TERC* and *hTERT* (which form telomerase) alterations and observed the amplification of *hTERT* in patients' leukocytes [118]. However, this finding was not confirmed subsequently [119,120]. In recent years, many alterations in the shelterin complex's genes have been reported. The shelterin complex is formed by six proteins (POT1, ACD, TINF2, TERF1, TERF2, and TERF2IP), and protects the telomere from DDR mechanisms. Along with telomerase, this complex is vital for genomic stability because telomeric ends resemble DNA double breaks. Telomeric repeat binding factor 1 (TERF1, also known as TRF1), telomeric repeat binding factor 2 (TERF2, also known TRF2), and protection of telomeres 1 (POT1) directly recognize TTAGGG repeats. In contrast, adrenocortical dysplasia protein homolog (ACD, also known as TPP1), TERF1-interacting nuclear factor 2 (TINF2, also known as TIN2), and telomeric repeat binding factor 2 interacting protein (TERF2IP, also known as RAP1) form a complex that differentiates telomeres from sites of DNA damage.

TINF2 mutation was described in a family with melanoma and thyroid cancer predisposition. Functional analysis showed that mutated *TINF2* was unable to activate *TERF2*, resulting in longer telomere lengths. All shelterin complex's genes were screened in a subsequent 24 families with FNMTC, and two missense variants in *TINF2* and *ACD* genes were found, but only the *ACD* variant was predicted as deleterious [121].

Another group reported a new mutation in *POT1* (c.85G>T; p.V29L) [122] in an Italian FNMTC. *POT1* disruptions can interfere with the interaction of the POT1-ACD complex. In agreement with these findings, another *POT1* mutation (c.268A>G, p.K90E) was described in a family with a predisposition to several tumors (melanoma, breast, kidney, and thyroid cancer, pituitary tumor, and Cushing syndrome) [123]. Moreover, an association between the increased risk of thyroid cancer and the presence of an intronic variant of *POT1* (rs58722976) was also observed in a cohort of childhood cancer survivors [124].

Altogether, it suggests that telomere abnormalities and shelterin complex genes alteration may influence the predisposition to the FNMTC.

3.2.7. miRNA

The miRNA-related SNPs affect the microRNA biogenesis and function. A large study evaluated approximately 80 families displaying Mendelian-like inheritance and found two candidate miRNA (*let-7e* and *miR-181b*). The variants of let-7e and miR-182b-2 were located at the 5′ end of 3p mature miRNA and the 3′ end of 5p mature miRNA, respectively, which downregulate the expression by impairing the miRNA processing [125]. The gain or loss of specific miRNAs is an important oncogenic event [69].

3.3. Whole Exome/Genome Sequence

The whole-exome sequence (WES) or the whole genome sequence (WGS) of family members with FNMTC is another strategy besides the GWAS in large populations of differentiated thyroid cancer (DTC). Using this approach, an enormous number of variants is detected, demanding some criteria to filter and select the candidate variants. In general, minor allele frequency (MAF), the expression in thyroid and predictor functions (i.e., SIFT, PolyPhen, CADD, and others) are used as filters. Variants related to cancer pathways can also be used as filters. Since the application of this strategy has been consolidated for genetic studies in recent years, some authors have proposed new variants involved in FNMTC. Many are still under validation.

3.3.1. *SRRM2*

The association of linkage analysis and WES identified an *SRRM2* variant in a family with FNMTC [126]. However, this variant was not exclusively present in FNMTC, as it was found in sporadic NMTC cases, implying the occurrence of FNMTC may also depend on environmental factors or other genes [126].

3.3.2. *NOP53*

The presence of rs78530808 (*NOP53*, c.91G>C, p.D31H) was observed in one family with FNMTC when using a less strict filter than other studies (MAF < 2%) [116]. NOP53 participates in ribosome biogenesis and regulates the p53 activation in the case of ribosome biogenesis perturbation. The variant c.91G>C was also identified in three out of 44 families with FNMTC [127]. In the tumor samples, NOP53 expression was increased when compared to the adjacent normal tissue. Furthermore, *NOP53* knockdown inhibited cell proliferation and colony formation in vitro [127]. Altogether, these findings suggested that this variant could have an oncogenic role in thyroid tumorigenesis [127].

3.3.3. *HABP2*

HABP2 variant is an excellent example to describe how careful we should be with possible false-positive findings. The variant G534E was described in a family with seven members with PTC [128]. However, this finding was severely criticized later by other researchers. Even though it seemed the right candidate in the beginning, further studies did not confirm it in other populations. Furthermore, since its MAF is high in the European population, we would expect a higher incidence of FNMTC [129]. Besides, the prevalence of this same variant was similar among patients with FNMTC, sporadic PTC, and controls [130,131].

3.4. *Candidate Variants Associated with FNMTC*

Recently, different groups have pinpointed a list of candidate variants in FNMTC. A Korean study identified seven candidate variants localized in *ANO7, CAV2, KANK1, PIK3CB, PKD1L1, PTPRF,* and *RHBDD2* genes in a family with four patients with PTC [132]. In addition, a Brazilian group reported seven new variants located in *FKBP10, PLEKHG5, P2RX5, SAPCD1, ANXA3, NTN4,* and *SERPINA1* [133].

In a large series including 17 families with isolated FNMTC and FNMTC associated with other malignancies, 41 rare candidate variants were identified in *TDRD6, IDE, TINF2, RNF213, AGK, NHLH1, TMCC1, ALB, THBS4, C5orf15, KLH3, FGFR4, SMARCD3, GPR107, NSMF, SVIL, EIF3, RNF169, NFRB, CIS, CDH11, EDC4, FOXA3, CDS2, NAPB, SALL4, ATG14, UNC79, LZTR1, ATP13A2, CTDSP1, MAPKAPK3, AARS, KDSR, ZNF302, ZNF17, ITGAD, FGD6, PDPR,* and *EFCAB8* genes. Cancer susceptibility genes (*CHEK2, PRF1, ATM, AKAP13, SLC26A11*) were also observed [11]. As described before, the authors further correlated the presence of *TINF2* (a shelterin gene) to families with PTC and melanoma.

It was also interesting to observe that some of these genes have already been associated with thyroid cancer predisposition [59,134]. Despite these promising findings, most of the variants need to be better investigated for its functional role in thyroid cancer risk.

4. Conclusions

It was expected that the advent of new technologies of genome study would shed new light on the genetic predisposition of FNMTC. The NGS certainly did shed light on a whole new spectrum of variants and pointed to the co-occurrence of several variants in FNMTC. However, the limiting point in this scenario is the lack of a detailed in vitro validation that could precisely identify the contribution of each variant for the complex FNMTC entity. Moreover, the expansion of already known genetic data in multiple cohorts is essential to establish their role in FNMTC carcinogenesis.

Author Contributions: E.T.K. conceived the idea; F.Y.M., C.S.F., G.A.d.C. and E.T.K. were involved in planning, writing, and editing the manuscript. All authors have read and agreed to the published version of the manuscript.

Acknowledgments: We gratefully acknowledge the CNPq by the grant 308331/2017-6 (E.T.K.), FAPESP (The São Paulo Research Foundation-Brazil) by the grant 2020/10403-9 (C.S.F.), and the scholarships from CAPES (Coordenação de Aperfeiçoamento de Pessoal de Nível Superior-Brazil): PDSE 88881.362254/2019-01 (F.Y.M.) and PNPD 88887.374682/2019-00 (C.S.F.).

Abbreviations

AD	autosomal dominant
AR	autosomal recessive
ATC	anaplastic thyroid cancer
CMVPTC	cribriform-morular variant of PTC
cPTC	classical PTC
DDR	DNA damage response
DTC	differentiated thyroid cancer
FA	follicular adenoma
FAP	familial adenomatous polyposis
FNMTC	familial nonmedullary thyroid cancer
FTC	follicular thyroid cancer
FVPTC	follicular variant of PTC
GWAS	genome-wide association studies
HR	hazard ratio
LOD	logarithm of odds
MAF	minor allele frequency
miRNAs	microRNAs
MNG	multinodular goiter
MTC	medullary thyroid cancer
NGS	next generation sequencing
NMTC	nonmedullary thyroid cancer
PTC	papillary thyroid cancer
SNPs	single nucleotide polymorphisms
TCGA	The Cancer Genome Atlas
VUS	variant of uncertain significance
WES	whole exome sequence
WGS	whole genome sequence

References

1. Hincza, K.; Kowalik, A.; Kowalska, A. Current Knowledge of Germline Genetic Risk Factors for the Development of Non-Medullary Thyroid Cancer. *Genes* **2019**, *10*, 482. [CrossRef] [PubMed]
2. Guilmette, J.; Nosé, V. Hereditary and familial thyroid tumours. *Histopathology* **2017**, *72*, 70–81. [CrossRef] [PubMed]
3. Firminger, H.I.; Skelton, F.R. Carcinoma of the thyroid: Papillary adenocarcinoma occurring in twins and a case of Hürthle cell carcinoma; tumor conference. *J. Kans. Med. Soc.* **1953**, *54*, 427–432. [PubMed]
4. Sippel, R.S.; Caron, N.R.; Clark, O.H. An evidence-based approach to familial nonmedullary thyroid cancer: Screening, clinical management, and follow-up. *World J. Surg.* **2007**, *31*, 924–933. [CrossRef] [PubMed]

5. Mazeh, H.; Sippel, R.S. Familial nonmedullary thyroid carcinoma. *Thyroid* **2013**, *23*, 1049–1056. [CrossRef]
6. Canzian, F.; Amati, P.; Harach, H.R.; Kraimps, J.-L.; Lesueur, F.; Barbier, J.; Levillain, P.; Romeo, G.; Bonneau, D. A gene predisposing to familial thyroid tumors with cell oxyphilia maps to chromosome 19p13.2. *Am. J. Hum. Genet.* **1998**, *63*, 1743–1748. [CrossRef]
7. Bignell, G.R.; Canzian, F.; Shayeghi, M.; Stark, M.; Shugart, Y.Y.; Biggs, P.; Mangion, J.; Hamoudi, R.; Rosenblatt, J.; Buu, P.; et al. Familial nontoxic multinodular thyroid goiter locus maps to chromosome 14q but does not account for familial nonmedullary thyroid cancer. *Am. J. Hum. Genet.* **1997**, *61*, 1123–1130. [CrossRef]
8. Malchoff, C.D.; Sarfarazi, M.; Tendler, B.; Forouhar, F.; Whalen, G.; Joshi, V.; Arnold, A.; Malchoff, D.M. Papillary thyroid carcinoma associated with papillary renal neoplasia: Genetic linkage analysis of a distinct heritable tumor syndrome. *J. Clin. Endocrinol. Metab.* **2000**, *85*, 1758–1764. [CrossRef]
9. McKay, J.D.; Lesueur, F.; Jonard, L.; Pastore, A.; Williamson, J.; Hoffman, L.; Burgess, J.; Duffield, A.; Papotti, M.; Stark, M.; et al. Localization of a susceptibility gene for familial nonmedullary thyroid carcinoma to chromosome 2q21. *Am. J. Hum. Genet.* **2001**, *69*, 440–446. [CrossRef]
10. Cavaco, B.M.; Batista, P.F.; Sobrinho, L.G.; Leite, V. Mapping a new familial thyroid epithelial neoplasia susceptibility locus to chromosome 8p23.1-p22 by high-density single-nucleotide polymorphism genome-wide linkage analysis. *J. Clin. Endocrinol. Metab.* **2008**, *93*, 4426–4430. [CrossRef]
11. Wang, Y.; Liyanarachchi, S.; Miller, K.E.; Nieminen, T.T.; Comiskey, D.F., Jr.; Li, W.; Brock, P.; Symer, D.E.; Akagi, K.; DeLap, K.E.; et al. Identification of Rare Variants Predisposing to Thyroid Cancer. *Thyroid* **2019**, *29*, 946–955. [CrossRef] [PubMed]
12. Saenko, V.A.; Rogounovitch, T.I. Genetic Polymorphism Predisposing to Differentiated Thyroid Cancer: A Review of Major Findings of the Genome-Wide Association Studies. *Endocrinol. Metab.* **2018**, *33*, 164–174. [CrossRef]
13. Carbone, M.; Arron, S.T.; Beutler, B.; Bononi, A.; Cavenee, W.; Cleaver, J.E.; Croce, C.M.; D'Andrea, A.; Foulkes, W.D.; Gaudino, G.; et al. Tumour predisposition and cancer syndromes as models to study gene-environment interactions. *Nat. Rev. Cancer* **2020**, *20*, 533–549. [CrossRef] [PubMed]
14. Haugen, B.R.; Alexander, E.K.; Bible, K.C.; Doherty, G.M.; Mandel, S.J.; Nikiforov, Y.E.; Pacini, F.; Randolph, G.W.; Sawka, A.M.; Schlumberger, M.; et al. 2015 American Thyroid Association Management Guidelines for Adult Patients with Thyroid Nodules and Differentiated Thyroid Cancer: The American Thyroid Association Guidelines Task Force on Thyroid Nodules and Differentiated Thyroid Cancer. *Thyroid* **2016**, *26*, 1–133. [CrossRef]
15. Van Os, N.J.; Roeleveld, N.; Weemaes, C.M.R.; Jongmans, M.C.J.; Janssens, G.O.; Taylor, A.M.R.; Hoogerbrugge, N.; Willemsen, M.A.A.P. Health risks for ataxia-telangiectasia mutated heterozygotes: A systematic review, meta-analysis and evidence-based guideline. *Clin. Genet.* **2016**, *90*, 105–117. [CrossRef] [PubMed]
16. Geoffroy-Perez, B.; Janin, N.; Ossian, K.; Laugé, A.; Croquette, M.F.; Griscelli, C.; Debré, M.; Bressac-de-Paillerets, B.; Aurias, A.; Stoppa-Lyonnet, D.; et al. Cancer risk in heterozygotes for ataxia-telangiectasia. *Int. J. Cancer* **2001**, *93*, 288–293. [CrossRef]
17. Kamilaris, C.D.C.; Faucz, F.R.; Voutetakis, A.; Stratakis, C.A. Carney Complex. *Exp. Clin. Endocrinol. Diabetes* **2019**, *127*, 156–164. [CrossRef]
18. Gammon, A.; Jasperson, K.; Champine, M. Genetic basis of Cowden syndrome and its implications for clinical practice and risk management. *Appl. Clin. Genet.* **2016**, *9*, 83–92. [CrossRef]
19. Yehia, L.; Keel, E.; Eng, C. The Clinical Spectrum of PTEN Mutations. *Annu. Rev. Med.* **2020**, *71*, 103–116. [CrossRef]
20. Frio, T.R.; Bahubeshi, A.; Kanellopoulou, C.; Hamel, N.; Niedziela, M.; Sabbaghian, N.; Pouchet, C.; Gilbert, L.; O'Brien, P.K.; Serfas, K.; et al. DICER1 Mutations in Familial Multinodular Goiter With and Without Ovarian Sertoli-Leydig Cell Tumors. *JAMA* **2011**, *305*, 68–77. [CrossRef]
21. Hill, D.A.; Ivanovich, J.; Priest, J.R.; Gurnett, C.A.; Dehner, L.P.; Desruisseau, D.; Jarzembowski, J.A.; Wikenheiser-Brokamp, K.A.; Suarez, B.K.; Whelan, A.J.; et al. DICER1 Mutations in Familial Pleuropulmonary Blastoma. *Science* **2009**, *325*, 965. [CrossRef] [PubMed]
22. Tomoda, C.; Miyauchi, A.; Uruno, T.; Takamura, Y.; Ito, Y.; Miya, A.; Kobayashi, K.; Matsuzuka, F.; Kuma, S.; Kuma, K.; et al. Cribriform-morular variant of papillary thyroid carcinoma: Clue to early detection of familial adenomatous polyposis-associated colon cancer. *World J. Surg.* **2004**, *28*, 886–889. [CrossRef] [PubMed]

23. Nieminen, T.T.; Walker, C.J.; Olkinuora, A.; Genutis, L.K.; O'Malley, M.; Wakely, P.E.; LaGuardia, L.; Koskenvuo, L.; Arola, J.; Lepistö, A.H.; et al. Thyroid Carcinomas That Occur in Familial Adenomatous Polyposis Patients Recurrently Harbor Somatic Variants in APC, BRAF, and KTM2D. *Thyroid* **2020**, *30*, 380–388. [CrossRef] [PubMed]
24. Formiga, M.N.D.C.; De Andrade, K.C.; Kowalski, L.P.; Achatz, M.I. Frequency of Thyroid Carcinoma in Brazilian TP53 p.R337H Carriers with Li Fraumeni Syndrome. *JAMA Oncol.* **2017**, *3*, 1400–1402. [CrossRef] [PubMed]
25. Oshima, J.; Sidorova, J.M.; Monnat, R.J., Jr. Werner syndrome: Clinical features, pathogenesis and potential therapeutic interventions. *Ageing Res. Rev.* **2017**, *33*, 105–114. [CrossRef] [PubMed]
26. Pereda, C.M.; Lesueur, F.; Pertesi, M.; Robinot, N.; Lence-Anta, J.J.; Turcios, S.; Velasco, M.; Chappe, M.; Infante, I.; Bustillo, M.; et al. Common variants at the 9q22.33, 14q13.3 and ATM loci, and risk of differentiated thyroid cancer in the Cuban population. *BMC Genet.* **2015**, *16*, 22. [CrossRef]
27. Maillard, S.; Damiola, F.; Clero, E.; Pertesi, M.; Robinot, N.; Rachédi, F.; Boissin, J.-L.; Sebbag, J.; Shan, L.; Bost-Bezeaud, F.; et al. Common variants at 9q22.33, 14q13.3, and ATM loci, and risk of differentiated thyroid cancer in the French Polynesian population. *PLoS ONE* **2015**, *10*, e0123700. [CrossRef]
28. Tan, M.-H.; Mester, J.; Peterson, C.; Yang, Y.; Chen, J.-L.; Rybicki, L.A.; Milas, K.; Pederson, H.; Remzi, B.; Orloff, M.S.; et al. A clinical scoring system for selection of patients for PTEN mutation testing is proposed on the basis of a prospective study of 3042 probands. *Am. J. Hum. Genet.* **2011**, *88*, 42–56. [CrossRef]
29. Schultz, K.A.P.; Rednam, S.P.; Kamihara, J.; Doros, L.; Achatz, M.I.; Wasserman, J.D.; Diller, L.R.; Brugières, L.; Druker, H.; Schneider, K.A.; et al. PTEN, DICER1, FH, and Their Associated Tumor Susceptibility Syndromes: Clinical Features, Genetics, and Surveillance Recommendations in Childhood. *Clin. Cancer Res.* **2017**, *23*, e76–e82. [CrossRef]
30. Ikeda, Y.; Kiyotani, K.; Yew, P.Y.; Kato, T.; Tamura, K.; Yap, K.L.; Nielsen, S.M.; Mester, J.L.; Eng, C.; Nakamura, Y.; et al. Germline PARP4 mutations in patients with primary thyroid and breast cancers. *Endocr. Relat. Cancer* **2016**, *23*, 171–179. [CrossRef]
31. Yehia, L.; Ni, Y.; Sesock, K.; Niazi, F.; Fletcher, B.; Chen, H.J.L.; LaFramboise, T.; Eng, C. Unexpected cancer-predisposition gene variants in Cowden syndrome and Bannayan-Riley-Ruvalcaba syndrome patients without underlying germline PTEN mutations. *PLoS Genet.* **2018**, *14*, e1007352. [CrossRef] [PubMed]
32. Ngeow, J.; Ni, Y.; Tohme, R.; Chen, F.S.; Bebek, G.; Eng, C. Germline alterations in RASAL1 in Cowden syndrome patients presenting with follicular thyroid cancer and in individuals with apparently sporadic epithelial thyroid cancer. *J. Clin. Endocrinol. Metab.* **2014**, *99*, E1316–E1321. [CrossRef] [PubMed]
33. Naderali, E.; Khaki, A.A.; Rad, J.S.; Ali-Hemmati, A.; Rahmati, M.; Charoudeh, H.N. Regulation and modulation of PTEN activity. *Mol. Biol. Rep.* **2018**, *45*, 2869–2881. [CrossRef] [PubMed]
34. Costa, H.A.; Leitner, M.G.; Sos, M.L.; Mavrantoni, A.; Rychkova, A.; Johnson, J.R.; Newton, B.W.; Yee, M.C.; De La Vega, F.M.; Ford, J.M.; et al. Discovery and functional characterization of a neomorphic PTEN mutation. *Proc. Natl. Acad. Sci. USA* **2015**, *112*, 13976–13981. [CrossRef] [PubMed]
35. Milella, M.; Falcone, I.; Conciatori, F.; Cesta Incani, U.; Del Curatolo, A.; Inzerilli, N.; Nuzzo, C.M.; Vaccaro, V.; Vari, S.; Cognetti, F.; et al. PTEN: Multiple Functions in Human Malignant Tumors. *Front. Oncol.* **2015**, *5*, 24. [CrossRef]
36. Ringel, M.D.; Hayre, N.; Saito, J.; Saunier, B.; Schuppert, F.; Burch, H.; Bernet, V.; Burman, K.D.; Kohn, L.D.; Saji, M. Overexpression and overactivation of Akt in thyroid carcinoma. *Cancer Res.* **2001**, *61*, 6105–6111.
37. Xing, M. Molecular pathogenesis and mechanisms of thyroid cancer. *Nat. Rev. Cancer* **2013**, *13*, 184–199. [CrossRef]
38. Liu, D.; Yang, C.; Bojdani, E.; Murugan, A.K.; Xing, M. Identification of RASAL1 as a major tumor suppressor gene in thyroid cancer. *J. Natl. Cancer Inst.* **2013**, *105*, 1617–1627. [CrossRef]
39. Pepe, S.; Korbonits, M.; Iacovazzo, D. Germline and mosaic mutations causing pituitary tumours: Genetic and molecular aspects. *J. Endocrinol.* **2019**, *240*, R21–R45. [CrossRef]
40. Griffin, K.J.; Kirschner, L.S.; Matyakhina, L.; Stergiopoulos, S.; Robinson-White, A.; Lenherr, S.; Weinberg, F.D.; Claflin, E.; Meoli, E.; Cho-Chung, Y.S.; et al. Down-regulation of regulatory subunit type 1A of protein kinase A leads to endocrine and other tumors. *Cancer Res.* **2004**, *64*, 8811–8815. [CrossRef]
41. Sandrini, F.; Matyakhina, L.; Sarlis, N.J.; Kirschner, L.S.; Farmakidis, C.; Gimm, O.; Stratakis, C.A. Regulatory subunit type I-α of protein kinase A (PRKAR1A): A tumor-suppressor gene for sporadic thyroid cancer. *Genes Chromosomes Cancer* **2002**, *35*, 182–192. [CrossRef] [PubMed]

42. Pringle, D.R.; Yin, Z.; Lee, A.A.; Manchanda, P.K.; Yu, L.; Parlow, A.F.; Jarjoura, D.; La Perle, K.M.D.; Kirschner, L.S. Thyroid-specific ablation of the Carney complex gene, PRKAR1A, results in hyperthyroidism and follicular thyroid cancer. *Endocrine-Related Cancer* **2012**, *19*, 435–446. [CrossRef] [PubMed]

43. Kari, S.; Vasko, V.V.; Priya, S.; Kirschner, L.S. PKA Activates AMPK Through LKB1 Signaling in Follicular *Thyroid Cancer. Front. Endocrinol.* **2019**, *10*, 769. [CrossRef] [PubMed]

44. Goto, M.; Miller, R.W.; Ishikawa, Y.; Sugano, H. Excess of rare cancers in Werner syndrome (adult progeria). *Cancer Epidemiol. Biomarkers Prev.* **1996**, *5*, 239–246. [PubMed]

45. Muftuoglu, M.; Oshima, J.; von Kobbe, C.; Cheng, W.H.; Leistritz, D.F.; Bohr, V.A. The clinical characteristics of Werner syndrome: Molecular and biochemical diagnosis. *Hum. Genet.* **2008**, *124*, 369–377. [CrossRef]

46. Shamanna, R.A.; Lu, H.; de Freitas, J.K.; Tian, J.; Croteau, D.L.; Bohr, V.A. WRN regulates pathway choice between classical and alternative non-homologous end joining. *Nat. Commun.* **2016**, *7*, 13785. [CrossRef]

47. Ishikawa, Y.; Sugano, H.; Matsumoto, T.; Furuichi, Y.; Miller, R.W.; Goto, M. Unusual features of thyroid carcinomas in Japanese patients with Werner syndrome and possible genotype-phenotype relations to cell type and race. *Cancer* **1999**, *85*, 1345–1352. [CrossRef]

48. Uchino, S.; Noguchi, S.; Yamashita, H.; Yamashita, H.; Watanabe, S.; Ogawa, T.; Tsuno, A.; Murakami, A.; Miyauchi, A. Mutational analysis of the APC gene in cribriform-morula variant of papillary thyroid carcinoma. *World J. Surg.* **2006**, *30*, 775–779. [CrossRef]

49. De Herreros, A.G.; Duñach, M. Intracellular Signals Activated by Canonical Wnt Ligands Independent of GSK3 Inhibition and β-Catenin Stabilization. *Cells* **2019**, *8*, 1148. [CrossRef]

50. Heinen, C.D. Genotype to phenotype: Analyzing the effects of inherited mutations in colorectal cancer families. *Mutat. Res.* **2010**, *693*, 32–45. [CrossRef]

51. Giannelli, S.M.; McPhaul, L.; Nakamoto, J.; Gianoukakis, A.G. Familial adenomatous polyposis-associated, cribriform morular variant of papillary thyroid carcinoma harboring a K-RAS mutation: Case presentation and review of molecular mechanisms. *Thyroid* **2014**, *24*, 1184–1189. [CrossRef]

52. Iwama, T.; Konishi, M.; Iijima, T.; Yoshinaga, K.; Tominaga, T.; Koike, M.; Miyaki, M. Somatic mutation of the APC gene in thyroid carcinoma associated with familial adenomatous polyposis. *Jpn. J. Cancer Res.* **1999**, *90*, 372–376. [CrossRef] [PubMed]

53. Miyaki, M.; Iijima, T.; Ishii, R.; Hishima, T.; Mori, T.; Yoshinaga, K.; Takami, H.; Kuroki, T.; Iwama, T. Molecular Evidence for Multicentric Development of Thyroid Carcinomas in Patients with Familial Adenomatous Polyposis. *Am. J. Pathol.* **2000**, *157*, 1825–1827. [CrossRef]

54. Syngal, S.; Brand, R.E.; Church, J.M.; Giardiello, F.M.; Hampel, H.L.; Burt, R.W. ACG clinical guideline: Genetic testing and management of hereditary gastrointestinal cancer syndromes. *Am. J. Gastroenterol.* **2015**, *110*, 223–262. [CrossRef] [PubMed]

55. Achatz, M.I.; Porter, C.C.; Brugières, L.; Druker, H.; Frebourg, T.; Foulkes, W.D.; Kratz, C.P.; Kuiper, R.P.; Hansford, J.R.; Hernandez, H.S.; et al. Cancer Screening Recommendations and Clinical Management of Inherited Gastrointestinal Cancer Syndromes in Childhood. *Clin. Cancer Res.* **2017**, *23*, e107–e114. [CrossRef]

56. Dombernowsky, S.L.; Weischer, M.; Allin, K.H.; Bojesen, S.E.; Tybjirg-Hansen, A.; Nordestgaard, B.G. Risk of cancer by ATM missense mutations in the general population. *J. Clin. Oncol.* **2008**, *26*, 3057–3062. [CrossRef]

57. Shiloh, Y. ATM: Expanding roles as a chief guardian of genome stability. *Exp. Cell Res.* **2014**, *329*, 154–161. [CrossRef]

58. Ribezzo, F.; Shiloh, Y.; Schumacher, B. Systemic DNA damage responses in aging and diseases. *Semin. Cancer Biol.* **2016**, *37–38*, 26–35. [CrossRef]

59. Akulevich, N.M.; Saenko, V.A.; Rogounovitch, T.I.; Drozd, V.M.; Lushnikov, E.F.; Ivanov, V.K.; Mitsutake, N.; Kominami, R.; Yamashita, S. Polymorphisms of DNA damage response genes in radiation-related and sporadic papillary thyroid carcinoma. *Endocr. Relat. Cancer* **2009**, *16*, 491–503. [CrossRef]

60. Xu, L.; Morari, E.C.; Wei, Q.; Sturgis, E.M.; Ward, L.S. Functional variations in the ATM gene and susceptibility to differentiated thyroid carcinoma. *J. Clin. Endocrinol. Metab.* **2012**, *97*, 1913–1921. [CrossRef]

61. Gu, Y.; Shi, J.; Qiu, S.; Qiao, Y.; Zhang, X.; Cheng, Y.; Liu, Y. Association between ATM rs1801516 polymorphism and cancer susceptibility: A meta-analysis involving 12,879 cases and 18,054 controls. *BMC Cancer* **2018**, *18*, 1060. [CrossRef]

62. Song, C.M.; Kwon, T.K.; Park, B.L.; Ji, Y.B.; Tae, K. Single nucleotide polymorphisms of ataxia telangiectasia mutated and the risk of papillary thyroid carcinoma. *Environ. Mol. Mutagen.* **2015**, *56*, 70–76. [CrossRef] [PubMed]
63. Wójcicka, A.; Czetwertyńska, M.; Świerniak, M.; Długosińska, J.; Maciąg, M.; Czajka, A.; Dymecka, K.; Kubiak, A.; Kot, A.; Płoski, R.; et al. Variants in the ATM-CHEK2-BRCA1 axis determine genetic predisposition and clinical presentation of papillary thyroid carcinoma. *Genes Chromosomes Cancer* **2014**, *53*, 516–523. [CrossRef] [PubMed]
64. Kitahara, C.M.; Farkas, D.K.R.; Jørgensen, J.O.L.; Cronin-Fenton, D.; Sørensen, H.T. Benign Thyroid Diseases and Risk of Thyroid Cancer: A Nationwide Cohort Study. *J. Clin. Endocrinol. Metab.* **2018**, *103*, 2216–2224. [CrossRef] [PubMed]
65. Smith, J.J.; Chen, X.; Schneider, D.F.; Broome, J.T.; Sippel, R.S.; Chen, H.; Solórzano, C.C. Cancer after Thyroidectomy: A Multi-Institutional Experience with 1,523 Patients. *J. Am. Coll. Surg.* **2013**, *216*, 571–577. [CrossRef] [PubMed]
66. Khan, N.E.; Bauer, A.J.; Schultz, K.A.P.; Doros, L.; DeCastro, R.M.; Ling, A.; Lodish, M.B.; Harney, L.A.; Kase, R.G.; Carr, A.G.; et al. Quantification of Thyroid Cancer and Multinodular Goiter Risk in the DICER1 Syndrome: A Family-Based Cohort Study. *J. Clin. Endocrinol. Metab.* **2017**, *102*, 1614–1622. [CrossRef]
67. Lin, S.; Gregory, R.I. MicroRNA biogenesis pathways in cancer. *Nat. Rev. Cancer* **2015**, *15*, 321–333. [CrossRef]
68. Poma, A.M.; Condello, V.; Denaro, M.; Torregrossa, L.; Elisei, R.; Vitti, P.; Basolo, F. DICER1 somatic mutations strongly impair miRNA processing even in benign thyroid lesions. *Oncotarget* **2019**, *10*, 1785–1797. [CrossRef]
69. Fuziwara, C.S.; Kimura, E.T. MicroRNAs in thyroid development, function and tumorigenesis. *Mol. Cell. Endocrinol.* **2017**, *456*, 44–50. [CrossRef]
70. Rodriguez, W.; Jin, L.; Janssens, V.; Pierreux, C.; Hick, A.-C.; Urizar, E.; Costagliola, S. Deletion of the RNaseIII Enzyme Dicer in Thyroid Follicular Cells Causes Hypothyroidism with Signs of Neoplastic Alterations. *PLoS ONE* **2012**, *7*, e29929. [CrossRef]
71. Frezzetti, D.; Reale, C.; Calì, G.; Nitsch, L.; Fagman, H.; Nilsson, O.; Scarfò, M.; De Vita, G.; Di Lauro, R. The microRNA-Processing Enzyme Dicer Is Essential for Thyroid Function. *PLoS ONE* **2011**, *6*, e27648. [CrossRef] [PubMed]
72. Schultz, K.A.P.; Williams, G.M.; Kamihara, J.; Stewart, D.R.; Harris, A.K.; Bauer, A.J.; Turner, J.; Shah, R.; Schneider, K.; Schneider, K.W.; et al. DICER1 and Associated Conditions: Identification of At-risk Individuals and Recommended Surveillance Strategies. *Clin. Cancer Res.* **2018**, *24*, 2251–2261. [CrossRef] [PubMed]
73. Rutter, M.M.; Jha, P.; Schultz, K.A.P.; Sheil, A.; Harris, A.K.; Bauer, A.J.; Field, A.L.; Geller, J.; Hill, D.A. DICER1Mutations and Differentiated Thyroid Carcinoma: Evidence of a Direct Association. *J. Clin. Endocrinol. Metab.* **2016**, *101*, 1–5. [CrossRef] [PubMed]
74. Cerami, E.; Gao, J.; Dogrusoz, U.; Gross, B.E.; Sumer, S.O.; Aksoy, B.A.; Jacobsen, A.; Byrne, C.J.; Heuer, M.L.; Larsson, E.; et al. The cBio Cancer Genomics Portal: An Open Platform for Exploring Multidimensional Cancer Genomics Data: Figure 1. *Cancer Discov.* **2012**, *2*, 401–404. [CrossRef] [PubMed]
75. Gao, J.; Aksoy, B.A.; Dogrusoz, U.; Dresdner, G.; Gross, B.; Sumer, S.O.; Sun, Y.; Jacobsen, A.; Sinha, R.; Larsson, E.; et al. Integrative Analysis of Complex Cancer Genomics and Clinical Profiles Using the cBioPortal. *Sci. Signal.* **2013**, *6*, pl1. [CrossRef]
76. cBioPortal for Cancer Genomics. Available online: https://www.cbioportal.org (accessed on 16 August 2020).
77. Cancer Genome Atlas Research Network. Integrated genomic characterization of papillary thyroid carcinoma. *Cell* **2014**, *159*, 676–690. [CrossRef]
78. Landa, I.; Ibrahimpasic, T.; Boucai, L.; Sinha, R.; Knauf, J.A.; Shah, R.H.; Dogan, S.; Ricarte-Filho, J.C.; Krishnamoorthy, G.P.; Xu, B.; et al. Genomic and transcriptomic hallmarks of poorly differentiated and anaplastic thyroid cancers. *J. Clin. Investig.* **2016**, *126*, 1052–1066. [CrossRef]
79. Chernock, R.D.; Rivera, B.; Borrelli, N.; Hill, D.A.; Fahiminiya, S.; Shah, T.; Chong, A.-S.; Aqil, B.; Mehrad, M.; Giordano, T.J.; et al. Poorly differentiated thyroid carcinoma of childhood and adolescence: A distinct entity characterized by DICER1 mutations. *Mod. Pathol.* **2020**, *33*, 1264–1274. [CrossRef]
80. Wasserman, J.D.; Sabbaghian, N.; Fahiminiya, S.; Chami, R.; Mete, O.; Acker, M.; Wu, M.K.; Shlien, A.; De Kock, L.; Foulkes, W.D. DICER1 Mutations Are Frequent in Adolescent-Onset Papillary Thyroid Carcinoma. *J. Clin. Endocrinol. Metab.* **2018**, *103*, 2009–2015. [CrossRef]
81. Canberk, S.; Ferreira, J.C.; Pereira, L.; Batısta, R.; Vieira, A.F.; Soares, P.; Simões, M.S.; Máximo, V. Analyzing the Role of DICER1 Germline Variations in Papillary Thyroid Carcinoma. *Eur. Thyroid J.* **2020**, 1–8. [CrossRef]

82. Rivera, B.; Nadaf, J.; Fahiminiya, S.; Apellaniz-Ruiz, M.; Saskin, A.; Chong, A.-S.; Sharma, S.; Wagener, R.; Revil, T.; Condello, V.; et al. DGCR8 microprocessor defect characterizes familial multinodular goiter with schwannomatosis. *J. Clin. Investig.* **2020**, *130*, 1479–1490. [CrossRef] [PubMed]

83. Kastenhuber, E.R.; Lowe, S.W. Putting p53 in Context. *Cell* **2017**, *170*, 1062–1078. [CrossRef] [PubMed]

84. Goldgar, D.E.; Easton, D.F.; Cannon-Albright, L.A.; Skolnick, M.H. Systematic Population-Based Assessment of Cancer Risk in First-Degree Relatives of Cancer Probands. *J. Natl. Cancer Inst.* **1994**, *86*, 1600–1608. [CrossRef] [PubMed]

85. Hemminki, K.; Eng, C.; Chen, B. Familial Risks for Nonmedullary Thyroid Cancer. *J. Clin. Endocrinol. Metab.* **2005**, *90*, 5747–5753. [CrossRef]

86. Bauer, A.J. Clinical Behavior and Genetics of Nonsyndromic, Familial Nonmedullary Thyroid Cancer. *Front. Horm. Res.* **2013**, *41*, 141–148. [CrossRef]

87. Capezzone, M.; Marchisotta, S.; Cantara, S.; Busonero, G.; Brilli, L.; Pazaitou-Panayiotou, K.; Carli, A.F.; Caruso, G.; Toti, P.; Capitani, S.; et al. Familial non-medullary thyroid carcinoma displays the features of clinical anticipation suggestive of a distinct biological entity. *Endocr. Relat. Cancer* **2008**, *15*, 1075–1081. [CrossRef]

88. He, H.; Bronisz, A.; Liyanarachchi, S.; Nagy, R.; Li, W.; Huang, Y.; Akagi, K.; Saji, M.; Kula, D.; Wojcicka, A.; et al. SRGAP1 Is a Candidate Gene for Papillary Thyroid Carcinoma Susceptibility. *J. Clin. Endocrinol. Metab.* **2013**, *98*, E973–E980. [CrossRef]

89. Suh, I.; Filetti, S.; Vriens, M.R.; Guerrero, M.A.; Tumino, S.; Wong, M.; Shen, W.T.; Kebebew, E.; Duh, Q.-Y.; Clark, O.H. Distinct loci on chromosome 1q21 and 6q22 predispose to familial nonmedullary thyroid cancer: A SNP array-based linkage analysis of 38 families. *Surgery* **2009**, *146*, 1073–1080. [CrossRef]

90. He, H.; Nagy, R.; Liyanarachchi, S.; Jiao, H.; Li, W.; Suster, S.; Kere, J.; De La Chapelle, A. A Susceptibility Locus for Papillary Thyroid Carcinoma on Chromosome 8q24. *Cancer Res.* **2009**, *69*, 625–631. [CrossRef]

91. He, H.; Li, W.; Wu, D.; Nagy, R.; Liyanarachchi, S.; Akagi, K.; Jendrzejewski, J.; Jiao, H.; Hoag, K.; Wen, B.; et al. Ultra-Rare Mutation in Long-Range Enhancer Predisposes to Thyroid Carcinoma with High Penetrance. *PLoS ONE* **2013**, *8*, e61920. [CrossRef]

92. Ngan, E.S.W.; Lang, B.H.H.; Liu, T.; Shum, C.K.Y.; So, M.-T.; Lau, D.K.C.; Leon, T.Y.Y.; Cherny, S.S.; Tsai, S.Y.; Lo, C.-Y.; et al. A Germline Mutation (A339V) in Thyroid Transcription Factor-1 (TITF-1/NKX2.1) in Patients with Multinodular Goiter and Papillary Thyroid Carcinoma. *J. Natl. Cancer Inst.* **2009**, *101*, 162–175. [CrossRef] [PubMed]

93. McKay, J.D.; Thompson, D.B.; Lesueur, F.; Stankov, K.; Pastore, A.; Watfah, C.; Strolz, S.; Riccabona, G.; Moncayo, R.C.; Romeo, G.; et al. Evidence for interaction between the TCO and NMTC1 loci in familial non-medullary thyroid cancer. *J. Med. Genet.* **2004**, *41*, 407–412. [CrossRef] [PubMed]

94. Medapati, M.R.; Dahlmann, M.; Ghavami, S.; Pathak, K.A.; Lucman, L.; Klonisch, T.; Hoang-Vu, C.; Stein, U.; Hombach-Klonisch, S. RAGE Mediates the Pro-Migratory Response of Extracellular S100A4 in Human Thyroid Cancer Cells. *Thyroid* **2015**, *25*, 514–527. [CrossRef] [PubMed]

95. Burgess, J.R.; Duffield, A.; Wilkinson, S.J.; Ware, R.; Greenaway, T.M.; Percival, J.; Hoffman, L. Two Families with an Autosomal Dominant Inheritance Pattern for Papillary Carcinoma of the Thyroid. *J. Clin. Endocrinol. Metab.* **1997**, *82*, 345–348. [CrossRef]

96. Bakhsh, A.; Kirov, G.; Gregory, J.W.; Williams, E.D.; Ludgate, M. A new form of familial multi-nodular goitre with progression to differentiated thyroid cancer. *Endocr.-Relat. Cancer* **2006**, *13*, 475–483. [CrossRef]

97. Franceschi, S.; Preston-Martin, S.; Maso, L.D.; Negri, E.; La Vecchia, C.; Mack, W.J.; McTiernan, A.; Kolonel, L.; Mark, S.D.; Mabuchi, K.; et al. A pooled analysis of case—Control studies of thyroid cancer. IV. Benign thyroid diseases. *Cancer Causes Control.* **1999**, *10*, 583–595. [CrossRef]

98. Gudmundsson, J.; Sulem, P.; Gudbjartsson, D.F.; Jonasson, J.G.; Sigurdsson, A.; Bergthorsson, J.T.; He, H.; Blondal, T.; Geller, F.; Jakobsdottir, M.; et al. Common variants on 9q22.33 and 14q13.3 predispose to thyroid cancer in European populations. *Nat. Genet.* **2009**, *41*, 460–464. [CrossRef]

99. Gudmundsson, J.; Sulem, P.; Gudbjartsson, D.F.; Jonasson, J.G.; Masson, G.; He, H.; Jonasdottir, A.; Sigurdsson, A.; Stacey, S.N.; Johannsdottir, H.; et al. Discovery of common variants associated with low TSH levels and thyroid cancer risk. *Nat. Genet.* **2012**, *44*, 319–322. [CrossRef]

100. Takahashi, M.; Saenko, V.A.; Rogounovitch, T.I.; Kawaguchi, T.; Drozd, V.M.; Takigawa-Imamura, H.; Akulevich, N.M.; Ratanajaraya, C.; Mitsutake, N.; Takamura, N.; et al. The FOXE1 locus is a major genetic determinant for radiation-related thyroid carcinoma in Chernobyl. *Hum. Mol. Genet.* **2010**, *19*, 2516–2523. [CrossRef]
101. Köhler, A.; Chen, B.; Gemignani, F.; Elisei, R.; Romei, C.; Figlioli, G.; Cipollini, M.; Cristaudo, A.; Bambi, F.; Hoffmann, P.; et al. Genome-Wide Association Study on Differentiated Thyroid Cancer. *J. Clin. Endocrinol. Metab.* **2013**, *98*, E1674–E1681. [CrossRef]
102. Son, H.-Y.; Hwangbo, Y.; Yoo, S.-K.; Im, S.-W.; Yang, S.D.; Kwak, S.-J.; Park, M.S.; Kwak, S.H.; Cho, S.W.; Ryu, J.S.; et al. Genome-wide association and expression quantitative trait loci studies identify multiple susceptibility loci for thyroid cancer. *Nat. Commun.* **2017**, *8*, 15966. [CrossRef] [PubMed]
103. Gudmundsson, J.; Thorleifsson, G.; Sigurdsson, J.K.; Stefansdottir, L.; Jonasson, J.G.; Gudjonsson, S.A.; Gudbjartsson, D.F.; Masson, G.; Johannsdottir, H.; Halldorsson, G.H.; et al. A genome-wide association study yields five novel thyroid cancer risk loci. *Nat. Commun.* **2017**, *8*, 14517. [CrossRef] [PubMed]
104. Nikitski, A.V.; Rogounovitch, T.I.; Bychkov, A.; Takahashi, M.; Yoshiura, K.-I.; Mitsutake, N.; Kawaguchi, T.; Matsuse, M.; Drozd, V.M.; Demidchik, Y.; et al. Genotype Analyses in the Japanese and Belarusian Populations Reveal Independent Effects of rs965513 and rs1867277 but Do Not Support the Role of FOXE1 Polyalanine Tract Length in Conferring Risk for Papillary Thyroid Carcinoma. *Thyroid* **2017**, *27*, 224–235. [CrossRef] [PubMed]
105. Landa, I.; Ruiz-Llorente, S.; Montero-Conde, C.; Inglada-Pérez, L.; Schiavi, F.; Leskelä, S.; Pita, G.; Milne, R.; Maravall, J.; Ramos, I.; et al. The Variant rs1867277 in FOXE1 Gene Confers Thyroid Cancer Susceptibility through the Recruitment of USF1/USF2 Transcription Factors. *PLoS Genet.* **2009**, *5*, e1000637. [CrossRef]
106. Nikitski, A.; Saenko, V.; Shimamura, M.; Nakashima, M.; Matsuse, M.; Suzuki, K.; Rogounovitch, T.I.; Bogdanova, T.; Shibusawa, N.; Yamada, M.; et al. Targeted Foxe1 Overexpression in Mouse Thyroid Causes the Development of Multinodular Goiter But Does Not Promote Carcinogenesis. *Endocrinology* **2016**, *157*, 2182–2195. [CrossRef]
107. Wang, Y.; He, H.; Li, W.; Phay, J.; Shen, R.; Yu, L.; Hancioglu, B.; De La Chapelle, A. MYH9 binds to lncRNA genePTCSC2and regulates FOXE1 in the 9q22 thyroid cancer risk locus. *Proc. Natl. Acad. Sci. USA* **2017**, *114*, 474–479. [CrossRef]
108. Jones, A.M.; Howarth, K.M.; Martin, L.; Gorman, M.; Mihai, R.; Moss, L.; Auton, A.; Lemon, C.; Mehanna, H.; Mohan, H.; et al. Thyroid cancer susceptibility polymorphisms: Confirmation of loci on chromosomes 9q22 and 14q13, validation of a recessive 8q24 locus and failure to replicate a locus on 5q24. *J. Med. Genet.* **2012**, *49*, 158–163. [CrossRef]
109. Jendrzejewski, J.; He, H.; Radomska, H.S.; Li, W.; Tomsic, J.; Liyanarachchi, S.; Davuluri, R.V.; Nagy, R.; De La Chapelle, A. The polymorphism rs944289 predisposes to papillary thyroid carcinoma through a large intergenic noncoding RNA gene of tumor suppressor type. *Proc. Natl. Acad. Sci. USA* **2012**, *109*, 8646–8651. [CrossRef]
110. Goedert, L.; Plaça, J.R.; Fuziwara, C.S.; Machado, M.C.R.; Plaça, D.R.; Almeida, P.P.; Sanches, T.P.; Dos Santos, J.F.; Corveloni, A.C.; Pereira, I.E.G.; et al. Identification of Long Noncoding RNAs Deregulated in Papillary Thyroid Cancer and Correlated with BRAFV600E Mutation by Bioinformatics Integrative Analysis. *Sci. Rep.* **2017**, *7*, 1662. [CrossRef]
111. Jendrzejewski, J.; Thomas, A.; Liyanarachchi, S.; Eiterman, A.; Tomsic, J.; He, H.; Radomska, H.S.; Li, W.; Nagy, R.; Sworczak, K.; et al. PTCSC3 Is Involved in Papillary Thyroid Carcinoma Development by Modulating S100A4 Gene Expression. *J. Clin. Endocrinol. Metab.* **2015**, *100*, E1370–E1377. [CrossRef]
112. Cantara, S.; Capuano, S.; Formichi, C.; Pisu, M.; Capezzone, M.; Pacini, F. Lack of germline A339V mutation in thyroid transcription factor-1 (TITF-1/NKX2.1) gene in familial papillary thyroid cancer. *Thyroid Res.* **2010**, *3*, 4. [CrossRef] [PubMed]
113. He, H.; Li, W.; Liyanarachchi, S.; Wang, Y.; Yu, L.; Genutis, L.K.; Maharry, S.; Phay, J.E.; Shen, R.; Brock, P.; et al. The Role of NRG1 in the Predisposition to Papillary Thyroid Carcinoma. *J. Clin. Endocrinol. Metab.* **2018**, *103*, 1369–1379. [CrossRef] [PubMed]
114. Coe, E.A.; Tan, J.Y.; Shapiro, M.; Louphrasitthiphol, P.; Bassett, A.R.; Marques, A.C.; Goding, C.R.; Vance, K.W. The MITF-SOX10 regulated long non-coding RNA DIRC3 is a melanoma tumour suppressor. *PLoS Genet.* **2019**, *15*, e1008501. [CrossRef] [PubMed]

115. Świerniak, M.; Wójcicka, A.; Czetwertyńska, M.; Długosińska, J.; Stachlewska, E.; Gierlikowski, W.; Kot, A.; Górnicka, B.; Koperski, Ł.; Bogdańska, M.; et al. Association between GWAS-Derived rs966423 Genetic Variant and Overall Mortality in Patients with Differentiated Thyroid Cancer. *Clin. Cancer Res.* **2016**, *22*, 1111–1119. [CrossRef]
116. Hińcza, K.; Kowalik, A.; Pałyga, I.; Walczyk, A.; Gąsior-Perczak, D.; Mikina, E.; Trybek, T.; Szymonek, M.; Gadawska-Juszczyk, K.; Zajkowska, K.; et al. Does the TT Variant of the rs966423 Polymorphism in DIRC3 Affect the Stage and Clinical Course of Papillary Thyroid Cancer? *Cancers* **2020**, *12*, 423. [CrossRef]
117. Liyanarachchi, S.; Gudmundsson, J.; Ferkingstad, E.; He, H.; Jonasson, J.G.; Tragante, V.; Asselbergs, F.W.; Xu, L.; Kiemeney, L.A.; Netea-Maier, R.T.; et al. Assessing thyroid cancer risk using polygenic risk scores. *Proc. Natl. Acad. Sci. USA* **2020**, *117*, 5997–6002. [CrossRef]
118. Capezzone, M.; Cantara, S.; Marchisotta, S.; Filetti, S.; De Santi, M.M.; Rossi, B.; Ronga, G.; Durante, C.; Pacini, F. Short Telomeres, Telomerase Reverse Transcriptase Gene Amplification, and Increased Telomerase Activity in the Blood of Familial Papillary Thyroid Cancer Patients. *J. Clin. Endocrinol. Metab.* **2008**, *93*, 3950–3957. [CrossRef]
119. He, M.; Bian, B.; Gesuwan, K.; Gulati, N.; Zhang, L.; Nilubol, N.; Kebebew, E. Telomere Length Is Shorter in Affected Members of Families with Familial Nonmedullary Thyroid Cancer. *Thyroid* **2013**, *23*, 301–307. [CrossRef]
120. Cantara, S.; Capuano, S.; Capezzone, M.; Benigni, M.; Pisu, M.; Marchisotta, S.; Pacini, F. Lack of Mutations of the Telomerase RNA Component in Familial Papillary Thyroid Cancer with Short Telomeres. *Thyroid* **2012**, *22*, 363–368. [CrossRef]
121. He, H.; Li, W.; Comiskey, D.F.; Liyanarachchi, S.; Nieminen, T.T.; Wang, Y.; DeLap, K.E.; Brock, P.; De La Chapelle, A. A Truncating Germline Mutation of TINF2 in Individuals with Thyroid Cancer or Melanoma Results in Longer Telomeres. *Thyroid* **2020**, *30*, 204–213. [CrossRef]
122. Srivastava, A.; Miao, B.; Skopelitou, D.; Kumar, V.; Kumar, A.; Paramasivam, N.; Bonora, E.; Hemminki, K.; Foersti, A.; Bandapalli, O.R. A Germline Mutation in the POT1 Gene Is a Candidate for Familial Non-Medullary Thyroid Cancer. *Cancers* **2020**, *12*, 1441. [CrossRef] [PubMed]
123. Wilson, T.L.-S.; Hattangady, N.; Lerario, A.M.; Williams, C.; Koeppe, E.; Quinonez, S.; Osborne, J.; Cha, K.B.; Else, T. A new POT1 germline mutation—expanding the spectrum of POT1-associated cancers. *Fam. Cancer* **2017**, *16*, 561–566. [CrossRef] [PubMed]
124. Richard, M.A.; Lupo, P.J.; Morton, L.M.; Yasui, Y.A.; Sapkota, Y.A.; Arnold, M.A.; Aubert, G.; Neglia, J.P.; Turcotte, L.M.; Leisenring, W.M.; et al. Genetic variation in POT1 and risk of thyroid subsequent malignant neoplasm: A report from the Childhood Cancer Survivor Study. *PLoS ONE* **2020**, *15*, e0228887. [CrossRef] [PubMed]
125. Tomsic, J.; Fultz, R.; Liyanarachchi, S.; Genutis, L.K.; Wang, Y.; Li, W.; Volinia, S.; Jazdzewski, K.; He, H.; Wakely, P.E., Jr.; et al. Variants in microRNA genes in familial papillary thyroid carcinoma. *Oncotarget* **2017**, *8*, 6475–6482. [CrossRef]
126. Tomsic, J.; He, H.; Akagi, K.; Liyanarachchi, S.; Pan, Q.; Bertani, B.; Nagy, R.; Symer, D.E.; Blencowe, B.J.; De La Chapelle, A. A germline mutation in SRRM2, a splicing factor gene, is implicated in papillary thyroid carcinoma predisposition. *Sci. Rep.* **2015**, *5*, 10566. [CrossRef]
127. Orois, A.; Gara, S.K.; Mora, M.; Halperin, I.; Martínez, S.; Alfayate, R.; Kebebew, E.; Oriola, J. NOP53 as A Candidate Modifier Locus for Familial Non-Medullary Thyroid Cancer. *Genes* **2019**, *10*, 899. [CrossRef]
128. Gara, S.K.; Jia, L.; Merino, M.J.; Agarwal, S.K.; Zhang, L.; Cam, M.; Patel, D.; Kebebew, E. Germline HABP2 Mutation Causing Familial Nonmedullary Thyroid Cancer. *N. Engl. J. Med.* **2015**, *373*, 448–455. [CrossRef]
129. Tomsic, J.; He, H.; de la Chapelle, A. HABP2 Mutation and Nonmedullary Thyroid Cancer. *N. Engl. J. Med.* **2015**, *373*, 2086. [CrossRef]
130. Tomsic, J.; Fultz, R.; Liyanarachchi, S.; He, H.; Senter, L.; De La Chapelle, A. HABP2 G534E Variant in Papillary Thyroid Carcinoma. *PLoS ONE* **2016**, *11*, e0146315. [CrossRef]
131. Kowalik, A.; Gąsior-Perczak, D.; Gromek, M.; Siołek, M.; Walczyk, A.; Pałyga, I.; Chłopek, M.; Kopczyński, J.; Mężyk, R.; Kowalska, A.; et al. The p.G534E variant of HABP2 is not associated with sporadic papillary thyroid carcinoma in a Polish population. *Oncotarget* **2017**, *8*, 58304–58308. [CrossRef]
132. Zhu, J.; Wu, K.; Lin, Z.; Bai, S.; Wu, J.; Li, P.; Xue, H.; Du, J.; Shen, B.; Wang, H.; et al. Identification of susceptibility gene mutations associated with the pathogenesis of familial nonmedullary thyroid cancer. *Mol. Genet. Genom. Med.* **2019**, *7*, e1015. [CrossRef] [PubMed]

133. Sarquis, M.; Moraes, D.C.; Bastos-Rodrigues, L.; Azevedo, P.G.; Ramos, A.V.; Reis, F.V.; Dande, P.V.; Paim, I.; Friedman, E.; De Marco, L. Germline Mutations in Familial Papillary Thyroid Cancer. *Endocr. Pathol.* **2020**, *31*, 14–20. [CrossRef] [PubMed]
134. Siołek, M.; Cybulski, C.; Gąsior-Perczak, D.; Kowalik, A.; Kozak-Klonowska, B.; Kowalska, A.; Chłopek, M.; Kluźniak, W.; Wokołorczyk, D.; Pałyga, I.; et al. CHEK2mutations and the risk of papillary thyroid cancer. *Int. J. Cancer* **2015**, *137*, 548–552. [CrossRef] [PubMed]

3

HER2 Analysis in Sporadic Thyroid Cancer of Follicular Cell Origin

Rosaria M. Ruggeri [1,*], Alfredo Campennì [2], Giuseppe Giuffrè [3], Luca Giovanella [4], Massimiliano Siracusa [2], Angela Simone [3], Giovanni Branca [3], Rosa Scarfì [3], Francesco Trimarchi [1], Antonio Ieni [3] and Giovanni Tuccari [3]

1 Department of Clinical and Experimental Medicine, Unit of Endocrinology, University of Messina, AOU Policlinico G. Martino, 98125 Messina, Italy; Francesco.Trimarchi@unime.it

2 Department of Biomedical Sciences and Morphological and Functional Images, Unit of Nuclear Medicine, University of Messina, AOU Policlinico G. Martino, 98125 Messina, Italy; acampenni@unime.it (A.C.); m.siracusadr@alice.it (M.S.)

3 Department of Human Pathology in Adult and Developmental Age "Gaetano Barresi", Unit of Pathological Anatomy, University of Messina, AOU Policlinico G. Martino, 98125 Messina, Italy; giuffre@unime.it (G.G.); asimone@unime.it (A.S.); giobranca81@gmail.com (G.B.); rscarfi@unime.it (R.S.); aieni@unime.it (A.I.); tuccari@unime.it (G.T.)

4 Department of Nuclear Medicine, Thyroid and PET/CT Center, Oncology Institute of Southern Switzerland, 6500 Bellinzona, Switzerland; luca.giovanella@eoc.ch

* Correspondence: rmruggeri@unime.it

Academic Editor: Daniela Gabriele Grimm

Abstract: The Epidermal Growth Factor Receoptor (EGFR) family member human epidermal growth factor receptor 2 (HER2) is overexpressed in many human epithelial malignancies, representing a molecular target for specific anti-neoplastic drugs. Few data are available on HER2 status in differentiated thyroid cancer (DTC). The present study was aimed to investigate HER2 status in sporadic cancers of follicular cell origin to better clarify the role of this receptor in the stratification of thyroid cancer. By immunohistochemistry and fluorescence in-situ hybridization, HER2 expression was investigated in formalin-fixed paraffin-embedded surgical specimens from 90 DTC patients, 45 follicular (FTC) and 45 papillary (PTC) histotypes. No HER2 immunostaining was recorded in background thyroid tissue. By contrast, overall HER2 overexpression was found in 20/45 (44%) FTC and 8/45 (18%) PTC, with a significant difference between the two histotypes ($p = 0.046$). Five of the six patients who developed metastatic disease during a median nine-year follow-up had a HER2-positive tumor. Therefore, we suggest that HER2 expression may represent an additional aid to identify a subset of patients who are characterized by a worse prognosis and are potentially eligible for targeted therapy.

Keywords: sporadic differentiated thyroid cancer; HER2 (Human Epidermal Growth Factor Receptor 2); immunohistochemistry; FISH (fluorescence in situ hybridization)

---

1. Introduction

The human epidermal growth factor receptor 2 (HER2) is a cell surface receptor belonging to the Epidermal growth factor receptor (EGFR) family of receptors, which includes four distinct, but closely related tyrosine kinase receptors: EGFR, HER2 (HER2/c-neu), HER3, and HER4 [1,2]. HER2 has no known cognate ligand and may become active upon hetero-dimerization with other family members, such as EGFR. Upon activation, EGFR and HER2 undergo dimerization and tyrosine auto-phosphorylation, thus leading to activation of proliferative and anti-apoptotic pathways, principally the MAPK, Akt, and JNK pathways. Through such effects on cell-cycle progression, apoptosis, angiogenesis, and tumor-cell motility, HER2 is implicated in the development and progression of cancer [1,2].

The HER2 gene is frequently amplified and the protein overexpressed in several human epithelial malignancies, including breast, gastric, ovarian, and colon-rectal cancers [3–9]. In such tumors, HER2 amplification/overexpression has been linked to a poor overall outcome and a poorly differentiated phenotype [3–7]. It has also been considered a useful indicator of response to specifically targeted therapies, such as trastuzumab, that inhibit the extracellular domain of HER2 [8,9]. Many studies have been addressed to determine the HER2-positive rate, mainly in breast and gastric carcinomas, utilizing a well codified scoring system [10,11], and HER2 status assessment is currently being used in such cancers to determine patient eligibility for treatment with trastuzumab [8,9,12,13].

Studies on HER2 have also been performed in thyroid cancer cells and tissues [14–26]. Interestingly, a wide variation in HER2 overexpression was reported in such studies, with positivity rates varying from 0% up to 70%, which may largely be attributed to inter-study technical and interpretive variations. Due to these conflicting findings, there is no consensus in the currently available literature regarding the potential prognostic and therapeutic value of this marker in thyroid cancer [16,18,23,24]. More recently, HER2 expression has been linked to the expression of estrogen receptors in thyroid tumor tissue [27] and associated with $BRAF^{V600E}$ mutation and a more aggressive phenotype in familial papillary thyroid cancers (PTCs) [28].

In the present study, we investigate HER2 expression status in a surgical series of sporadic differentiated thyroid carcinomas of follicular cell origin to better clarify the role of this receptor in the stratification of thyroid cancer.

2. Results

2.1. Clinical-Pathological Findings

The clinical-pathological features of the 90 differentiated thyroid cancer (DTC) patients (73 F and 17 M, mean age 51.6 ± 12.7 years, median 49 years) are summarized in Table 1. The 45 patients with PTC comprised 34 females and 11 males who ranged in ages from 28 to 71 years (median age, 49 years). Histologically, the papillary carcinomas were as follows: 16 classic variant, 21 follicular variant, 4 Hürthle cell variant, and 4 sclerosing variant. The 45 patients with follicular thyroid cancer (FTC) comprised 39 females and 6 males aged 22–76 years (median age, 55 years). The follicular carcinomas included 34 that were minimally invasive and 11 that were widely invasive.

All patients had undergone total or subtotal thyroidectomy. In 61% of the patients, the tumor was <2 cm, pT1 according to TNM classification [29], and 11% had lymph node metastases (Table 1). No patient exhibited distant metastases at the time of surgery.

All patients were followed up for at least five years after thyroidectomy at our Endocrine Unit (median follow-up duration 8.7 years, range 5–20 years). During follow-up, 6 out of 90 (6.7%) patients (all females, aged 43–76 years, median 45 years) developed metastases: one was affected by PTC in the classic variant pT1b stage, two by PTC follicular variant in the pT2 stage, and three by FTC in the pT3 stage. All PTC metastatic patients except for one (with lung metastases) had lymph-nodes metastases, located in the right lateral neck (n = 1), left lateral neck (n = 1), anterior central compartment (n = 3), and upper mediastinum (n = 1). The three FTC patients had lung and skeletal metastases.

Table 1. Clinical and pathological features of the 90 differentiated thyroid cancer (DTC) patients at the time of surgery.

Variables	PTC Cases (n = 45)	FTC Cases (n = 45)
Age (years, mean ± SD)	50.6 ± 12.3	52.7 ± 13.2
Sex		
Male	11	6
Female	34	39
M:F	1:3	1:6.5
Histological features	Classic variant, n = 16 Follicular variant, n = 21 Hürtle cell variant, n = 4 Sclerosing variant, n = 4	Minimally invasive, n = 34 Widely invasive, n = 11
Primary Tumour pT [29]		
T1	34 (13 T1a and 21 T1b)	21 (9 T1a and 12 T1b)
T2	10	13
T3	1	11
T4	/	/
Node metastasis (NX/N0/N1) [29]		
pNX	12	20
pN0	23	25
pN1	10 (N1a)	/

The symbol/means no case.

2.2. *Immunohistochemical (IHC) and Fluorescence In Situ Hybridization (FISH) Results*

Twenty-seven specimens (17 PTC and 10 FTC) presented unamplified HER2 status and were therefore scored 0. The remaining 63 cases (28 PTC and 35 FTC) stained for HER2 with a variable intensity ranging from 1+ to 3+ (Table 2). A not negligible number of tumors, mostly papillary histotype (15 cases, 13 PTC and 2 FTC), exhibited a low (1+) and patchy expression of HER2, with a granular or diffuse cytoplasmic distribution of the staining. Such cases with no membranous staining were considered negative.

Table 2. Human epidermal growth factor receptor 2 (HER2) expression in thyroid cancer tissue *.

HER2 Status	FTC (n = 45)	PTC (n = 45)	p
IHC Negative/low (0, 1+)	12 (26.6%)	30 (66.6%)	0.020
Equivocal (2+)	15	7	
Positive (3+)	18	8	
IHC/FISH Positive cases (3+ and amplified)	20 (44.4%)	8 (17.7%)	0.046

* HER2 status has been assessed by using immunohistochemistry (IHC) to detect protein expression. Fluorescence in situ hybridization (FISH) was also performed in cases that tested 2+ at IHC, as specified in the Materials and Methods section to detect gene amplification.

HER2 was clearly overexpressed (3+) at IHC with membranous staining in 26 cases: 18 FTC, of which 6 were widely invasive (see example in Figure 1A), and 8 PTC (2 classic, 5 follicular variant, and 1 Hürthle cell variant) (see example in Figure 1B). Twenty-two tumors (15 FTC and 7 PTC) were scored as 2+ by IHC for HER2. All 2+ cases (Figure 2A) were evaluated by FISH: two FTC revealed HER2 amplification (Figure 2B), while the others were unamplified (Figure 2C). Therefore, the overall rate of HER2-positive cases was 31% (28/90 cases). Specifically, HER2 amplification/overexpression was found in 20/45 (44%) FTC and 8/45 (18%) PTC, with a significant difference between the two histotypes (x^2 = 3.96; p = 0.046) (Figure 3). Normal thyroid parenchyma surrounding the tumor lacked expression of HER2.

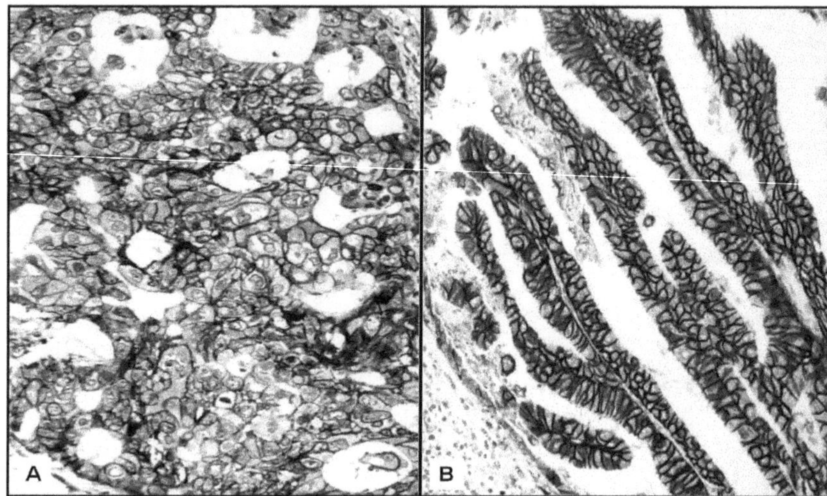

Figure 1. An evident diffuse membranous HER2 immunopositivity was seen in FTC (**A**, ×400) as well as in the classic variant of papillary thyroid cancer (PTC) (**B**, ×400) (Mayer's hemalum counterstain).

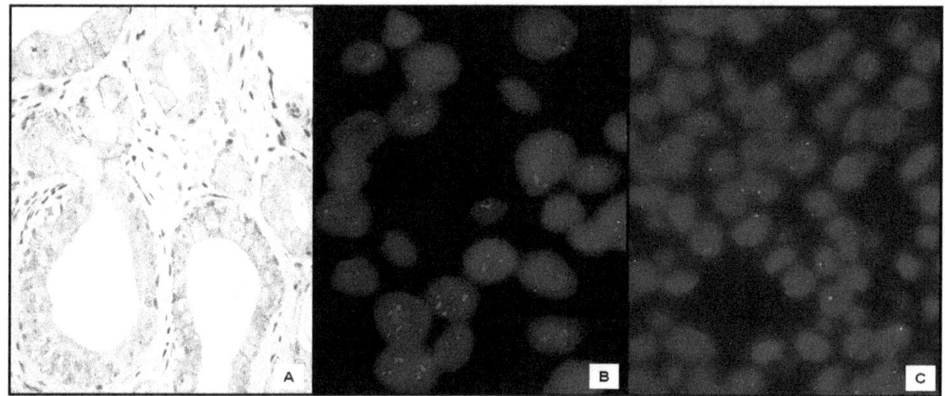

Figure 2. IHC equivocal (2+) follicular thyroid cancer (FTC) case (**A**, ×400) (Mayer's hemalum counterstain) that showed a corresponding HER2 amplification by FISH (**B**, ×660). Another unamplified HER2 FTC case (**C**, ×460).

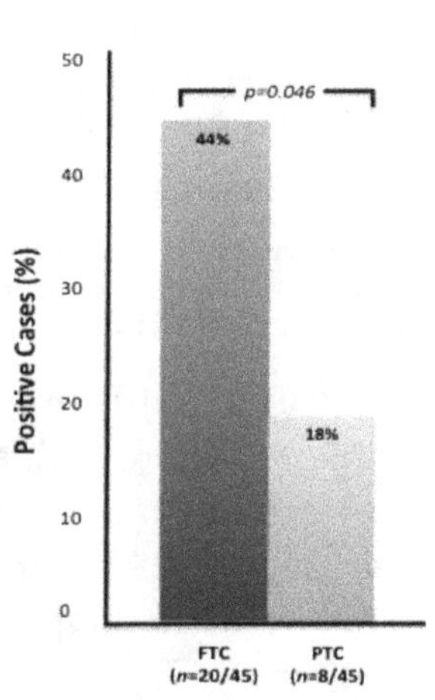

Figure 3. Percentages of FTC and PTC cases which tested positive for HER2 at both FISH and IHC (3+).

No significant correlation was found between HER2 expression and tumor size, as well as lymph node metastases at the time of surgery. However, among the six patients who developed metastatic disease during follow-up, five had a HER2-positive tumor. Three tumors (2 PTC and 1 FTC) stained 3+ at IHC; and the remaining two FTCs stained 2+ at IHC and revealed HER2 amplification at FISH. Thus, 5 out of 28 HER2-positive tumors and 1 out of the remaining 62 HER2-negative tumors developed metastatic disease during the follow-up ($x^2 = 8.18$; $p = 0.004$).

None of our cancers was iodine refractory. Concerning iodine uptake, in our cohort of DTC patients, the intensity of 131-radioiodine uptake observed (visual analysis) in thyroid remnant and, mainly, in lymph-node metastases at post-therapy whole body scan (pT-WBS) did not differ in cases overexpressing HER2 compared to negative ones.

3. Discussion

In the present study, we assessed HER2 status in a series of sporadic differentiated thyroid cancers (DTCs) and found that HER2 was overall overexpressed in about one-third of cases; in particular, the expression rate was significantly higher in the follicular (FTC) histotype compared to the papillary (PTC) one.

To date, many studies have evaluated HER2 expression in thyroid cancer with controversial results, largely due to inter-study differences in the size and setting of the examined series and, most of all, to the subjective assessment and lack of uniform methodology [14–26]. Indeed, studies reported in the literature in the past several decades markedly differ by the methodological approach used to assess HER2 status [14–26]. Moreover, the criteria for scoring HER2 expression were different, and, in many studies, cytoplasmic staining patterns were reported as positive immunostaining for HER2 [16–18,22,23,26]. As a consequence, the results of these studies are not comparable and therefore not conclusive.

The present study aimed to evaluate HER2 status using a method as reproducible and as standardized as possible, similar to other cancers. Indeed, a similarly wide variation in HER2 overexpression has been reported in many other tumor types [3–8]. Therefore, as the prognostic and therapeutic relevance of HER2 status has grown, the need to achieve a standardized HER2 assessment method has also arisen in neoplastic sites different from the stomach and breast [11]. In the present study, we utilized the updated ASCO-CAP scoring system reported in breast cancer [10]. Applying such strict criteria to our DTC series, we reported an overall HER2 expression of 31%. In detail, both PTC (18%) and FTC (44%) cases were found to overexpress HER2 in our series, and the expression rate was significantly different between the two histotypes in favor of the follicular one. These data may suggest a prognostic impact of HER2 status in DTC, further supported by the finding that, in nearly all patients who had metastases diagnosed during follow-up, HER2 was overexpressed in the primary tumor. Obviously, such results should be confirmed in a larger series to better determine whether HER2 amplification/overexpression can be considered an additional prognostic aid to identify cases characterized by a more aggressive disease, such as in other epithelial cancers [3,8–10,13].

Other studies have shown the absence of HER2 amplification in normal thyroid tissue, as well as increased expression during malignant progression in DTC [18,19,21,22]. These findings are in agreement with ours, although the importance of a standardized scoring methodology should be emphasized in order to explain the partially contradictory results on DTC. In detail, Sugishita et al. [24] investigated HER2 expression in a surgical series of 69 DTC, including 61 PTC and only 8 FTC, and found that 14 PTC and 2 FTC had a score 3+ at IHC. Amplification of HER2 gene was confirmed via FISH in 10 PTC 3+ plus 4 PTC cases 2+, and in one FTC, with an overall expression rate of 21.7% (23% considering the sole PTC). Therefore, the highest rate of HER2 expression was recorded in PTC. However, there are some limitations in the above-mentioned study [24]. First of all, the authors set an arbitrary cut-off value for the FISH ratio of 1.3 to score their cases because of the low rate of HER2 gene amplification they had found. If they had applied the HER2 amplification criteria for breast and gastric cancer (i.e., FISH ratio > 2.0) strictly to thyroid cancer, as we did, all cases would be judged as negative. Thus, these data are not comparable to ours. Secondly, the series from Sugishita et al. included only

8 FTC, without any morphological evidence of HER2 expression [24]. Successively, another surgical series of 69 DTC has been investigated for HER2 expression [25], but again a low number of FTC was included (11 cases). Although the authors utilized a HER2 scoring methodology equivalent to ours, they reported a very low rate of HER2 overexpression, since no FTC and only four (6.9%) PTCs showed HER-2 overexpression [25]. Therefore, the rate of HER2 expression in PTC was definitely lower than that previously reported elsewhere [24]; in addition, Mdah et al. [25] failed to find HER2 expression in FTC. More recently, Caria and co-workers reported a scattered HER2 expression, restricted to less than 10% of tumor cells, in a few cases of familial PTC [28]. In particular, 5/13 (38.5%) of familial PTC cases showed 5.1%–10% $HER2^{+}$ cells, while no sporadic PTC cases exceeded the cut-off value [28]. Moreover, when familial PTCs were analyzed via IHC using an anti-c-erbB2 antibody to detect HER2 protein expression, inconsistent results compared to the FISH analysis were obtained, also possibly biased by the age of the available histological sections (7–20 years) [28]. Finally, no data about HER2 expression were recorded about different varieties present in PTC, nor in relation to the metastatic event in PTC [28].

In the present study, we analyzed a large sporadic DTC registry including the same number of PTC and FTC cases. Consequently, our data appear to be statistically more significant in comparison to the reported studies [24,25,28] and reveal a significant HER2 expression related to histotype, greatly favoring FTC. Moreover, its overexpression is more evident in metastatic DTC compared to non-metastatic ones. These findings might have potential practical implications. HER2 may be helpful in identifying a subset of DTC patients characterized by a worse prognosis, but eligible for potential targeted therapies with HER2 inhibitors, such as trastuzumab. This may be relevant in iodine-refractory cancers, since novel molecular targets and therapeutic strategies are currently under investigation for these tumors, whose treatment is still a major challenge [30,31]. Moreover, HER2 expression may be used for prognostic application in the context of other well-accepted clinic-pathological prognostic parameters for DTC (age, gender, pTNM stage, histological subtype), since very few new markers revealed prognostic value *per se* [32,33]. If our observations are confirmed in a larger series, HER2 overexpression may play a role not only in the development and progression of a subset of thyroid carcinomas, but also in their prognostic and therapeutic stratification.

4. Materials and Methods

4.1. Sample Collection

Ninety sporadic differentiated thyroid tumors (DTCs) (45 papillary (PTCs) and 45 follicular (FTCs) thyroid cancers) with available formalin-fixed paraffin-embedded tissue blocks were selected from the files of the Department of Pathology of our University Hospital. The surgical samples were from 90 patients (73 F and 17 M, aged 28–76 years) who were diagnosed and followed up at the Endocrine Unit of our University Hospital over the last twenty years. The clinical records of the 90 patients were reviewed.

Histological classification was performed by two pathologists with experience in thyroid pathology (Giovanni Tuccari, Antonio Ieni and Giovanni Branca), according to the World Health Organization guidelines [34]. Institutional review board approval was obtained.

4.2. Immunohistochemistry

For each case, 5-μm-thick sections from representative tissue blocks of the tumor were obtained. Immunohistochemistry (IHC) was performed twice on each specimen using, firstly, the monoclonal antibody against HER2-pY-1248 (Phosphorylation site specific) (clone PN2A, Dako; w.d. 1:100) and, successively, the Hercep Test (Dako, Glostrup, Denmark), with an automated procedure (DAKO Autostainer Link48), according to the manufacturer's instructions. An antigen retrieval pre-treatment was performed in 3 cycles in a 0.01 M citrate buffer, pH 6.0, in a microwave oven at 750 W. Staining intensity, the percentage of positive cells, and cellular localization were evaluated both in the tumor and in the adjacent non-neoplastic thyroid tissue.

Since there are no established criteria for thyroid cancer, we adapted the current breast criteria for scoring HER2 in our DTC. Staining intensity and cellular localization in the tumor were evaluated and scored according to the updated ASCO-CAP scoring system for breast cancer [10]. Accordingly, the degree of HER2 staining was scored from 0 to 3+. HER2 positivity was defined as 3+ when strong membranous staining was noted in at least 10% of cells, 2+ when weak to moderate complete membranous staining was evident in 10% of tumor cells, 1+ when a faint or weak and incomplete membrane staining was observed, and 0 when no staining was observed or when staining was present in less than 10% of neoplastic cells.

Immunohistochemical evaluations were carried out twice and blindly by two pathologists (Giovanni Tuccari, Antonio Ieni and Giovanni Branca). In the case of disagreement, cases were jointly discussed using a double-headed microscope until agreement was reached.

4.3. Fluorescence In Situ Hybridization

In cases showing 2+ immunostaining, as determined by IHC with the Hercept test, fluorescence in situ hybridization (FISH) analysis was performed using a HER2 FISH PharmDx™ kit (Dako, Glostrup, Denmark), according to the manufacturer's instructions, to detect amplification of the *HER2* gene, as for breast cancer [35]. Gene amplification was recorded when the ratio HER2/centromeric probe for chromosome 17 (CEP17) signal was $\geq$2.0.

Specimens of breast carcinoma were used as appropriate positive controls for both IHC and FISH analysis (Figure 4A). Negative controls were obtained either by omitting the primary antiserum or by replacing the primary antiserum with normal mouse serum, in a parallel section of the same cases (Figure 4B).

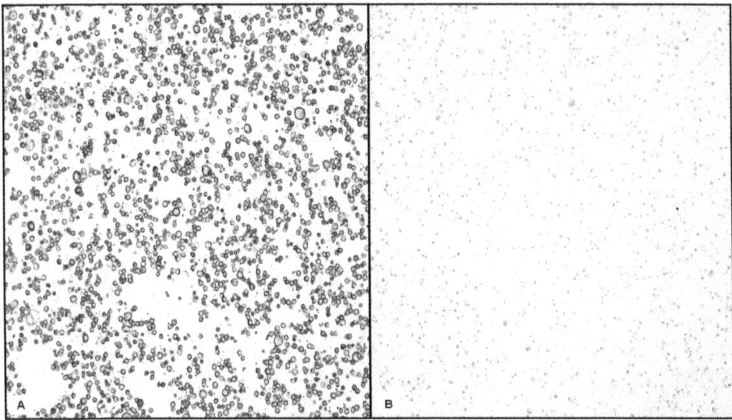

Figure 4. Breast carcinoma tissue section as positive control (**A**, 200×) and negative control (**B**, 200×).

4.4. Statistical Analysis

Once tested for normal distribution and variance, data (mean ± standard deviation) were analyzed by the two-tailed Student's *t*-test, a chi-square test with Yates' correction for continuity, and linear regression analysis. The level of statistical significance was always set at $p < 0.05$.

Acknowledgments: We thank Massimo Bongiovanni from the Institute of Pathology, Lausanne University Hospital, (Lausanne, Switzerland) for his useful suggestions.

Author Contributions: Rosaria M. Ruggeri and Giovanni Tuccari conceived of the study, participated in its design and coordination, and drafted the manuscript. Alfredo Campennì and Francesco Trimarchi participated in the design of the study and took care of the clinical approach to patients. Giuseppe Giuffrè and Angela Simone carried out the FISH studies. Angela Simone and Rosi Scarfì carried out the immunohistochemistry analysis. Massimiliano Siracusa was responsible for data collection and database management. Giovanni Branca and Antonio Ieni performed the histopatological and immunohistochemical evaluations of the specimens and data interpretation along with Giovanni Tuccari, and drafted the manuscript. Luca Giovanella participated in writing and critical reviewing of the manuscript. All authors read and approved the final version.

References

1. Yarden, Y. The EGFR family and its ligands in human cancer. Signaling mechanisms and therapeutic opportunities. *Eur. J. Cancer* **2001**, *4*, S3–S8. [CrossRef]
2. Salomon, D.S.; Brandt, R.; Ciardiello, F.; Normanno, N. Epidermal growth factor-related peptides and their receptors in human malignancies. *Crit. Rev. Oncol. Hematol.* **1995**, *19*, 183–232. [CrossRef]
3. Ieni, A.; Barresi, V.; Giuffrè, G.; Caruso, R.A.; Lanzafame, S.; Villari, L.; Salomone, E.; Roz, E.; Cabibi, D.; Franco, V.; et al. HER2 status in advanced gastric carcinoma: A retrospective multicentric analysis from Sicily. *Oncol. Lett.* **2013**, *6*, 1591–1594. [PubMed]
4. Ieni, A.; Barresi, V.; Caltabiano, R.; Caleo, A.; Bonetti, L.R.; Lanzafame, S.; Zeppa, P.; Caruso, R.A.; Tuccari, G. Discordance rate of HER2 status in primary gastric carcinomas and synchronous lymph node metastases: A multicenter retrospective analysis. *Int. J. Mol. Sci.* **2014**, *15*, 22331–22341. [CrossRef] [PubMed]
5. Ieni, A.; Barresi, V.; Caltabiano, R.; Cascone, A.M.; del Sordo, R.; Cabibi, D.; Zeppa, P.; Lanzafame, S.; Sidoni, A.; Franco, V.; et al. Discordance rate of HER2 status in primary breast carcinomas versus synchronous axillary lymph node metastases: A multicenter retrospective investigation. *Onco. Targets Ther.* **2014**, *7*, 1267–1272. [PubMed]
6. Slamon, D.J.; Clark, G.M.; Wong, S.G.; Levin, W.J.; Ullrich, A.; McGuire, W.L. Human breast cancer: Correlation of relapse and survival with amplification of the HER-2/neu oncogene. *Science* **1987**, *235*, 177–182. [CrossRef] [PubMed]
7. Allgayer, H.; Babic, R.; Gruetzner, K.U.; Tarabichi, A.; Schildberg, F.W.; Heiss, M.M. c-erbB-2 is of independent prognostic relevance in gastric cancer and is associated with the expression of tumor-associated protease systems. *J. Clin. Oncol.* **2000**, *18*, 2201–2209. [PubMed]
8. Ieni, A.; Barresi, V.; Rigoli, L.; Caruso, R.A.; Tuccari, G. HER2 Status in Premalignant, Early, and Advanced Neoplastic Lesions of the Stomach. *Dis. Markers* **2015**, *2015*, 234851. [CrossRef] [PubMed]
9. Ieni, A.; Giuffrè, G.; Lanzafame, S.; Nuciforo, G.; Curduman, M.; Villari, L.; Roz, E.; Certo, G.; Cabibi, D.; Salomone, E.; et al. Morphological and biomolecular characteristics of subcentimetric invasive breast carcinomas in Sicily: A multicentre retrospective study in relation to trastuzumab treatment. *Oncol. Lett.* **2012**, *3*, 141–146. [CrossRef] [PubMed]
10. Rakha, E.A.; Starczynski, J.; Lee, A.H.; Ellis, I.O. The updated ASCO/CAP guideline recommendations for HER2 testing in the management of invasive breast cancer: A critical review of their implications for routine practice. *Histopathology* **2014**, *64*, 609–615. [CrossRef] [PubMed]
11. Valtorta, E.; Martino, C.; Sartore-Bianchi, A.; Penaullt-Llorca, F.; Viale, G.; Risio, M.; Rugge, M.; Grigioni, W.; Bencardino, K.; Lonardi, S.; et al. Assessment of a HER2 scoring system for colorectal cancer: Results from a validation study. *Mod. Pathol.* **2015**, *28*, 481–1491. [CrossRef] [PubMed]
12. Baselga, J.; Lewis Phillips, G.D.; Verma, S.; Ro, J.; Huober, J.; Guardino, A.E.; Samant, M.K.; Olsen, S.; de Haas, S.L.; Pegram, M.D. Relationship between Tumor Biomarkers and Efficacy in EMILIA, a Phase III Study of Trastuzumab Emtansine in HER2-Positive Metastatic Breast Cancer. *Clin. Cancer Res.* **2016**, *22*, 3755–3763. [CrossRef] [PubMed]
13. Bang, Y.J.; van Cutsem, E.; Feyereislova, A.; Chung, H.C.; Shen, L.; Sawaki, A.; Lordick, F.; Ohtsu, A.; Omuro, Y.; Satoh, T.; et al. Trastuzumab in combination with chemotherapy versus chemotherapy alone for treatment of HER2-positive advanced gastric or gastro-oesophageal junction cancer (ToGA): A phase 3, open-label, randomised controlled trial. *Lancet* **2010**, *376*, 687–697. [CrossRef]
14. Lemoine, N.K.; Wyllie, F.S.; Lillehaug, J.R.; Staddon, S.L.; Hughes, C.M.; Aasland, R.; Shaw, J.; Varhaug, J.E.; Brown, C.L.; Gullick, W.J.; et al. Absence of abnormalities of the c-erbB-1 and c-erbB-2 proto-oncogenes in human thyroid neoplasia. *Eur. J. Cancer* **1990**, *26*, 777–779. [CrossRef]
15. Haugen, D.R.; Akslen, L.A.; Varhaug, J.E.; Lillehaug, J.R. Expression of c-erbB-2 protein in papillary thyroid carcinomas. *Br. J. Cancer* **1992**, *65*, 832–837. [CrossRef] [PubMed]
16. Sugg, S.L.; Ezzat, S.; Zheng, L.; Rosen, I.B.; Freeman, J.L.; Asa, S.L. Cytoplasmic staining of erbB-2 but not mRNA levels correlates with differentiation in human thyroid neoplasia. *Clin. Endocrinol.* **1998**, *49*, 629–637. [CrossRef]

17. Utrilla, J.C.; Martin-Lacave, I.; San Martin, M.V.; Fernandez-Santos, J.M.; Galera-Davidson, H. Expression of c-erbB-2 oncoprotein in human thyroid tumours. *Histopathology* **1999**, *34*, 60–65. [CrossRef] [PubMed]
18. Kremser, R.; Obrist, P.; Spizzo, G.; Erler, H.; Kendler, D.; Kemmler, G.; Mikuz, G.; Ensinger, C. Her2/neu overexpression in differentiated thyroid carcinomas predicts metastatic disease. *Virchows. Arch.* **2003**, *442*, 322–328. [PubMed]
19. Ensinger, C.; Prommegger, R.; Kendler, D.; Gabriel, M.; Spizzo, G.; Mikuz, G.; Kremser, R. Her2/neu expression in poorly-differentiated and anaplastic thyroid carcinomas. *Anticancer Res.* **2003**, *23*, 2349–2353. [PubMed]
20. Mondi, M.M.; Rich, R.; Ituarte, P.; Wong, M.; Bergman, S.; Clark, O.H.; Perrier, N.D. HER2 expression in thyroid tumors. *Am. Surg.* **2003**, *69*, 1100–1103. [PubMed]
21. Murakawa, T.; Tsuda, H.; Tanimoto, T.; Tanabe, T.; Kitahara, S.; Matsubara, O. Expression of KIT, EGFR, HER2/NEU and tyrosine phosphorylation in undifferentiated thyroid carcinoma: Implication for a new therapeutic approach. *Pathol. Int.* **2005**, *55*, 757–765. [CrossRef] [PubMed]
22. Elliott, D.D.; Sherman, S.I.; Busaidy, N.L.; Williams, M.D.; Santarpia, L.; Clayman, G.L.; El-Naggar, A.K. Growth factor receptors expression in anaplastic thyroid carcinoma: Potential markers for therapeutic stratification. *Hum. Pathol.* **2008**, *39*, 15–20. [CrossRef] [PubMed]
23. Qin, C.; Cau, W.; Zhang, Y.; Mghanga, F.P.; Lan, X.; Gao, Z.; An, R. Correlation of clinic-pathological features and expression of molecular markers with prognosis after 131I treatment of differentiated thyroid carcinoma. *Clin. Nucl. Med.* **2012**, *37*, e40–e46. [CrossRef] [PubMed]
24. Sugishita, Y.; Kammori, M.; Yamada, O.; Poon, S.S.; Kobayashi, M.; Onoda, N.; Yamazaki, K.; Fukumori, T.; Yoshikawa, K.; Onose, H.; et al. Amplification of the human epidermal growth factor receptor 2 gene in differentiated thyroid cancer correlates with telomere shortening. *Int. J. Oncol.* **2013**, *42*, 1589–1596. [PubMed]
25. Mdah, W.; Mzalbat, R.; Gilbey, P.; Stein, M.; Sharabi, A.; Zidan, J. Lack of HER-2 gene amplification and association with pathological and clinical characteristics of differentiated thyroid cancer. *Mol. Clin. Oncol.* **2014**, *2*, 1107–1110. [CrossRef] [PubMed]
26. Wu, G.; Wang, J.; Zhou, Z.; Li, T.; Tang, F. Combined staining for immunohistochemical markers in the diagnosis of papillary thyroid carcinoma: Improvement in the sensitivity or specificity? *J. Int. Med. Res.* **2013**, *41*, 975–983. [CrossRef] [PubMed]
27. Kavanagh, D.O.; McIlroy, M.; Myers, E.; Bane, F.; Crotty, T.B.; McDermott, E.; Hill, A.D.; Young, L.S. The role of oestrogen receptor α in human thyroid cancer: Contributions from coregulatory proteins and the tyrosine kinase receptor HER2. *Endocr. Relat. Cancer* **2010**, *17*, 255–264. [CrossRef] [PubMed]
28. Caria, P.; Cantara, S.; Frau, D.V.; Pacini, F.; Vanni, R.; Dettori, T. Genetic Heterogeneity of HER2 Amplification and Telomere Shortening in Papillary Thyroid Carcinoma. *Int. J. Mol. Sci.* **2016**, *17*, e1759. [CrossRef] [PubMed]
29. The American Joint Committee on Cancer. Thyroid. In *AJCC Cancer Staging Manual*, 7th ed.; Edge, S.B., Byrd, D.R., Compton, C.C., Eds.; Springer: New York, NY, USA, 2010; pp. 87–96.
30. Alonso-Gordoa, T.; Díez, J.J.; Durán, M.; Grande, E. Advances in thyroid cancer treatment: Latest evidence and clinical potential. *Ther. Adv. Med. Oncol.* **2015**, *7*, 22–38. [CrossRef] [PubMed]
31. Bulotta, S.; Celano, M.; Costante, G.; Russo, D. Emerging strategies for managing differentiated thyroid cancers refractory to radioiodine. *Endocrine* **2016**, *52*, 214–221. [CrossRef] [PubMed]
32. Soares, P.; Celestino, R.; Melo, M.; Fonseca, E.; Sobrinho-Simões, M. Prognostic biomarkers in thyroid cancer. *Virchows. Arch.* **2014**, *464*, 333–346. [CrossRef] [PubMed]
33. Ruggeri, R.M.; Campennì, A.; Baldari, S.; Trimarchi, F.; Trovato, M. What is New on Thyroid Cancer Biomarkers. *Biomark. Insights* **2008**, *3*, 237–252. [PubMed]
34. De Lellis, R.A. *WHO Classification of Tumours, Pathology and Genetics of Tumours of Endocrine Organs*, 3rd ed.; Ronald, A., de Lellis, R.A., Riccardo, V.L., Philipp, U.H., Charis, E., Eds.; IARC Press: Lyon, France, 2004; Volume 8, p. 230.
35. La, P.; Salazar, P.A.; Hudis, C.A.; Ladanyi, M.; Chen, B. HER-2 testing in breast cancer using immunohistochemical analysis and fluorescence in situ hybridization: A single-institution experience of 2279 cases and comparison of dual-color and single-color scoring. *Am. J. Clin. Pathol.* **2004**, *121*, 631–636.

4

Actions of L-Thyroxine (T4) and Tetraiodothyroacetic Acid (Tetrac) on Gene Expression in Thyroid Cancer Cells

Paul J. Davis [1,2,*], Hung-Yun Lin [3,4,5], Aleck Hercbergs [6] and Shaker A. Mousa [2]

1 Department of Medicine, Albany Medical College, Albany, NY 12208, USA
2 Pharmaceutical Research Institute, Albany College of Pharmacy and Health Sciences, Rensselaer, NY 12144, USA; shaker.mousa@acphs.edu
3 Ph.D. Program for Cancer Molecular Biology and Drug Discovery, College of Medical Science and Technology, Taipei Medical University, Taipei 11031, Taiwan; linhy@tmu.edu.tw
4 Cancer Center, Wan Fang Hospital, Taipei Medical University, Taipei 11031, Taiwan
5 Traditional Herbal Medicine Research Center of Taipei Medical University Hospital, Taipei Medical University, Taipei 11031, Taiwan
6 Department of Radiation Oncology, The Cleveland Clinic, Cleveland, OH 44195, USA; hercbergs@gmail.com
* Correspondence: pdavis.ordwayst@gmail.com

Abstract: The clinical behavior of thyroid cancers is seen to reflect inherent transcriptional activities of mutated genes and trophic effects on tumors of circulating pituitary thyrotropin (TSH). The thyroid hormone, L-thyroxine (T4), has been shown to stimulate proliferation of a large number of different forms of cancer. This activity of T4 is mediated by a cell surface receptor on the extracellular domain of integrin αvβ3. In this brief review, we describe what is known about T4 as a circulating trophic factor for differentiated (papillary and follicular) thyroid cancers. Given T4's cancer-stimulating activity in differentiated thyroid cancers, it was not surprising to find that genomic actions of T4 were anti-apoptotic. Transduction of the T4-generated signal at the integrin primarily involved mitogen-activated protein kinase (MAPK). In thyroid C cell-origin medullary carcinoma of the thyroid (MTC), effects of thyroid hormone analogues, such as tetraiodothyroacetic acid (tetrac), include pro-angiogenic and apoptosis-linked genes. Tetrac is an inhibitor of the actions of T4 at αvβ3, and it is assumed, but not yet proved, that the anti-angiogenic and pro-apoptotic actions of tetrac in MTC cells are matched by T4 effects that are pro-angiogenic and anti-apoptotic. We also note that papillary thyroid carcinoma cells may express the leptin receptor, and circulating leptin from adipocytes may stimulate tumor cell proliferation. Transcription was stimulated by leptin in anaplastic, papillary, and follicular carcinomas of genes involved in invasion, such as matrix metalloproteinases (MMPs). In summary, thyroid hormone analogues may act at their receptor on integrin αvβ3 in a variety of types of thyroid cancer to modulate transcription of genes relevant to tumor invasiveness, apoptosis, and angiogenesis. These effects are independent of TSH.

Keywords: apoptosis; angiogenesis; integrin αvβ3; L-thyroxine (T4); thyroid cancer; tetraiodothyroacetic acid (tetrac)

---

1. Introduction

The clinical behavior of thyroid gland cancers is seen to reflect gene mutation and/or epigenetic changes [1,2], and effects of circulating or local trophic factors [3,4]. Circulating trophic factors include target tissue-specific thyrotropin (TSH) secreted by the pituitary gland and adipose tissue-source leptin, which enhances growth of a variety of tumors, including those of the thyroid gland [5]. In the clinical management of differentiated thyroid cancers, host pituitary TSH secretion is suppressed with exogenous L-thyroxine (T4) in conjunction with tumor surgery and radioablation of the cancers.

Discovery of a cell surface thyroid hormone analogue receptor on plasma membrane integrin αvβ3 has provided additional information about the biological activity of T4. T4 has been viewed primarily as a source of 3,3′,5-triiodo-L-thyronine (T3), the principally active form of the hormone at nuclear thyroid hormone receptors (TRs) [6,7]. At physiological concentrations, however, T4 is the primary ligand of the cell surface iodothyronine receptor on the plasma membrane [8]. The integrin is generously expressed by cancer cells and rapidly dividing endothelial cells [6] and at this site, T4 promotes proliferation of tumor cells and supports angiogenesis [8]. T4 may also be a factor that contributes to metastasis of cancer cells [9].

Reverse T3 (3,3′,5′-triiodo-L-thyronine, rT3) has also been thought to have little bioactivity but is known to affect the state of actin in cells [10] and, recently, to stimulate proliferation of cancer cells [11]. In contrast to T4 and to rT3, tetraiodothyroacetic acid (tetrac), a derivative of T4, has anti-proliferative and anti-angiogenic properties at αvβ3 [6,8,12]. Prior to recognition of anti-tumor activity of tetrac at the cell surface integrin, tetrac was seen to have low-grade T3-like activity at the nuclear receptors [6].

Against this background, we examine in the present review the actions of T4 and tetrac, and chemical derivatives of tetrac on the biology of human thyroid cancer cells, including expression of a number of genes relevant to proliferation, apoptosis, and angiogenesis. These actions of T4 and tetrac are initiated at the hormone receptor on integrin αvβ3 (Figure 1). The signals generated at the integrin by thyroid hormone analogues involve early transduction within the cell primarily by mitogen-activated protein kinase (MAPK) [6,8].

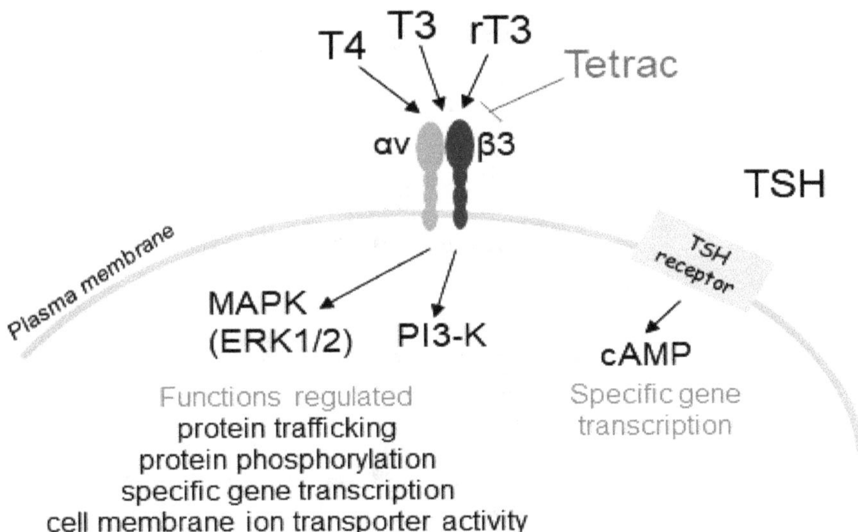

Figure 1. Cancer-relevant actions of thyroid hormones and pituitary thyrotropin (TSH) at thyroid carcinoma cells. Plasma membrane integrin αvβ3 contains a cell surface receptor for thyroid hormones and is overexpressed by cancer cells. T4 is the principal ligand for this receptor and the T4 signal is transduced by mitogen-activated protein kinase (MAPK/ERK1/2) or phosphatidylinositol 3-kinase (PI3-K) into cancer-linked gene transcription. A deaminated analogue of T4, tetrac, blocks actions of T4 at the integrin and is under development as an anticancer agent. At physiological concentrations, T3 is not active at the integrin, but reverse T3 (rT3) has cancer cell-stimulating activity at this plasma membrane receptor. T3 is the principal ligand of nuclear thyroid hormone receptors (TRs) in normal cells; TRs are not shown in the figure. Pituitary TSH acts at a specific cAMP-generating receptor on the plasma membrane of thyroid cancer cells. TRs and the TSH receptor are not structurally related to the T4 binding site on αvβ3. 2. T4 Actions at the Integrin αvβ3 in Papillary and Follicular Thyroid Carcinoma Cells.

2. T4 Actions at the Integrin αvβ3 in Papillary and Follicular Thyroid Carcinoma Cells

The physiological loops that connect the components of the normal hypothalamic-pituitary-thyroid gland axis have been assumed to be intact when the axis is disrupted by thyroid cancer [3,6,13–15]. In differentiated thyroid cancers, the tumor cells are usually TSH-responsive in terms of proliferation and pharmacologic administration of thyroid hormone—as T4, serving as a source of T3 at the level of nuclear TRs in the pituitary—and can take advantage of the thyro-pituitary feedback loop and suppress endogenous thyrotropin. The reduction of circulating TSH frequently contributes to arrest of the thyroid cancer. The amounts of exogenous T4 that are required to fully suppress host TSH via generated T3 are, by the nature of the definition of the feedback loop, supraphysiologic. The thyroid hormone receptors involved are exclusively nuclear TRs.

Lin et al. [16] showed in 2007 that differentiated papillary and follicular human thyroid carcinoma cells in vitro proliferated in response to physiological levels of T4. The index of cell division was expression of proliferating cell nuclear antigen (PCNA) (see Figure 2). The proliferative effect of T4 was inhibited by tetrac that, as noted above, blocks actions of T4 that are initiated at integrin αvβ3. An Arg-Gly-Asp (RGD) peptide that acts on a number of integrins and has a receptor close to the T4 receptor on αvβ3, also blocked the action of T4 on thyroid cancer cells, but a control Arg-Gly-Glu (RGE) peptide did not affect the action of T4. This report, thus, documented a local and primary effect of the principal hormonal product of the thyroid gland on thyroid gland cancer cells. TSH was not involved. The cell lines in this work had been well-studied by other endocrine laboratories and were the subjects of more than 20 publications.

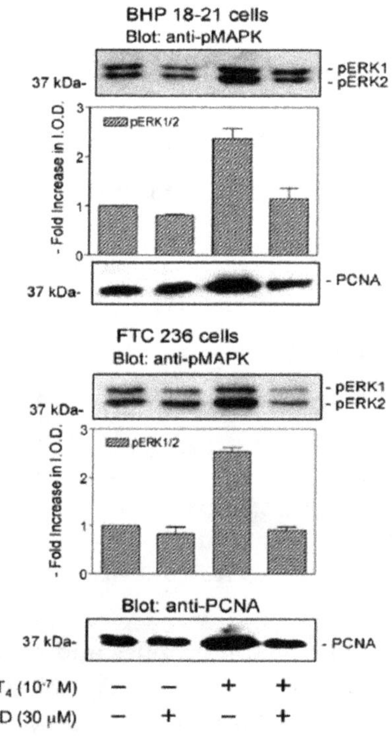

Figure 2. Proliferative activity of T4 in vitro on differentiated human papillary (BHP 18-21; upper panel) and follicular (FTC 236: lower panel) thyroid carcinoma cells. Proliferation was measured by immunoblotting of proliferative cell nuclear antigen (PCNA) from cultured cells. The 2.5-fold increase in PCNA in both cell lines was achieved with 10^{-7} M total T4 concentration (10^{-10} M free T4 in medium) [17]. The proliferative effect of the hormone required activation of ERK1/2 (MAPK). Inhibition of activation of ERK1/2 with PD98059 (PD) prevented enhancement of proliferation in both cell lines. T4 activates MAPK via the thyroid hormone analogue receptor on the extracellular domain of plasma membrane integrin αvβ3 [8,17]. Reprinted with permission from Elsevier from Lin et al. [16]. ERK1/2, extracellular signal-regulated kinases 1 and 2; MAPK, mitogen-activated protein kinase.

Another feature of the Lin et al. study was to define molecular components of the mechanism, downstream of its receptor on the integrin [8,16,17] by which T4 stimulated cell proliferation. That activation of MAPK was essential to the induction of proliferation was shown with the use of pharmacologic inhibitor of MAPK [18] (Figure 2), which eliminated the stimulatory T4 action on PCNA. The requirement for MAPK participation in T4's action on proliferation has been shown in a number of cancer cells [19–25]. Only at supraphysiologic concentrations was T3 effective as a proliferative factor [16] and this is a feature of cancer cell responses that are mediated by the receptor for thyroid hormone on integrin αvβ3 [17].

To define the specific genes whose transcription is affected by T4, Lin and co-workers [16] studied the effects of T4 on pharmacologically induced apoptosis in papillary and follicular thyroid cancer cells. The stilbene, resveratrol, induces apoptosis in differentiated thyroid cancer cells by a complex molecular mechanism that involves *p21*, *c-Jun*, and *c-Fos* expression [26]. As shown in Figure 3, resveratrol activated pro-apoptotic p53 and increased cancer cell expression of *p21*, *c-Fos*, and *c-Jun* genes. Addition of T4 to the cells cultured with resveratrol prevented p53 activation and apoptosis and also blocked induction of expression of *p21*, *c-Jun*, and *c-Fos*. Thus, T4 has anti-apoptotic activity in thyroid cancer cells by multiple mechanisms, including expression of multiple genes and reversing activation of p53. It is also important to note that tetrac inhibited resveratrol-induced apoptosis, as shown in nucleosome ELISA studies [16]. The anti-apoptosis effects of T4 in these studies, like those on cell proliferation, are initiated at the cell surface thyroid hormone receptor on integrin αvβ3.

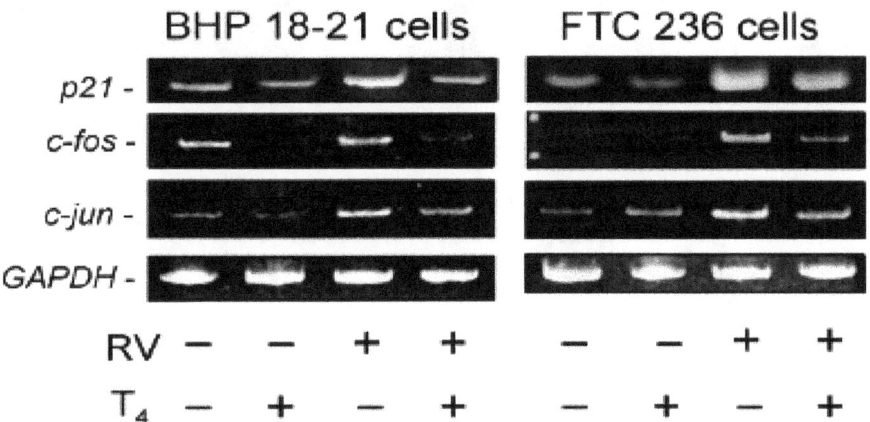

Figure 3. Effects of T4 on mRNA abundance (RT-PCR) of pro-apoptotic *p21*, *c-fos*, and *c-jun* in human differentiated papillary (BHP 18-2) and follicular (FTC 236) thyroid carcinoma cells. Cells were treated in vitro for 24 h with resveratrol (RV) (10 μM) or T4 (10^{-7} M total hormone concentration, 10^{-10} M free hormone) or with both agents. T4 inhibited the expression of RV-induced pro-apoptotic genes and did not affect control *GAPDH* gene. *GAPDH*, glyceraldehyde 3-phosphate dehydrogenase. Reprinted with permission from Elsevier from Lin et al. [16].

Poorly differentiated or anaplastic thyroid carcinoma cells were not studied by Lin et al. in terms of possible responsiveness to T4.

3. Gene Expression in Thyroid Cancer Cells Exposed to Leptin

In the clinical setting of overweight, adipose tissue is expected to secrete leptin protein [27,28]. An endogenous anti-appetite factor, leptin has also been shown to support the growth of certain tumors, including papillary thyroid carcinoma, that express the leptin receptor [4]. There are a variety of other observations that link leptin and thyroid hormone together at cancer cells. Thyroid hormone may increase adipocyte secretion of leptin [29], and circulating leptin levels may be increased in papillary thyroid cancer patients [30]. Leptin variably modulates iodide uptake by thyroid cells [31]. Migration in vitro of papillary thyroid carcinoma cells is increased by leptin [32]. Finally, stimulation of epithelial-to-mesenchymal transition (EMT) is obtained with leptin [33] and with thyroid hormone [34], suggesting that both factors may support cancer metastasis.

Lin and co-workers have identified certain genes whose transcription is modulated in papillary thyroid carcinoma cells by leptin (Figure 4) [5]. Leptin and its derivative, OB3, both significantly reduce abundance of MMP9 mRNA in follicular thyroid cancer cells (Figure 4B), but do not affect expression of *MMP9* in papillary thyroid carcinoma cells (Figure 4A). In the latter cells, however, OB3 and leptin both reduce cell proliferation. Thus, leptin has thyroid cancer-type-specific actions on gene transcription. Such observations raise the possibility that body mass index with changes in endogenous leptin production may be associated with different clinical behaviors of papillary vs. follicular thyroid carcinomas.

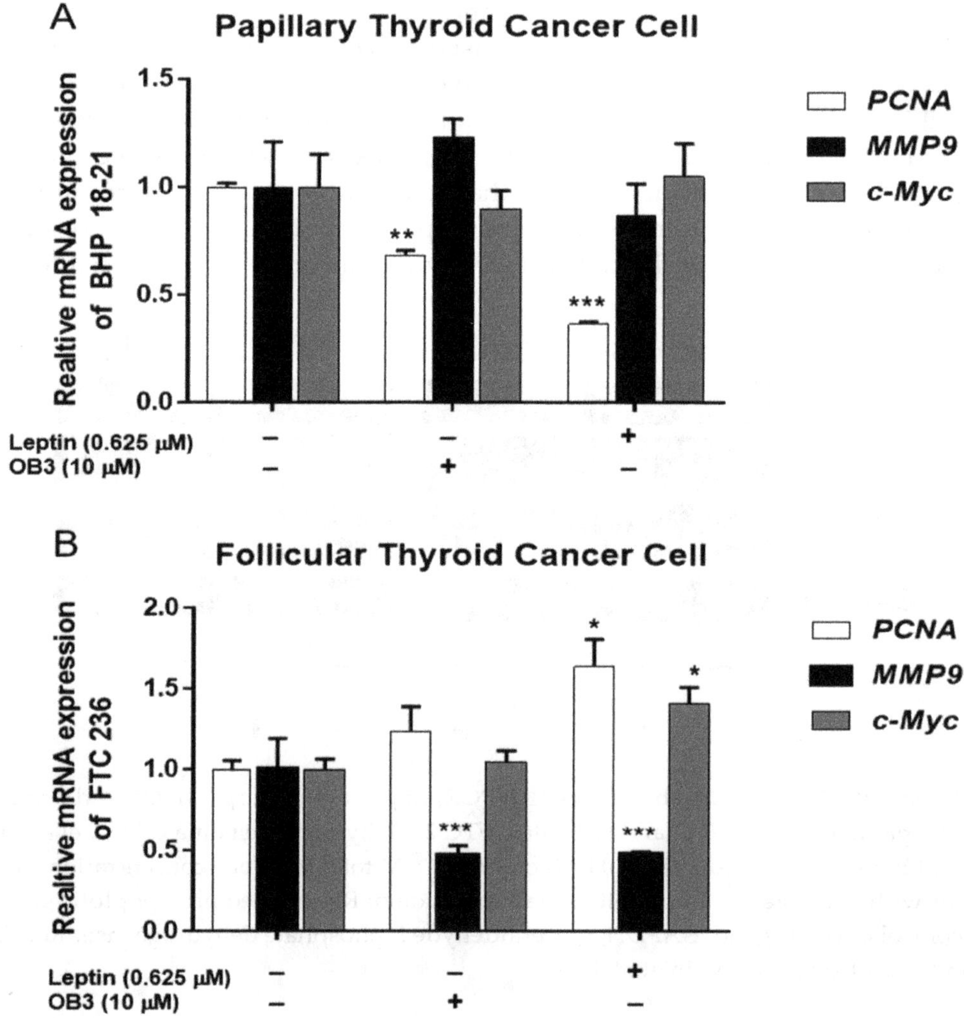

Figure 4. Effect of OB3 and leptin peptides on expression of genes relevant to invasion and cell proliferation in thyroid cancer cell lines. (**A**) Papillary and (**B**) follicular thyroid cancer cells were treated with either 0.625 μM leptin or 10 μM OB3 for 24 h. Cells were harvested, and total RNA was extracted. qPCR for *PCNA, MMP9* and *c-Myc* was conducted as described in Yang et al. [5]. Data were expressed as mean ± S.D. in triplicate. * $p < 0.05$, ** $p < 0.01$, *** $p < 0.001$, were compared with control.

4. Actions of Thyroid Hormone Analogues on Cells of Medullary Thyroid Carcinoma (MTC)

Medullary carcinoma originates in thyroid gland C cells, is thus distinct from papillary and follicular thyroid cancers and is an aggressive, non-TSH-dependent form of thyroid cancer. MTC may occur sporadically or conjunctively as a component of genetic multiple endocrine adenomatosis type 2 [35].

Gene expression that is subject to regulation in MTC cells by certain thyroid hormone analogues has been studied by Yalcin and co-workers [36]. In these studies, tetrac was the thyroid hormone analogue used to probe for thyroid hormone sensitivity of gene expression. Because tetrac, in various non-thyroidal cancer cells studied to-date, is anti-proliferative, pro-apoptotic, and anti-angiogenic [8,37]—the antithesis of T4 [19,21–24,38]—several implications of tetrac studies are clear. First, when it may be studied in the same cells, T4 is likely to have effects that are the direct opposite of tetrac and chemically modified tetrac. Tetrac is an antagonist of T4 at the integrin. Second, the panel of tetrac effects conveys the prospect of effectiveness as an anticancer agent. Third, the effects downstream on a) signal transduction and b) consequent gene expression of the αvβ3 thyroid hormone receptor are extensive.

Acting on MCT cells grafted into the chick chorioallantoic membrane (CAM) model system, tetrac or tetrac analogues reduced tumor weight and tumor hemoglobin content—an index of angiogenesis—by more than 60% at 3 weeks [36]. This anti-angiogenic effect was then studied with q-PCR and RNA microarray in cultured MTC cells. Here, tetrac or a formulation of tetrac downregulated expression of vascular endothelial growth factor A (VEGFA) and upregulated anti-angiogenic thrombospondin 1 (*THSB1*) genes. The tumor shrinkage in the CAM studies reflected anti-angiogenesis, but in addition pro-apoptosis gene expression was observed. For example, significant increases in transcription of *DFFA*, *FAF1* and *CASP2* were induced by tetrac molecules. Thus, thyroid hormone analogues have access to control mechanisms via αvβ3 for MCT angiogenesis- and apoptosis-relevant gene expression. Because tetrac is a specific inhibitor of the actions of T4 at integrin αvβ3, we propose that T4 has actions in MCT cells that are anti-apoptotic, as has been shown to be the case in papillary and follicular thyroid cancer cells.

5. Discussion

Clinical activity of the various forms of thyroid carcinoma is largely a function of specific gene mutations and epigenetic changes that are the subjects of other papers in this issue of the journal. Endogenous TSH may be a trophic factor, particularly in differentiated thyroid cancers and, as pointed out above and elsewhere in this symposium, pharmacologic administration of T4 to suppress host pituitary TSH production may be therapeutically helpful. When differentiated thyroid carcinomas recur in the context of T4-conditioned suppression of TSH, we have suggested that the tumors are no longer TSH-dependent and, in fact, may be T4-dependent [3]. This possibility has not been systematically examined.

T4 is a growth factor for human carcinomas, including thyroid cancers, and a number of studies have concluded that a receptor for thyroid hormone analogues is involved on the extracellular domain of cancer cell integrin αvβ3 [8,37,39,40]. Transduction of the T4 or other thyroid hormone analogue signal at the integrin results in the downstream modulation of transcription of a number of genes in a variety of cancers [8,37]. These genes are relevant to cancer cell division, to apoptosis, to invasiveness, and to tumor-relevant angiogenesis in a large panel of carcinomas of various organs. We have reviewed here the evidence for the trophic action of T4 on various forms of thyroid cancer. It is clear, however, that additional investigation is needed to confirm the extent of such action of T4. It is also of some importance to deal with the possibility that thyroid hormone analogues may act via integrin αvβ3 to alter thyroid tumor radiosensitivity as they have been shown to do in other forms of cancers [41,42]. Also needed are studies that assess the possibility of effects of T4 on anaplastic thyroid carcinomas.

When differentiated thyroid carcinomas remain clinically active, despite full suppression of host TSH, we would suggest the possibility that the tumor is now T4-responsive [3]. A therapeutic option in this setting is induction of euthyroid hypothyroxinemia that we have tested clinically in a variety of advanced, T4-responsive (non-thyroid) cancers [43]. The limited genetic data we have reviewed in the current paper indicates a need for comparing genotypic information from differentiated, but now aggressive, thyroid cancers that (1) are and are not TSH-responsive and (2) are and are not T4-responsive in vitro. Genotyping of aspiration biopsies might then be useful in considering interruption of T4-suppression of TSH.

We have noted above that rT3—another thyroid hormone analogue thought to have little or no biological activity—is capable of stimulating cancer cell proliferation [11]. This proliferative effect has not yet been sought experimentally in differentiated thyroid carcinoma. However, the Type 3 deiodinase that generates rT3 from T4 [44] is present in papillary thyroid carcinoma cells [45].

Finally, we have also pointed out in the current review that leptin may be a trophic factor for papillary thyroid carcinoma, a form of cancer known to express the leptin receptor [5]. These interesting preclinical studies are of potential relevance to suboptimal clinical response of well-differentiated papillary thyroid cancer to TSH suppression in overweight patients. The genes whose expression was affected by leptin include those linked to angiogenesis and invasiveness.

Author Contributions: Conceptualization, P.J.D.; writing—original draft preparation, P.J.D.; writing—review and editing, P.J.D., H.-Y.L., A.H., and S.A.M. All authors have read and agreed to the published version of the manuscript.

Acknowledgments: We thank Kelly A. Keating of the Pharmaceutical Research Institute for editing the manuscript and for constructing Figure 1.

References

1. Xing, M. Molecular pathogenesis and mechanisms of thyroid cancer. *Nat. Rev. Cancer* **2013**, *13*, 184–199. [CrossRef] [PubMed]
2. Roth, M.Y.; Witt, R.L.; Steward, D.L. Molecular testing for thyroid nodules: Review and current state. *Cancer* **2018**, *124*, 888–898. [CrossRef] [PubMed]
3. Davis, P.J.; Hercbergs, A.; Luidens, M.K.; Lin, H.Y. Recurrence of differentiated thyroid carcinoma during full tsh suppression: Is the tumor now thyroid hormone dependent? *Horm. Cancer* **2015**, *6*, 7–12. [CrossRef] [PubMed]
4. Celano, M.; Maggisano, V.; Lepore, S.M.; Sponziello, M.; Pecce, V.; Verrienti, A.; Durante, C.; Maranghi, M.; Lucia, P.; Bulotta, S.; et al. Expression of leptin receptor and effects of leptin on papillary thyroid carcinoma cells. *Int. J. Endocrinol.* **2019**, *2019*, 5031696. [CrossRef] [PubMed]
5. Yang, Y.C.; Chin, Y.T.; Hsieh, M.T.; Lai, H.Y.; Ke, C.C.; Crawford, D.R.; Lee, O.K.; Fu, E.; Mousa, S.A.; Grasso, P.; et al. Novel leptin OB3 peptide-induced signaling and progression in thyroid cancers: Comparison with leptin. *Oncotarget* **2016**, *7*, 27641–27654. [CrossRef]
6. Cheng, S.Y.; Leonard, J.L.; Davis, P.J. Molecular aspects of thyroid hormone actions. *Endocr. Rev.* **2010**, *31*, 139–170. [CrossRef]
7. Brent, G.A. Mechanisms of thyroid hormone action. *J. Clin. Investig.* **2012**, *122*, 3035–3043. [CrossRef]
8. Davis, P.J.; Goglia, F.; Leonard, J.L. Nongenomic actions of thyroid hormone. *Nat. Rev. Endocrinol.* **2016**, *12*, 111–121. [CrossRef]
9. Mousa, S.A.; Glinsky, G.V.; Lin, H.Y.; Ashur-Fabian, O.; Hercbergs, A.; Keating, K.A.; Davis, P.J. Contributions of thyroid hormone to cancer metastasis. *Biomedicines* **2018**, *6*, 89. [CrossRef]
10. Leonard, J.L.; Farwell, A.P. Thyroid hormone-regulated actin polymerization in brain. *Thyroid* **1997**, *7*, 147–151. [CrossRef]
11. Lin, H.Y.; Tang, H.Y.; Leinung, M.; Mousa, S.A.; Hercbergs, A.; Davis, P.J. Action of reverse T3 on cancer cells. *Endocr. Res.* **2019**, *44*, 148–152. [CrossRef] [PubMed]
12. Davis, P.J.; Mousa, S.A.; Cody, V.; Tang, H.Y.; Lin, H.Y. Small molecule hormone or hormone-like ligands of integrin $\alpha V\beta 3$: Implications for cancer cell behavior. *Horm. Cancer* **2013**, *4*, 335–342. [CrossRef]
13. Cabanillas, M.E.; McFadden, D.G.; Durante, C. Thyroid cancer. *Lancet* **2016**, *388*, 2783–2795. [CrossRef]
14. Haugen, B.R.; Alexander, E.K.; Bible, K.C.; Doherty, G.M.; Mandel, S.J.; Nikiforov, Y.E.; Pacini, F.; Randolph, G.W.; Sawka, A.M.; Schlumberger, M.; et al. 2015 American Thyroid Association management guidelines for adult patients with thyroid nodules and differentiated thyroid cancer: The American Thyroid

Association Guidelines Task Force on Thyroid Nodules and Differentiated Thyroid Cancer. *Thyroid* **2016**, *26*, 1–133. [CrossRef]

15. Schmidbauer, B.; Menhart, K.; Hellwig, D.; Grosse, J. Differentiated thyroid cancer-treatment: State of the art. *Int. J. Mol. Sci.* **2017**, *18*, 1292. [CrossRef]
16. Lin, H.Y.; Tang, H.Y.; Shih, A.; Keating, T.; Cao, G.; Davis, P.J.; Davis, F.B. Thyroid hormone is a MAPK-dependent growth factor for thyroid cancer cells and is anti-apoptotic. *Steroids* **2007**, *72*, 180–187. [CrossRef]
17. Bergh, J.J.; Lin, H.Y.; Lansing, L.; Mohamed, S.N.; Davis, F.B.; Mousa, S.; Davis, P.J. Integrin αVβ3 contains a cell surface receptor site for thyroid hormone that is linked to activation of mitogen-activated protein kinase and induction of angiogenesis. *Endocrinology* **2005**, *146*, 2864–2871. [CrossRef]
18. Davis, P.J.; Shih, A.; Lin, H.Y.; Martino, L.J.; Davis, F.B. Thyroxine promotes association of mitogen-activated protein kinase and nuclear thyroid hormone receptor (TR) and causes serine phosphorylation of TR. *J. Biol. Chem.* **2000**, *275*, 38032–38039. [CrossRef]
19. Chen, Y.R.; Chen, Y.S.; Chin, Y.T.; Li, Z.L.; Shih, Y.J.; Yang, Y.S.H.; ChangOu, C.A.; Su, P.Y.; Wang, S.H.; Wu, Y.H.; et al. Thyroid hormone-induced expression of inflammatory cytokines interfere with resveratrol-induced anti-proliferation of oral cancer cells. *Food Chem. Toxicol.* **2019**, *132*, 110693. [CrossRef]
20. Hercbergs, A.; Mousa, S.A.; Leinung, M.; Lin, H.Y.; Davis, P.J. Thyroid hormone in the clinic and breast cancer. *Horm. Cancer* **2018**, *9*, 139–143. [CrossRef] [PubMed]
21. Lee, Y.S.; Chin, Y.T.; Shih, Y.J.; Nana, A.W.; Chen, Y.R.; Wu, H.C.; Yang, Y.S.H.; Lin, H.Y.; Davis, P.J. Thyroid hormone promotes β-catenin activation and cell proliferation in colorectal cancer. *Horm. Cancer* **2018**, *9*, 156–165. [CrossRef] [PubMed]
22. Shinderman-Maman, E.; Cohen, K.; Weingarten, C.; Nabriski, D.; Twito, O.; Baraf, L.; Hercbergs, A.; Davis, P.J.; Werner, H.; Ellis, M.; et al. The thyroid hormone-avb3 integrin axis in ovarian cancer: Regulation of gene transcription and MAPK-dependent proliferation. *Oncogene* **2016**, *35*, 1977–1987. [CrossRef] [PubMed]
23. Cohen, K.; Ellis, M.; Khoury, S.; Davis, P.J.; Hercbergs, A.; Ashur-Fabian, O. Thyroid hormone is a MAPK-dependent growth factor for human myeloma cells acting via αvβ3 integrin. *Mol. Cancer Res.* **2011**, *9*, 1385–1394. [CrossRef]
24. Davis, F.B.; Tang, H.Y.; Shih, A.; Keating, T.; Lansing, L.; Hercbergs, A.; Fenstermaker, R.A.; Mousa, A.; Mousa, S.A.; Davis, P.J.; et al. Acting via a cell surface receptor, thyroid hormone is a growth factor for glioma cells. *Cancer Res.* **2006**, *66*, 7270–7275. [CrossRef]
25. Lin, H.Y.; Chin, Y.T.; Nana, A.W.; Shih, Y.J.; Lai, H.Y.; Tang, H.Y.; Leinung, M.; Mousa, S.A.; Davis, P.J. Actions of L-thyroxine and nano-diamino-tetrac (Nanotetrac) on PD-L1 in cancer cells. *Steroids* **2016**, *114*, 59–67. [CrossRef]
26. Shih, A.; Davis, F.B.; Lin, H.Y.; Davis, P.J. Resveratrol induces apoptosis in thyroid cancer cell lines via a MAPK- and p53-dependent mechanism. *J. Clin. Endocrinol. Metab.* **2002**, *87*, 1223–1232. [CrossRef]
27. Zhang, Y.; Chua, S., Jr. Leptin function and regulation. *Compr. Physiol.* **2017**, *8*, 351–369.
28. Klok, M.D.; Jakobsdottir, S.; Drent, M.L. The role of leptin and ghrelin in the regulation of food intake and body weight in humans: A review. *Obes. Rev.* **2007**, *8*, 21–34. [CrossRef]
29. Yoshida, T.; Monkawa, T.; Hayashi, M.; Saruta, T. Regulation of expression of leptin mRNA and secretion of leptin by thyroid hormone in 3T3-L1 adipocytes. *Biochem. Biophys. Res. Commun.* **1997**, *232*, 822–826. [CrossRef]
30. Hedayati, M.; Yaghmaei, P.; Pooyamanesh, Z.; Zarif Yeganeh, M.; Hoghooghi Rad, L. Leptin: A correlated peptide to papillary thyroid carcinoma? *J. Thyroid Res.* **2011**, *2011*, 832163. [CrossRef]
31. de Oliveira, E.; Teixeira Silva Fagundes, A.; Teixeira Bonomo, I.; Curty, F.H.; Fonseca Passos, M.C.; de Moura, E.G.; Lisboa, P.C. Acute and chronic leptin effect upon in vivo and in vitro rat thyroid iodide uptake. *Life Sci.* **2007**, *81*, 1241–1246. [CrossRef]
32. Cheng, S.P.; Yin, P.H.; Chang, Y.C.; Lee, C.H.; Huang, S.Y.; Chi, C.W. Differential roles of leptin in regulating cell migration in thyroid cancer cells. *Oncol. Rep.* **2010**, *23*, 1721–1727. [PubMed]
33. Peng, C.; Sun, Z.; Li, O.; Guo, C.; Yi, W.; Tan, Z.; Jiang, B. Leptin stimulates the epithelialmesenchymal transition and proangiogenic capability of cholangiocarcinoma cells through the miR122/PKM2 axis. *Int. J. Oncol.* **2019**, *55*, 298–308. [PubMed]

34. Weingarten, C.; Jenudi, Y.; Tshuva, R.Y.; Moskovich, D.; Alfandari, A.; Hercbergs, A.; Davis, P.J.; Ellis, M.; Ashur-Fabian, O. The interplay between epithelial-mesenchymal transition (EMT) and the thyroid hormones-αvβ3 axis in ovarian cancer. *Horm. Cancer* **2018**, *9*, 22–32. [CrossRef]
35. Raue, F.; Frank-Raue, K. Multiple endocrine neoplasia type 2: 2007 update. *Horm. Res.* **2007**, *68*, 101–104. [CrossRef]
36. Yalcin, M.; Dyskin, E.; Lansing, L.; Bharali, D.J.; Mousa, S.S.; Bridoux, A.; Hercbergs, A.H.; Lin, H.Y.; Davis, F.B.; Glinsky, G.V.; et al. Tetraiodothyroacetic acid (tetrac) and nanoparticulate tetrac arrest growth of medullary carcinoma of the thyroid. *J. Clin. Endocrinol. Metab.* **2010**, *95*, 1972–1980. [CrossRef]
37. Davis, P.J.; Glinsky, G.V.; Lin, H.Y.; Leith, J.T.; Hercbergs, A.; Tang, H.Y.; Ashur-Fabian, O.; Incerpi, S.; Mousa, S.A. Cancer cell gene expression modulated from plasma membrane integrin αvβ3 by thyroid hormone and nanoparticulate tetrac. *Front. Endocrinol. (Lausanne)* **2014**, *5*, 240.
38. Meng, R.; Tang, H.Y.; Westfall, J.; London, D.; Cao, J.H.; Mousa, S.A.; Luidens, M.; Hercbergs, A.; Davis, F.B.; Davis, P.J.; et al. Crosstalk between integrin αvβ3 and estrogen receptor-α is involved in thyroid hormone-induced proliferation in human lung carcinoma cells. *PLoS ONE* **2011**, *6*, e27547. [CrossRef]
39. Latteyer, S.; Christoph, S.; Theurer, S.; Hones, G.S.; Schmid, K.W.; Fuhrer, D.; Moeller, L.C. Thyroxine promotes lung cancer growth in an orthotopic mouse model. *Endocr. Relat. Cancer* **2019**, *26*, 565–574. [CrossRef]
40. Cayrol, F.; Sterle, H.A.; Díaz Flaqué, M.C.; Barreiro Arcos, M.L.; Cremaschi, G.A. Non-genomic actions of thyroid hormones regulate the growth and angiogenesis of T cell lymphomas. *Front. Endocrinol.* **2019**, *10*, 63. [CrossRef]
41. Leith, J.T.; Mousa, S.A.; Hercbergs, A.; Lin, H.Y.; Davis, P.J. Radioresistance of cancer cells, integrin αvβ3 and thyroid hormone. *Oncotarget* **2018**, *9*, 37069–37075. [CrossRef] [PubMed]
42. Leith, J.T.; Hercbergs, A.; Kenney, S.; Mousa, S.A.; Davis, P.J. Activation of tumor cell integrin αvβ3 by radiation and reversal of activation by chemically modified tetraiodothyroacetic acid (tetrac). *Endocr. Res.* **2018**, *43*, 215–219. [CrossRef] [PubMed]
43. Hercbergs, A.; Johnson, R.E.; Ashur-Fabian, O.; Garfield, D.H.; Davis, P.J. Medically induced euthyroid hypothyroxinemia may extend survival in compassionate need cancer patients: An observational study. *Oncologist* **2015**, *20*, 72–76. [CrossRef] [PubMed]
44. Sibilio, A.; Ambrosio, R.; Bonelli, C.; De Stefano, M.A.; Torre, V.; Dentice, M.; Salvatore, D. Deiodination in cancer growth: The role of type III deiodinase. *Minerva Endocrinol.* **2012**, *37*, 315–327.
45. Romitti, M.; Wajner, S.M.; Ceolin, L.; Ferreira, C.V.; Ribeiro, R.V.; Rohenkohl, H.C.; Weber Sde, S.; Lopez, P.L.; Fuziwara, C.S.; Kimura, E.T.; et al. MAPK and SHH pathways modulate type 3 deiodinase expression in papillary thyroid carcinoma. *Endocr. Relat. Cancer* **2016**, *23*, 135–146. [CrossRef]

5

Molecular Signature of Indeterminate Thyroid Lesions: Current Methods to Improve Fine Needle Aspiration Cytology (FNAC) Diagnosis

Silvia Cantara *, Carlotta Marzocchi, Tania Pilli, Sandro Cardinale, Raffaella Forleo, Maria Grazia Castagna and Furio Pacini

Department of Medical, Surgical and Neurological Sciences, University of Siena, 53100 Siena, Italy; carlottamarzocchi@libero.it (C.M.); t.pilli.e@ao-siena.toscana.it (T.P.); sandro.cardinale@gmail.com (S.C.); forleo.r@gmail.com (R.F.); m.g.castagna@ao-siena.toscana.it (M.G.C.); furio.pacini@unisi.it (F.P.)

* Correspondence: cantara@unisi.it

Academic Editor: Daniela Gabriele Grimm

Abstract: Fine needle aspiration cytology (FNAC) represents the gold standard for determining the nature of thyroid nodules. It is a reliable method with good sensitivity and specificity. However, indeterminate lesions remain a diagnostic challenge and researchers have contributed molecular markers to search for in cytological material to refine FNAC diagnosis and avoid unnecessary surgeries. Nowadays, several "home-made" methods as well as commercial tests are available to investigate the molecular signature of an aspirate. Moreover, other markers (i.e., microRNA, and circulating tumor cells) have been proposed to discriminate benign from malignant thyroid lesions. Here, we review the literature and provide data from our laboratory on mutational analysis of FNAC material and circulating microRNA expression obtained in the last 6 years.

Keywords: fine needle aspiration cytology (FNAC); indeterminate lesions; next generation sequencing; gene expression classifier; microRNAs (miRNAs)

---

1. Thyroid Nodules

In countries where iodine deficiency has been corrected by iodine prophylaxis, thyroid nodules are found in approximately 4–7% of the population [1]. However, in countries affected by moderate or severe iodine deficiency, the prevalence is even greater [2]. Subclinical nodules, detected by thyroid ultrasound, are found in over 50% of women older than 60 years, a number similar to that reported in autopsy series.

Any type of nodule may be found as a single lump in an otherwise normal thyroid gland or in the context of a multinodular goitre. Regardless of the presentation, the large majority are benign hyperplastic nodules, frequently an expression of underlying nodular goitre or autoimmune thyroiditis. Thyroid cancer is found in less than 10% of hypo-functioning nodules that are solid or mixed on thyroid ultrasound (US) and more than 80% of them are differentiated thyroid cancer of the follicular epithelium.

Surgical treatment of thyroid nodules without selection would expose millions of people annually to surgery. Since only a small proportion of these nodules finally result malignant at histology, this approach would imply a tremendous number of unnecessary surgeries and high financial costs. Thyroid nodules must therefore undergo rigorous selection based on a rational diagnostic protocol.

2. Diagnostic Evaluation of Thyroid Nodules: Fine-Needle Aspiration Cytology (FNAC)

The ultimate objective of the diagnostic protocol is to differentiate between benign and malignant nodules. Nowadays, the problem has largely been solved by fine-needle aspirate cytology. In expert hands, FNAC has an overall accuracy of 95%. The sensitivity is between 43% and 98% and the specificity is between 72% and 100%, with positive and negative predictive values of 89–98% and 94–99%, respectively [3]. False positive and false negative results are between 1–11% and 0–7%, respectively.

The Bethesda Classification System [4], a six diagnostic category system, is at present the most widespread reporting system for thyroid fine needle aspiration (FNA) cytology. The categories are: (I) non-diagnostic/unsatisfactory; (II) benign; (III) atypia of undetermined significance/follicular lesion of undetermined significance (AUS/FLUS); (IV) follicular neoplasm/suspicious for follicular neoplasm (FN); (V) suspicious for malignancy (SUSP) and (VI) malignant.

Category I refers to samples where inadequate or insufficient material is present for a diagnosis or the interpretation is precluded by technical artefacts. In different series, the rate of inadequate cytologies varies between 15% and 20% and in these cases it is recommended to repeat the procedure after some weeks or months [5–8]. Around 70% (range 53–90%) of aspirates are classified as category II, meaning that the features are consistent with a nodular goitre or thyroiditis. Meanwhile 4% (1–10%) are classified as category VI when unequivocal features of papillary, medullary or anaplastic carcinoma or lymphoma are present, and 10% (5–23%) are classified as category V. A particular issue is represented by category III and IV, representing nearly 20% of FNACs. In this case, the aspirate is represented by a monotonous population of follicular cells arranged on cohesive groups, whose cellular and nuclear features are similar whether the nodule is benign or malignant. The distinction is based on the presence of vascular and capsular invasion, which is detectable only at histology. In a meta-analysis of 25,445 thyroid FNAC [4] cases reported from eight studies using the Bethesda System, 9.6% of all samples were diagnosed as AUS/FLUS (category III) and 10.1% were diagnosed as follicular neoplasm/suspicious for follicular neoplasm (FN/SFN) (category IV) with an average cancer risk at final histology of 15.9% and 26.1%, respectively. It is evident that, both the AUS/FLUS and FN/SFN have a cancer risk that cannot be ignored. However, at final histology, only about 25% of the lesions result malignant, so the risk of cancer is not high enough to definitely support surgery as treatment of all indeterminate lesions.

3. Protein-Based Assays to Increase FNAC Performance

To avoid unnecessary surgeries and to increase FNAC performance especially for Categories III and IV, several markers have been proposed in the past years. Among those studied by immunocytochemistry, galectin-3 is one of the most reliable. Galectins are carbohydrate-binding proteins that are members of the β-galactoside binding lectin family. Galectin-3, (Gal-3) appears to be necessary for the maintenance of transformed thyroid papillary cancer (PTC) cell lines in vitro [9]. The use of Gal-3 in the detection of thyroid malignancy in indeterminate or suspicious FNA has a sensitivity that ranges from 20% to 100% and a specificity ranging from 62% to 100% [10–17]. In case of indeterminate FNAC with a positive staining for Gal-3, surgery is strongly recommended, however no specific suggestions can be made in case of Gal-3 negative staining [14]. Similar results have been described with the Hector Battiflora Mesothelial-1 (HBME-1), a monoclonal antibody developed against the microvillous surface of mesothelial cells, which has shown a sensitivity of 79–87% and a specificity of 83–96% [12,13,18–20] in Bethesda categories III and IV. Another proposed marker is CD44v6, a polymorphic family of immunologically related cell-surface glycoproteins, which have a functional role in regulating cell–cell and cell–matrix interactions, cell migration, tumor growth and progression [21–24]. The combined use of CD44v6 and Galectin-3 in indeterminate lesions showed 88% sensitivity, 98% specificity with a positive predictive value (PPV) of 91%, and a diagnostic accuracy of 97% [15].

Although the usage of different markers has been tested to improve the diagnostic efficacy in FNAC, so far none of the tested molecules has provided sufficient sensitivity and specificity to advocate its use in routine practice (not recommended by the America Thyroid Association (ATA).

4. Use of Molecular Markers in the Differential Diagnosis of Thyroid Nodules

The discovery of genetic alterations specific for differentiated thyroid cancer have provided molecular markers to be searched for in the material obtained by FNA, thus increasing the diagnostic accuracy of traditional cytology. The need to search for genetic alterations in FNAC sample should be considered especially for Bethesda categories III and IV. However, the revised guidelines for the management of thyroid cancer published by ATA in 2015 [25] do not provide strong recommendation in support of the use of molecular markers to help the management of patients with indeterminate cytology.

The most frequent genetic alterations detected in papillary and follicular thyroid carcinoma (PTC and FTC, respectively) are B-Raf proto-oncogene, serine/threonine kinase (BRAF), rat sarcoma (N-H-KRAS) point mutations, and REarranged during Transfection proto-oncogene (RET)/PTC, and Paired box 8/Peroxisome proliferator activated receptor gamma (PAX8/PPARγ) rearrangements [26,27]. Telomerase reverse transcriptase (TERT) promoter and Tumor protein 53 (TP53) mutations are more frequent in less differentiated carcinomas [28–30]. Nowadays, there are three diffuse approaches to investigating the molecular profile of FNA: (1) the seven genes panel; (2) the Afirma classifier and (3) next generation sequencing (NGS) assays.

4.1. Seven Genes Mutational Panel

The first study analyzing the contribution of molecular testing to thyroid fine-needle aspiration cytology was published in 2010 [31]. In this work, the authors considered BRAF and RAS gene mutations, as well as RET/PTC, and PAX8/PPAR-γ gene rearrangements in 117 indeterminate cytologies. Among these, 35 (29.9%) cases had a neoplastic outcome and 20 (17.1%) cases were found to be carcinoma. Positive molecular results were found in 12 cases, all of which were PTC. The authors found that the cancer probability for AUS/FLUS and FN/SFN with molecular alteration was 100%, while the probability for AUS/FLUS and FN/SFN without molecular alteration was 7.6%.

In the same year, another study [32] analyzed 174 consecutive FNAC (all categories) for BRAF, RAS, RET, TRK, and PPAR-γ alterations. Mutations were found in 67/235 (28.5%) cytological samples. Of the 67 mutated samples, 23 (34.3%) were mutated by RAS, 33 (49.3%) by BRAF, and 11 (16.4%) by RET/PTC. The presence of mutations at cytology was associated with cancer in 91.1% of the cases and with follicular adenoma in 8.9% of the time. The accuracy of molecular analysis was 90.2%, with a sensitivity of 78.2%, specificity of 96.2%, PPV of 91% and negative predictive value (NPV) of 89.9%. Considering only categories III and IV (n = 41), the authors found that 7/41 (17%) samples were mutated (2 BRAF, 2 RET-PTC, 3 RAS). At final histology, all but one (follicular adenoma) were PTC. Of the 34 samples with no mutation, 33 were benign lesions and only one was PTC. Specificity was 97%, sensitivity was 85% and accuracy 95%.

The most complete work aimed to disclose the clinical utility of molecular testing of thyroid FNA samples with indeterminate cytology was published in 2011 [33]. Nikiforov and co-workers analyzed the presence of BRAF, N-H and K-RAS point mutations and RET/PTC1-3, PAX8/PPARγ rearrangements in 1056 consecutive thyroid FNA samples with indeterminate cytology. In 967/1056 (92%) cytologies, the material was adequate for molecular analysis. They found 87 mutations including 62 RAS (71.3%), 19 BRAF (21.8%), 1 RET/PTC (1.1%) and 5 PAX8/PPARγ rearrangements (5.8%). In the AUS/FLUS category, sensitivity was 63%, specificity 99%, PPV 88%, NPV 94% and accuracy 94%. For the FN/SFN group, sensitivity was 57%, specificity 97%, PPV 87%, NPV 86% and accuracy 86%. In AUS/FLUS, FN/SFN categories the detection of any mutation conferred the risk of histological malignancy of 88 and 87%, respectively. The risk of cancer in mutation-negative nodules was 6%, 14%, and 28%, respectively.

In conclusion, mutation panels intended to identify malignancies in indeterminate lesions must include at least BRAF and RAS point mutations (H, K and NRAS), and RET/PTC, PAX8/PPAR-γ rearrangements. Several "homemade" methods comprising PCR with final Sanger sequencing and some commercial kits are available to screen for these alterations with the limitation that they cannot rule out malignancy with a NPV > 95%.

Since the publication of our previous work [32], we applied molecular testing in clinical routine, especially for FNAC categories III and IV. We collected 197 consecutive indeterminate samples and searched for BRAF, RAS (H, K and NRAS), and TERT point mutations, and RET/PTC1-3 and PAX8/PPAR-γ rearrangements. End point PCR, real time PCR, denaturing high performance liquid chromatography (DHPLC) and direct sequencing were used for the analysis [32]. The exam was performed on 176/197 (89.4%) of the sample as in 21/197 (10.6%) the collected material was inadequate for the investigation. We found 17 mutations (9.6%) including 3 BRAF, 2 HRAS, 5 NRAS, 1 KRAS and 6 RET/PTCs. These 17 patients were subjected to surgery and 15/17 (88.2%) were confirmed malignant at final histology (3 FTC, 5 PTC and 7 follicular variant PTC) whereas 2/17 (11.7%) were follicular adenoma (1 NRAS and 1 RET/PTC). Among the 159 nodules negative for mutations, 23 underwent surgery for other reasons (i.e., ultrasound characteristics, patient's decision, increased nodule size over time) and 21/23 (91.3%) were confirmed benign lesions at histology whereas 2/23 (8.6%) were malignant (2 microcarcinomas). The PPV was 88.2% and the NPV was 91.3%, with an accuracy of 90% (Table 1). One-hundred and thirty-six nodules/176 (77.2%) negative for mutation and not subjected to surgery are still under follow up. In a period of time from 1 up to 6 years, no increase in nodule size or changes in ultrasound features were observed. Twenty-two/136 (16.2%) samples repeated a second FNAC and a category II was found for these lesions confirming the results of molecular test. Despite the encouraging results, the method of the "seven genes" has the limitation that collected material can be inadequate to perform the complete panel, thus increasing the number of false negative results.

Table 1. Results from mutation analysis on indeterminate lesions treated with surgery.

Atypia of Undetermined Significance/Follicular Lesions of Undetermined Significance (AUS/FLUS)			
Follicular neoplasma/suspicious for follicular neoplasma (FN/SFN) (n = 40)			
	Histology Malignant	**Histology Benign**	
Mutation positive (n = 17)	7 RAS (6 FVPTC, 1 FTC) 3 BRAF (3 PTC) 5 RET/PTC (1 FVPTC, 2 PTC, 2 FTC)	1 NRAS (FA) 1 RET/PTC (FA)	Sensitivity 88.2% Specificity 91.3% PPV 88.2% NPV 91.3% Accuracy 90%
Mutation negative (n = 23)	2 microcarcinoma	21 (9 FA, 12 HN)	

PTC = papillary thyroid cancer; FTC = follicular thyroid cancer; FVPTC = follicular variant of PTC; FA = follicular adenoma; HN = hyperplastic nodules; PPV = positive predictive value; NPV = negative predictive value.

4.2. Afirma Classifier

The Afirma test is a gene expression classifier (GEC) [34] which uses the expression of 142 genes to categorize thyroid nodules into benign or suspicious (rule out method). The test was validated in a multi-institutional (for a total of 49 clinical sites) prospective double-blind study funded by industry (Veracyte) in indeterminate nodules [35]. Authors obtained 577 cytologically-indeterminate aspirates, 413 of which had corresponding histopathological specimens from excised lesions. After inclusion criteria were met, only 265 aspirated were allocated to GEC and were included in the final analysis [35]. Of these 265, 85 (32%) were confirmed to be malignant at histology. In the 265 indeterminate cytology nodules, the sensitivity of the Afirma test was 92% (95% confidence interval (CI), 84%, 97%, 78/85) and the specificity was 52% (95% CI, 44%, 59%, 93/180). In another study by same authors [36] on 339 cytologically-indeterminate nodules (165 AUS/FLUS; 161 FN; 13 suspicious for malignancy), 174/339 (51%) were GEC benign and 148/339 (44%) were GEC suspicious. Among GEC-suspicious nodules, 121 were surgically removed and 53 (44%) were malignant, confirming the previous study in terms of sensitivity and specificity. Recent studies, have shown results from the GEC classifier in indeterminate cytologies obtaining high sensitivity but lower specificity compared to previous reports thus stressing the need of additional, independent, non-industry supported studies to establish the performance of the classifier [37–39]. In summary, based on the above studies, Afirma test sensitivity has been reported to range from 83% to 100% and specificity from 7 to 52%, where the prevalence of malignancy in histopathologically confirmed study populations has ranged from 17% to 51% [35,37,38,40].

4.3. Thyroseq and Other NGS Platform

Targeted next generation sequencing (NGS) is a promising method to simultaneously examine multiple genes with high sensitivity potentially achieving not only high PPV but also high negative predictive value (NPV) [41] and with low input of starting material (5 to 10 ng).

ThyroSeq is a NGS-based gene mutation and fusion panel initially designed to target 12 cancer genes with 284 mutational hot spots [41], showing 100% accuracy with a sensitivity of 3–5% of mutant alleles. In the first work reporting data from Thyroseq, the authors analyzed 229 thyroid neoplastic and non-neoplastic samples and found mutation in 70% of PTCs (19/27), 83% of papillary thyroid cancer follicular variant (PTCFV) (25/30), 59% of FTC (21/36), 30% of poorly differentiated thyroid carcinoma (3/10), 74% of anaplastic thyroid cancer (ATC) (20/27) and in 73% of medullary thyroid carcinomas (11/15). The majority of samples were mutated for BRAF and RAS. Other studies confirmed the high PPV of the ThyroSeq (88% and 87% for AUS/FLUS and FN, respectively) [42,43] and indicate that the test could potentially be used as a "rule in" test.

In 2014, results from ThyroSeq v2, an enhanced version of the test, on AUS/FLUS and FN cytologies were published [44]. ThyroSeq v2 allowed the analysis of 14 genes (more than 1000 mutations) and RNA alterations (approximately 42 fusions) reaching a sensitivity and specificity of 90% and 93%, respectively, a PPV of 83%, an NPV of 96%, and accuracy of 92% [44]. These results suggested that ThyroSeq v2 may potentially works as both "rule out" and "rule in" test for nodules with indeterminate cytology. Finally, owing to the limited studies and data from literature, the value of ThyroSeq v2 needs further investigation. Moreover, clinical validation results are not available yet, whereas data for lung and other tumors show that next generation sequencing is as robust as Sanger sequencing in routine diagnostics and, in addition, is able to reveal mutations in low percentage and screen the mutational status of different critical samples offering innovative diagnostic opportunities [45–48]. Furthermore, methodological problems like result interpretation (e.g., for unknown mutations), definition of cut offs for mutation calling, and bioinformatics analysis need to be solved and common standard operation procedures (SOPs) need to be defined. On the matter of bioinformatics analysis, a recent report describes a solution called "SeqReport" [49]. This module automatically imports patient data and related NGS run information and allows comprehensive review of all variants by users linking to both COSMIC and dbSNP databases and manual review of variants. In addition, the program automatically locates variants with low frequency or coverage and compares the status of Sanger sequencing confirmation. In this method, the cut off values are determined for each multigene panel during validation. Human errors are minimized and the creation of clinical report is automatic also with appropriate clinical comments.

Le Mercier and colleagues [50] performed a pilot study with a commercially available NGS-based 50-gene panel kit (Ion AmpliSeq Cancer Hotspot Panel version 2; Thermo Fisher Scientific, Gent, Belgium) to evaluate 34 indeterminate FNA samples. The panel is designed to amplify 207 amplicons covering approximately 2800 COSMIC mutations from 50 oncogenes and tumor suppressor genes. The authors identified cytologies with a "molecular test negative" (including patients carrying germline polymorphisms, mutations of unknown clinical significance, or no mutation) or "molecular test positive" for patients carrying pathogenic mutations reaching a sensitivity and specificity of 71% and 89%, respectively. The PPV and NPV were 63% and 92%, respectively, with an accuracy of 85%.

ThyroSeq v2 actually has shown the best results in terms of sensitivity, specificity, PPV and NPV but further studies including a larger number of cases are required for the Ion AmpliSeq Panel.

5. Role of miRNAs in the Differential Diagnosis of Thyroid Lesions

MicroRNA (miRNAs) are small molecules of RNA (approximately 22 nt), non-encoding for protein which negatively regulate gene expression-targeting specific mRNAs [51]. miRNAs can be detected in plasma and serum as they circulate in the blood in a stable, cell-free form [52]. Furthermore, tumor cells have been shown to release miRNAs into the circulation [52] and profiles of miRNAs in plasma and serum have been found to be altered in cancer and other disease states [53–55]. Larger scale miRNA analysis has proven that miRNA expression enables the distinction of benign tissues from their malignant counterparts [56,57]. The mechanisms of miRNA implication in cancer development are linked to downregulation of tumor suppressor genes or upregulation of oncogenes.

Several studies have demonstrated a different miRNA signature between benign and malignant thyroid tissues [58–65] unfortunately using different detection systems (microarray and/or Quantative RT-PCR (Q-RT-PCR) and producing inconsistent results in terms of selected miRNAs, sensitivity and specificity. However, all authors concluded that a limited set of miRNAs can be used for the differential diagnosis between benign and malignant lesions in the surgical samples with high accuracy, implying the potential role of miRNAs in differentiating the nature of thyroid nodules in FNAC. Again, the most important question is question is whether the analysis of miRNAs in cytological samples can improve FNAC results, particularly for indeterminate lesions [61,66–74]. All the studies which addressed this issue obtained a similar diagnostic odds ratio (mean 20.3) and concluded that a set of multiple miRNAs seems to be more sensitive (sensitivity of 87%) than a single miRNA (sensitivity of 71%) although there is discrepancy in terms of set of miRNA proposed. Pooling together the results from these studies, however, a relative small set of 15 miRNAs emerge as the more powerful diagnostic panel for indeterminate lesions. The panel is composed of miRNA7, -146, -146b, -155, -221, -222, -21, -31, -187, -30a-3p, -30d, -146b-5p, -199b-5p, -328 and miRNA197. Future prospective and retrospective research are recommended on a large cohort of indeterminate lesions to validate the diagnostic value of this panel.

As pointed out previously, FNAC represents the gold standard for the differential diagnosis of thyroid nodules, however it is an invasive technique compared to blood sampling. Thus, the idea is to use miRNAs as a serological marker for thyroid cancer (TC) diagnosis from the moment that TC releases miRNAs into the bloodstream. Three studies addressed this issue [75–77], two of them in the Chinese population [77,78] and only one study in the Caucasian population [77]. Although these studies found different set of miRNAs, the preliminary results are promising for future research showing a good sensitivity (ranging from 61.4 to 94%) and specificity (ranging from 57.9% to 98.7%).

We performed a study on serum miRNA expression (miRNA95 and miRNA190) on 982 consecutive patients undergoing FNAC at our institute. We collected serum from 114/982 (11.6%) subjects with a Bethesda III and IV FNAC result. Seventy-five/114 (65.7%) underwent surgery and at final histology we had 11 follicular adenomas (FA), 32 hyperplastic nodules (HN), 27 PTCs, 4 FTCs and 1 Hurthle cell carcinoma (HC). miRNAs were extracted from 200 μL of serum using the miRNeasy Serum/Plasma Kit (Qiagen, Milan, Italy) and retro-transcribed by miScript II RT Kit (Qiagen). Two μL of cDNA was used as template for real time PCR (RT-PCR) to measure miRNA expression levels with the miScript SYBR Green PCR Kit (Qiagen) with specific primers for miRNA-95 and -190 (Qiagen). RT-PCR was performed in duplicate on the Rotor-gene Q MDx (Qiagen) under the following cycling conditions: 95 °C for 15 min, 40 cycles at 94 °C for 15 s, 55 °C for 30 s and 70 °C for 30 s. Relative expression levels were calculated using the $2^{-\Delta\Delta Ct}$ method with the miRNA-16 as endogenous control. miRNA expression correctly identified 38/43 (specificity of 88.4%) of the benign lesions and 27/32 (sensitivity of 84.3%) of malignant sample. We had 5 false positive (FP) (5 HNs) and 5 false negative (FN) (4 PTCs, 1 FTC) results, obtaining a final accuracy of 86.7% (Table 2). Despite the promising results, molecular analysis on FNAC has a better performance and further studies are required to identify the optimal set of circulating miRNAs specific for indeterminate lesions.

Table 2. Results from microRNA (miRNA) expression analysis on indeterminate lesions treated with surgery.

Histology	miRNA Expression Negative for Malignancy	miRNA Expression Positive for Malignancy	Performance
Benign at histology	38 (11 FA, 27 HN)	5 (5 HN)	Sensitivity 84.3% Specificity 88.4% PPV 88.4% NPV 84.3% Accuracy 86.7%
Malignant at histology	5 (1 FTC, 4 PTC)	27 (23 PTC, 3 FTC, 1 HC)	

PTC = papillary thyroid cancer, FTC = follicular thyroid cancer, FA = follicular adenoma, HN = hyperplastic nodules, HC = Hurtlhe cell carcinoma, PPV = positive predictive value, NPV = negative predictive value.

Serum normally contains low amounts of total RNA, of which miRNAs only constitute 0.4–0.5%. In addition, serum samples may be affected by technical problems, such as hemolysis and it is not known whether circulating serum expression can be influenced by other comorbidities. In this view, the analysis on FNAC may be preferable.

In 2016 two studies [78,79] were published on clinical validation of the RosettaGX Reveal test, a miRNA-based assay which evaluates a set of 24 miRNAs (by real time PCR) specific for cytologically indeterminate thyroid nodules. The assay can be used directly on FNA smears and it is able to categorize benign or suspicious nodules even when as little as 1% of thyroid cells is present or less than 5 ng RNA are extracted. The overall NPV reported was 99%, with sensitivity of 98% and specificity of 78%.

6. Proteomics: An Interesting Alternative Approach to Stratify Thyroid FNAC

Proteomics is the large-scale study of proteins and it is widely used to discover cancer biomarkers. In the field of thyroid cancer, proteomics has been initially applied on thyroid tissue specimens and cancer cell lines [80–89], using different techniques such as surface-enhanced laser desorption/ionization-time-of-flight-mass spectrometry (SELDI-TOF-MS), liquid chromatography–mass spectrometry (LC/MS) and MS alone. All these studies ended by identifying specific protein signatures for malignant and benign lesions with a final selection of clusters of proteins with discriminating abilities. In particular, proteins involved in oxidative stress, metabolic pathways, nuclear stability, turnover of thyroglobulin, and kinase signaling are those more represented in thyroid cancer. Techniques such as matrix-assisted laser desorption/ionization (MALDI)-TOF-MS and MALDI-imaging mass spectrometry (MALDI-IMS) have been applied in several studies [90–95] to cytological thyroid specimens. Most of these studies used ex vivo FNA [90,91,93–95] and one study [94] used pre-surgical FNAC obtaining an overall sensitivity of 87% and specificity of 94% in discriminating benign from suspicious samples, with a good reproducibility among studies. Proteomics could serve to improve the preoperative diagnosis of indeterminate lesions, but some aspects such as the limitation in the availability of these technologies and the lack of uniformity among techniques, need to be addressed before its introduction in clinical practice.

7. Conclusions

In summary, the purpose of thyroid molecular testing is to discriminate the nature of thyroid nodules and reduce the diagnostic uncertainty of cytologically indeterminate lesions prior to surgery. Mutation panels intended to identify malignancies must include at least BRAF, and RAS point mutations as well as RET/PTC, NTRK, and PAX8/PPARγ rearrangements. Several "home-made" methods and some commercial kits are available to screen for these alterations with the limitation that they cannot rule out malignancy with an NPV >95%. GEC recognizes benign lesions on the basis of an expression pattern of mRNA extracted from one or two dedicated FNA needle passes. A negative result in the Afirma test has resulted in a major decrease in the number of surgeries performed in samples classified as Bethesda categories III and IV. However, Afirma shows a low PPV. On the other hand, the risk of malignancy calculated by ThyroSeq or other NGS platforms is superior to that of the Afirma, reaching an NPV of 95% or more, with good sensitivity and high PPV. The identification of new biomarkers (i.e., miRNA, proteomic profiles) in the thyroid needs to be corroborated in larger studies with final histology as a gold standard and adequate follow up before use in the clinical routine [96]. Therefore, molecular testing must be always performed in specialized laboratories and results interpreted within the context of the clinical, radiographic, and cytological findings. In addition, clinicians may take into account that the interpretation of molecular testing and its utility are strongly influenced by the prevalence of cancer in each cytological category [96] which can differ among centers. Due to this aspect, molecular test performance may vary significantly.

Acknowledgments: Italian Ministry of Health RF-2011-02350673.

Author Contributions: Silvia Cantara performed molecular analysis, designed and performed experiments on miRNA and wrote the paper. Carlotta Marzocchi performed experiments on miRNA expression. Tania Pilli and Sandro Cardinale review data on miRNA expression. Raffaella Forleo and Maria Grazia Castagna identified indeterminate lesions for molecular analysis and review the data base with results. Furio Pacini review the manuscript.

References

1. Aschebrook-Kilfoy, B.; Ward, M.H.; Sabra, M.M.; Devesa, S.S. Thyroid cancer incidence patterns in the United States by histologic type, 1992–2006. *Thyroid* **2011**, *21*, 125–134. [CrossRef] [PubMed]
2. Belfiore, A.; La Rosa, G.L.; La Porta, G.A.; Giuffrida, D.; Milazzo, G.; Lupo, L.; Regalbuto, C.; Vigneri, R. Cancer risk in patients with cold thyroid nodules: Relevance of iodine intake, sex, age, and multinodularity. *Am. J. Med.* **1992**, *93*, 363–369. [CrossRef]
3. Gharib, H.; Goellner, J.R.; Johnson, D.A. Fine needle aspiration of the thyroid. A 12 year experience with 11,000 biopsies. *Clin. Lab. Med.* **1993**, *13*, 699–709. [PubMed]
4. Bongiovanni, M.; Spitale, A.; Faquin, W.C.; Mazzucchelli, L.; Baloch, Z.W. The Bethesda System for Reporting Thyroid Cytopathology: A meta-analysis. *Acta Cytol.* **2012**, *56*, 333–339. [CrossRef] [PubMed]
5. Hamming, J.F.; Goslings, B.M.; Van Steenis, G.J.; van Ravenswaay Claasen, H.; Hermans, J.; van de Velde, C.J.H. The value of one-needle aspiration biopsy in patients with nodular thyroid disease divided into groups of suspicion of malignant neoplasms on clinical grounds. *Arch. Intern. Med.* **1990**, *150*, 113–116. [CrossRef] [PubMed]
6. Caruso, D.; Mazzaferri, E.L. Fine-needle aspiration in the management of thyroid nodules. *Endocrinologist* **1991**, *1*, 194–202. [CrossRef]
7. Caplan, R.H.; Kisken, W.A.; Strutt, P.J.; Wester, S.M. Fine-needle aspiration biopsy of thyroid nodules: A cost-effective diagnostic plan. *Postgrad. Med.* **1991**, *90*, 183–190. [CrossRef] [PubMed]
8. Hamburger, J.I. Extensive personal experience. Diagnosis of thyroid nodules by fine needle biopsy: Use and abuse. *JCEM* **1994**, *79*, 335–339. [PubMed]
9. Yoshii, T.; Inohara, H.; Takenaka, Y.; Honjo, Y.; Akahani, S.; Nomura, T.; Raz, A.; Kubo, T. Galectin-3 maintains the transformed phenotype of thyroid papillary carcinoma cells. *Int. J. Oncol.* **2001**, *18*, 787–792. [CrossRef] [PubMed]
10. Sapio, M.R.; Guerra, A.; Posca, D.; Limone, P.P.; Deandrea, M.; Motta, M.; Troncone, G.; Caleo, A.; Vallefuoco, P.; Rossi, G.; et al. Combined analysis of galectin-3 and BRAFV600E improves the accuracy of fine-needle aspiration biopsy with cytological findings suspicious for papillary thyroid carcinoma. *Endocr. Relat. Cancer* **2007**, *14*, 1089–1097. [CrossRef] [PubMed]
11. Bryson, P.C.; Shores, C.G.; Hart, C.; Thorne, L.; Patel, M.R.; Richey, L.; Farag, A.; Zanation, A.M. Immunohistochemical distinction of follicular thyroid adenomas and follicular carcinomas. *Arch. Otolaryngol. Head Neck Surg.* **2008**, *134*, 581–586. [CrossRef] [PubMed]

12. Torregrossa, L.; Faviana, P.; Filice, M.E.; Materazzi, G.; Miccoli, P.; Vitti, P.; Fontanini, G.; Melillo, R.M.; Santoro, M.; Basolo, F. CXC chemokine receptor 4 immunodetection in the follicular variant of papillary thyroid carcinoma: Comparison to galectin-3 and hector battifora mesothelial cell-1. *Thyroid* **2010**, *20*, 495–504. [CrossRef] [PubMed]
13. Saggiorato, E.; de Pompa, R.; Volante, M.; Cappia, S.; Arecco, F.; Dei Tos, A.P.; Orlandi, F.; Papotti, M. Characterization of thyroid 'follicular neoplasms' in fine-needle aspiration cytological specimens using a panel of immunohistochemical markers: A proposal for clinical application. *Endocr. Relat. Cancer* **2005**, *12*, 305–317. [CrossRef] [PubMed]
14. Raggio, E.; Camandona, M.; Solerio, D.; Martino, P.; Franchello, A.; Orlandi, F.; Gasparri, G. The diagnostic accuracy of the immunocytochemical markers in the pre-operative evaluation of follicular thyroid lesions. *J. Endocrinol. Investig.* **2010**, *33*, 378–381. [CrossRef]
15. Bartolazzi, A.; Gasbarri, A.; Papotti, M.; Bussolati, G.; Lucante, T.; Khan, A.; Inohara, H.; Marandino, F.; Orlandi, F.; Nardi, F.; et al. Application of an immunodiagnostic method for improving preoperative diagnosis of nodular thyroid lesions. *Lancet* **2001**, *357*, 1644–1650. [CrossRef]
16. Zhang, L.; Krausz, T.; DeMay, R.M. A pilot study of galectin-3, HBME-1, and p27 triple immunostaining pattern for diagnosis of indeterminate thyroid nodules in cytology with correlation to histology. *Appl. Immunohistochem. Mol. Morphol.* **2015**, *23*, 481–490. [CrossRef] [PubMed]
17. Carpi, A.; Naccarato, A.G.; Iervasi, G.; Nicolini, A.; Bevilacqua, G.; Viacava, P.; Collecchi, P.; Lavra, L.; Marchetti, C.; Sciacchitano, S.; et al. Large needle aspiration biopsy and galectin-3 determination in selected thyroid nodules with indeterminate FNA-cytology. *Br. J. Cancer* **2006**, *95*, 204–209. [CrossRef] [PubMed]
18. Franco, C.; Martínez, V.; Allamand, J.P.; Medina, F.; Glasinovic, A.; Osorio, M.; Schachter, D. Molecular markers in thyroid fine-needle aspiration biopsy: A prospective study. *Appl. Immunohistochem. Mol. Morphol.* **2009**, *17*, 211–215. [CrossRef] [PubMed]
19. Das, D.K.; Al-Waheeb, S.K.; George, S.S.; Haji, B.I.; Mallik, MK. Contribution of immunocytochemical stainings for galectin-3, CD44, and HBME1 to fine-needle aspiration cytology diagnosis of papillary thyroid carcinoma. *Diagn. Cytopathol.* **2014**, *42*, 498–505. [CrossRef] [PubMed]
20. Trimboli, P.; Guidobaldi, L.; Amendola, S.; Nasrollah, N.; Romanelli, F.; Attanasio, D.; Ramacciato, G.; Saggiorato, E.; Valabrega, S.; Crescenzi, A. Galectin-3 and HBME-1 improve the accuracy of core biopsy in indeterminate thyroid nodules. *Endocrine* **2016**, *52*, 39–45. [CrossRef] [PubMed]
21. Naor, D.; Sionov, R.V.; Ish-Shalom, D. CD44: Structure, function, and association with the malignant process. *Adv. Cancer Res.* **1997**, *71*, 241–319. [PubMed]
22. Günthert, U.; Hofmann, M.; Rudy, W.; Reber, S.; Zöller, M.; Haussmann, I.; Matzku, S.; Wenzel, A.; Ponta, H.; Herrlich, P. A new variant of glycoprotein CD44 confers metastatic potential to rat carcinoma cells. *Cell* **1991**, *65*, 13–24. [CrossRef]
23. Matesa, N.; Samija, I.; Kusić, Z. Accuracy of fine needle aspiration biopsy with and without the use of tumor markers in cytologically indeterminate thyroid lesions. *Coll. Antropol.* **2010**, *34*, 53–57. [PubMed]
24. Maruta, J.; Hashimoto, H.; Yamashita, H.; Yamashita, H.; Noguchi, S. Immunostaining of galectin-3 and CD44v6 using fine-needle aspiration for distinguishing follicular carcinoma from adenoma. *Diagn. Cytopathol.* **2004**, *31*, 392–396. [CrossRef] [PubMed]
25. Haugen, B.R.; Alexander, E.K.; Bible, K.C.; Doherty, G.M.; Mandel, S.J.; Nikiforov, Y.E.; Pacini, F.; Randolph, G.W.; Sawka, A.M.; Schlumberger, M.; et al. 2015 American thyroid association management guidelines for adult patients with thyroid nodules and differentiated thyroid cancer: The American thyroid association guidelines task force on thyroid nodules and differentiated thyroid cancer. *Thyroid* **2016**, *26*, 1–133. [CrossRef] [PubMed]
26. Sobrinho-Simões, M.; Máximo, V.; Rocha, A.S.; Trovisco, V.; Castro, P.; Preto, A.; Lima, J.; Soares, P. Intragenic mutations in thyroid cancer. *Endocrinol. Metab. Clin. N. Am.* **2008**, *37*, 333–362. [CrossRef] [PubMed]
27. Xing, M. Molecular pathogenesis and mechanisms of thyroid cancer. *Nat. Rev. Cancer* **2013**, *13*, 184–199. [CrossRef] [PubMed]
28. Nikiforova, M.N.; Kimura, E.T.; Gandhi, M.; Biddinger, P.W.; Knauf, J.A.; Basolo, F.; Zhu, Z.; Giannini, R.; Salvatore, G.; Fusco, A.; et al. BRAF mutations in thyroid tumors are restricted to papillary carcinomas and anaplastic or poorly differentiated carcinomas arising from papillary carcinomas. *J. Clin. Endocrinol. Metab.* **2003**, *88*, 5399–5404. [CrossRef] [PubMed]

29. Vinagre, J.; Almeida, A.; Pópulo, H.; Batista, R.; Lyra, J.; Pinto, V.; Coelho, R.; Celestino, R.; Prazeres, H.; Lima, L.; et al. Frequency of TERT promoter mutations in human cancers. *Nat. Commun.* **2013**, *4*, 2185. [CrossRef] [PubMed]
30. Melo, M.; da Rocha, A.G.; Vinagre, J.; Batista, R.; Peixoto, J.; Tavares, C.; Celestino, R.; Almeida, A.; Salgado, C.; Eloy, C.; et al. TERT promoter mutations are a major indicator of poor outcome in differentiated thyroid carcinomas. *J. Clin. Endocrinol. Metab.* **2014**, *99*, E754–E765. [CrossRef] [PubMed]
31. Ohori, N.P.; Nikiforova, M.N.; Schoedel, K.E.; LeBeau, S.O.; Hodak, S.P.; Seethala, R.R.; Carty, S.E.; Ogilvie, J.B.; Yip, L.; Nikiforov, Y.E. Contribution of molecular testing to thyroid fine-needle aspiration cytology of "follicular lesion of undetermined significance/atypia of undetermined significance". *Cancer Cytopathol.* **2010**, *118*, 17–23. [CrossRef] [PubMed]
32. Cantara, S.; Capezzone, M.; Marchisotta, S.; Capuano, S.; Busonero, G.; Toti, P.; Di Santo, A.; Caruso, G.; Carli, A.F.; Brilli, L.; et al. Impact of proto-oncogene mutation detection in cytological specimens from thyroid nodules improves the diagnostic accuracy of cytology. *JCEM* **2010**, *95*, 1365–1369. [CrossRef] [PubMed]
33. Nikiforov, Y.E.; Ohori, N.P.; Hodak, S.P.; Carty, S.E.; LeBeau, S.O.; Ferris, R.L.; Yip, L.; Seethala, R.R.; Tublin, M.E.; Stang, M.T.; et al. Impact of mutational testing on the diagnosis and management of patients with cytologically indeterminate thyroid nodules: A prospective analysis of 1056 FNA samples. *JCEM* **2011**, *96*, 3390–3397. [CrossRef] [PubMed]
34. Chudova, D.; Wilde, J.I.; Wang, E.T.; Wang, H.; Rabbee, N.; Egidio, C.M.; Reynolds, J.; Tom, E.; Pagan, M.; Rigl, C.T.; et al. Molecular classification of thyroid nodules using high-dimensionality genomic data. *JCEM* **2010**, *95*, 5296–5304. [CrossRef] [PubMed]
35. Alexander, E.K.; Kennedy, G.C.; Baloch, Z.W.; Cibas, E.S.; Chudova, D.; Diggans, J.; Friedman, L.; Kloos, R.T.; LiVolsi, V.A.; Mandel, S.J.; et al. Preoperative diagnosis of benign thyroid nodules with indeterminate cytology. *N. Eng. J. Med.* **2012**, *367*, 705–715. [CrossRef] [PubMed]
36. Alexander, E.K.; Schorr, M.; Klopper, J.; Kim, C.; Sipos, J.; Nabhan, F.; Parker, C.; Steward, D.L.; Mandel, S.J.; Haugen, B.R. Multicenter clinical experience with the Afirma gene expression classifier. *JCEM* **2014**, *99*, 119–125. [CrossRef] [PubMed]
37. Harrell, R.M.; Bimston, D.N. Surgical utility of Afirma: Effects of high cancer prevalence and oncocytic cell types in patients with indeterminate thyroid cytology. *Endocr. Pract.* **2014**, *20*, 364–369. [CrossRef] [PubMed]
38. Lastra, R.R.; Pramick, M.R.; Crammer, C.J.; LiVolsi, V.A.; Baloch, Z.W. Implications of a suspicious afirma test result in thyroid fine-needle aspiration cytology: An institutional experience. *Cancer Cytopathol.* **2014**, *122*, 737–744. [CrossRef] [PubMed]
39. Marti, J.L.; Avadhani, V.; Donatelli, L.A.; Niyogi, S.; Wang, B.; Wong, R.J.; Shaha, A.R.; Ghossein, R.A.; Lin, O.; Morris, L.G.; et al. Wide inter-institutional variation in performance of a molecular classifier for indeterminate thyroid nodules. *Ann. Surg. Oncol.* **2015**, *22*, 3996–4001. [CrossRef] [PubMed]
40. McIver, B.; Castro, M.R.; Morris, J.C.; Bernet, V.; Smallridge, R.; Henry, M.; Kosok, L.; Reddi, H. An independent study of a gene expression classifier (Afirma) in the evaluation of cytologically indeterminate thyroid nodules. *JCEM* **2014**, *99*, 4069–4077. [CrossRef] [PubMed]
41. Nikiforova, M.N.; Wald, A.I.; Roy, S.; Durso, M.B.; Nikiforov, Y.E. Targeted next-generation sequencing panel (ThyroSeq) for detection of mutations in thyroid cancer. *JCEM* **2013**, *98*, E1852–E1860. [CrossRef] [PubMed]
42. Beaudenon-Huibregtse, S.; Alexander, E.K.; Guttler, R.B.; Hershman, J.M.; Babu, V.; Blevins, T.C.; Moore, P.; Andruss, B.; Labourier, E. Centralized molecular testing for oncogenic gene mutations complements the local cytopathologic diagnosis of thyroid nodules. *Thyroid* **2014**, *24*, 1479–1487. [CrossRef] [PubMed]
43. Eszlinger, M.; Krogdahl, A.; Münz, S.; Rehfeld, C.; Precht Jensen, E.M.; Ferraz, C.; Bösenberg, E.; Drieschner, N.; Scholz, M.; Hegedüs, L.; et al. Impact of molecular screening for point mutations and rearrangements in routine air-dried fine-needle aspiration samples of thyroid nodules. *Thyroid* **2014**, *24*, 305–313. [CrossRef] [PubMed]
44. Nikiforov, Y.E.; Carty, S.E.; Chiosea, S.I.; Coyne, C.; Duvvuri, U.; Ferris, R.L.; Gooding, W.E.; Hodak, S.P.; LeBeau, S.O.; Ohori, N.P.; et al. Highly accurate diagnosis of cancer in thyroid nodules with follicular neoplasm/suspicious for a follicular neoplasm cytology by ThyroSeq v2 next-generation sequencing assay. *Cancer* **2014**, *120*, 3627–3634. [CrossRef] [PubMed]
45. Coco, S.; Truini, A.; Vanni, I.; Dal Bello, M.G.; Alama, A.; Rijavec, E.; Genova, C.; Barletta, G.; Sini, C.; Burrafato, G.; et al. Next generation sequencing in non-small cell lung cancer: New avenues toward the personalized medicine. *Curr. Drug Targets* **2015**, *16*, 47–59. [CrossRef] [PubMed]

46. Malapelle, U.; Vigliar, E.; Sgariglia, R.; Bellevicine, C.; Colarossi, L.; Vitale, D.; Pallante, P.; Troncone, G. Ion Torrent next-generation sequencing for routine identification of clinically relevant mutations in colorectal cancer patients. *J. Clin. Pathol.* **2015**, *68*, 64–68. [CrossRef] [PubMed]
47. Chevrier, S.; Arnould, L.; Ghiringhelli, F.; Coudert, B.; Fumoleau, P.; Boidot, R. Next-generation sequencing analysis of lung and colon carcinomas reveals a variety of genetic alterations. *Int. J. Oncol.* **2014**, *45*, 1167–1174. [CrossRef] [PubMed]
48. Ross, J.S.; Badve, S.; Wang, K.; Sheehan, C.E.; Boguniewicz, A.B.; Otto, G.A.; Yelensky, R.; Lipson, D.; Ali, S.; Morosini, D.; et al. Genomic profiling of advanced-stage, metaplastic breast carcinoma by next-generation sequencing reveals frequent, targetable genomic abnormalities and potential new treatment options. *Arch. Pathol. Lab. Med.* **2015**, *139*, 642–649. [CrossRef] [PubMed]
49. Roy, S.; Durso, M.B.; Wald, A.; Nikiforov, Y.E.; Nikiforova, M.N. SeqReporter: Automating next-generation sequencing result interpretation and reporting workflow in a clinical laboratory. *J. Mol. Diagn.* **2014**, *16*, 11–22. [CrossRef] [PubMed]
50. Le Mercier, M.; D'Haene, N.; de Nève, N.; Blanchard, O.; Degand, C.; Rorive, S.; Salmon, I. Next-generation sequencing improves the diagnosis of thyroid FNA specimens with indeterminate cytology. *Histopathology* **2015**, *66*, 215–224. [CrossRef] [PubMed]
51. Carthew, R.W.; Sontheimer, E.J. Origins and Mechanisms of miRNAs and siRNAs. *Cell* **2009**, *136*, 642–655. [CrossRef] [PubMed]
52. Mitchell, P.S.; Parkin, R.K.; Kroh, E.M.; Fritz, B.R.; Wyman, S.K.; Pogosova-Agadjanyan, E.L.; Peterson, A.; Noteboom, J.; O'Briant, K.C.; Allen, A.; et al. Circulating microRNAs as stable blood-based markers for cancer detection. *Proc. Natl. Acad. Sci. USA* **2008**, *105*, 10513–10518. [CrossRef] [PubMed]
53. Chen, X.; Ba, Y.; Ma, L.; Cai, X.; Yin, Y.; Wang, K.; Guo, J.; Zhang, Y.; Chen, J.; Guo, X.; et al. Characterization of microRNAs in serum: A novel class of biomarkers for diagnosis of cancer and other diseases. *Cell Res.* **2008**, *18*, 997–1006. [CrossRef] [PubMed]
54. Lawrie, C.H.; Gal, S.; Dunlop, H.M.; Pushkaran, B.; Liggins, A.P.; Pulford, K.; Banham, A.H.; Pezzella, F.; Boultwood, J.; Wainscoat, J.S.; et al. Detection of elevated levels of tumour-associated microRNAs in serum of patients with diffuse large B-cell lymphoma. *Br. J. Haematol.* **2008**, *141*, 672–675. [CrossRef] [PubMed]
55. Taylor, D.D.; Gercel-Taylor, C. MicroRNA signatures of tumor-derived exosomes as diagnostic biomarkers of ovarian cancer. *Gynecol. Oncol.* **2008**, *110*, 13–21. [CrossRef] [PubMed]
56. Lu, J.; Getz, G.; Miska, E.A.; Alvarez-Saavedra, E.; Lamb, J.; Peck, D.; Sweet-Cordero, A.; Ebert, B.L.; Mak, R.H.; Ferrando, A.A.; et al. MicroRNA expression profiles classify human cancers. *Nature* **2005**, *435*, 834–838. [CrossRef] [PubMed]
57. Volinia, S.; Calin, G.A.; Liu, C.G.; Ambs, S.; Cimmino, A.; Petrocca, F.; Visone, R.; Iorio, M.; Roldo, C.; Ferracin, M.; et al. A microRNA expression signature of human solid tumors defines cancer gene targets. *Proc. Natl. Acad. Sci. USA* **2006**, *103*, 2257–2261. [CrossRef] [PubMed]
58. Tetzlaff, M.T.; Liu, A.; Xu, X.; Master, S.R.; Baldwin, D.A.; Tobias, J.W.; Livolsi, V.A.; Baloch, Z.W. Differential expression of miRNAs in papillary thyroid carcinoma compared to multinodular goiter using formalin fixed paraffin embedded tissues. *Endocr. Pathol.* **2007**, *18*, 163–173. [CrossRef] [PubMed]
59. Chen, Y.T.; Kitabayashi, N.; Zhou, X.K.; Fahey, T.J., 3rd; Scognamiglio, T. MicroRNA analysis as a potential diagnostic tool for papillary thyroid carcinoma. *Mod. Pathol.* **2008**, *21*, 1139–1146. [CrossRef] [PubMed]
60. He, H.; Jazdzewski, K.; Li, W.; Liyanarachchi, S.; Nagy, R.; Volinia, S.; Calin, G.A.; Liu, C.G.; Franssila, K.; Suster, S.; et al. The role of microRNA genes in papillary thyroid carcinoma. *Proc. Natl. Acad. Sci. USA* **2005**, *102*, 19075–19080. [CrossRef] [PubMed]
61. Nikifororva, M.N.; Tseng, G.C.; Steward, D.; Diorio, D.; Nikiforov, Y. MicroRNA expression profiling of thyroid tumors: Biological significance and diagnostic utility. *JCEM* **2008**, *93*, 1600–1608.
62. Swierniak, M.; Wojcicka, A.; Czetwertynska, M.; Stachlewska, E.; Maciag, M.; Wiechno, W.; Gornicka, B.; Bogdanska, M.; Koperski, L.; de la Chapelle, A.; et al. In-depth characterization of the microRNA transcriptome in normal thyroid and papillary thyroid carcinoma. *JCEM* **2013**, *98*, E1401–E1409. [CrossRef] [PubMed]
63. Mancikova, V.; Castelblanco, E.; Pineiro-Yanez, E.; Perales-Paton, J.; de Cubas, A.A.; Inglada-Perez, L.; Matias-Guiu, X.; Capel, I.; Bella, M.; Lerma, E.; et al. MicroRNA deep-sequencing reveals master regulators of follicular and papillary thyroid tumors. *Mod. Pathol.* **2015**, *28*, 748–757. [CrossRef] [PubMed]

64. Kitano, M.; Rahbari, R.; Patterson, E.E.; Xiong, Y.; Prasad, N.B.; Wang, Y.; Zeiger, M.A.; Kebebew, E. Expression profiling of difficult-to-diagnose thyroid histologic subtypes shows distinct expression profiles and identify candidate diagnostic microRNAs. *Ann. Surg. Oncol.* **2011**, *18*, 3443–3452. [CrossRef] [PubMed]
65. Yip, L.; Kelly, L.; Shuai, Y.; Armstrong, M.J.; Nikiforov, Y.E.; Carty, S.E.; Nikiforova, M.N. MicroRNA signature distinguishes the degree of aggressiveness of papillary thyroid carcinoma. *Ann. Surg. Oncol.* **2011**, *18*, 2035–2041. [CrossRef] [PubMed]
66. Mazeh, H.; Levy, Y.; Mizrahi, I.; Appelbaum, L.; Ilyayev, N.; Halle, D.; Freund, H.R.; Nissan, A. Differentiating benign from malignant thyroid nodules using micro ribonucleic acid amplification in residual cells obtained by fine needle aspiration biopsy. *J. Surg. Res.* **2013**, *180*, 216–221. [CrossRef] [PubMed]
67. Agretti, P.; Ferrarini, E.; Rago, T.; Candelieri, A.; de Marco, G.; Dimida, A.; Niccolai, F.; Molinaro, A.; Di Coscio, G.; Pinchera, A.; et al. MicroRNA expression profile helps to distinguish benign nodules from papillary thyroid carcinomas starting from cells of fine-needle aspiration. *Eur. J. Endocrinol.* **2012**, *167*, 393–400. [CrossRef] [PubMed]
68. Wei, W.J.; Shen, C.T.; Song, H.J.; Qiu, Z.L.; Luo, Q.Y. MicroRNAs as a potential tool in the differential diagnosis of thyroid cancer: A systematic review and meta-analysis. *Clin. Endocrinol.* **2016**, *84*, 127–133. [CrossRef] [PubMed]
69. Kitano, M.; Rahbari, R.; Patterson, E.E.; Steinberg, S.M.; Prasad, N.B.; Wang, Y.; Zeiger, M.A.; Kebebew, E. Evaluation of candidate diagnostic microRNAs in thyroid fine-needle aspiration biopsy samples. *Thyroid* **2012**, *22*, 285–291. [CrossRef] [PubMed]
70. Keutgen, X.M.; Filicori, F.; Crowley, M.J.; Wang, Y.; Scognamiglio, T.; Hoda, R.; Buitrago, D.; Cooper, D.; Zeiger, M.A.; Zarnegar, R.; et al. A panel of four miRNAs accurately differentiates malignant from benign indeterminate thyroid lesions on fine needle aspiration. *Clin. Cancer Res.* **2012**, *18*, 2032–2038. [CrossRef] [PubMed]
71. Mazeh, H.; Mizrahi, I.; Halle, D.; Ilyayev, N.; Stojadinovic, A.; Trink, B.; Mitrani-Rosenbaum, S.; Roistacher, M.; Ariel, I.; Eid, A.; et al. Development of a microRNA-based molecular assay for the detection of papillary thyroid carcinoma in aspiration biopsy samples. *Thyroid* **2011**, *21*, 111–118. [CrossRef] [PubMed]
72. Panebianco, F.; Mazzanti, C.; Tomei, S.; Aretini, P.; Franceschi, S.; Lessi, F.; Di Coscio, G.; Bevilacqua, G.; Marchetti, I. The combination of four molecular markers improves thyroid cancer cytologic diagnosis and patient management. *BMC Cancer* **2015**, *19*, 918. [CrossRef] [PubMed]
73. Vriens, M.R.; Weng, J.; Suh, I.; Huynh, N.; Guerrero, M.A.; Shen, W.T.; Duh, Q.Y.; Clark, O.H.; Kebebew, E. MicroRNA expression profiling is a potential diagnostic tool for thyroid cancer. *Cancer* **2012**, *118*, 3426–3432. [CrossRef] [PubMed]
74. Ludvíková, M.; Kalfeřt, D.; Kholová, I. Pathobiology of MicroRNAs and Their Emerging Role in Thyroid Fine-Needle Aspiration. *Acta Cytol.* **2015**, *59*, 435–444. [CrossRef] [PubMed]
75. Lee, Y.S.; Lim, Y.S.; Lee, J.C.; Wang, S.G.; Park, H.Y.; Kim, S.Y.; Lee, B.J. Differential expression levels of plasma-derived miR-146b and miR-155 in papillary thyroid cancer. *Oral Oncol.* **2015**, *51*, 77–83. [CrossRef] [PubMed]
76. Yu, S.; Liu, Y.; Wang, J.; Guo, Z.; Zhang, Q.; Yu, F.; Zhang, Y.; Huang, K.; Li, Y.; Song, E.; et al. Circulating microRNA profiles as potential biomarkers for diagnosis of papillary thyroid carcinoma. *JCEM* **2012**, *97*, 2084–2092. [CrossRef] [PubMed]
77. Cantara, S.; Pilli, T.; Sebastiani, G.; Cevenini, G.; Busonero, G.; Cardinale, S.; Dotta, F.; Pacini, F. Circulating miRNA95 and miRNA190 are sensitive markers for the differential diagnosis of thyroid nodules in a Caucasian population. *JCEM* **2014**, *99*, 4190–4198. [CrossRef] [PubMed]
78. Lithwick-Yanai, G.; Dromi, N.; Shtabsky, A.; Morgenstern, S.; Strenov, Y.; Feinmesser, M.; Kravtsov, V.; Leon, M.; Hajdúch, M.; Ali, S.Z.; et al. Multicentre validation of a microRNA-based assay for diagnosing indeterminate thyroid nodules utilising fine needle aspirate smears. *J. Clin. Pathol.* **2016**. [CrossRef] [PubMed]
79. Benjamin, H.; Schnitzer-Perlman, T.; Shtabsky, A.; VandenBussche, C.J.; Ali, S.Z.; Kolar, Z.; Pagni, F.; Rosetta Genomics Group; Bar, D.; Meiri, E. Analytical validity of a microRNA-based assay for diagnosing indeterminate thyroid FNA smears from routinely prepared cytology slides. *Cancer Cytopathol.* **2016**, *124*, 711–721. [CrossRef] [PubMed]
80. Suriano, R.; Lin, Y.; Ashok, B.T.; Schaefer, S.D.; Schantz, S.P.; Geliebter, J.; Tiwari, R.K. Pilot study using SELDI-TOF-MS based proteomic profile for the identification of diagnostic biomarkers of thyroid proliferative diseases. *J. Proteome Res.* **2006**, *5*, 856–861. [CrossRef] [PubMed]

81. Torres-Cabala, C.; Bibbo, M.; Panizo-Santos, A.; Barazi, H.; Krutzsch, H.; Roberts, D.D.; Merino, M.J. Proteomic identification of new biomarkers and application in thyroid cytology. *Acta Cytol.* **2006**, *50*, 518–528. [CrossRef] [PubMed]
82. Brown, L.M.; Helmke, S.M.; Hunsucker, S.W.; Netea-Maier, R.T.; Chiang, S.A.; Heinz, D.E.; Shroyer, K.R.; Duncan, M.W.; Haugen, B.R. Quantitative and qualitative differences in protein expression between papillary thyroid carcinoma and normal thyroid tissue. *Mol. Carcinog.* **2006**, *45*, 613–626. [CrossRef] [PubMed]
83. Krause, K.; Karger, S.; Schierhorn, A.; Poncin, S.; Many, M.C.; Fuhrer, D. Proteomic profiling of cold thyroid nodules. *Endocrinology* **2007**, *148*, 1754–1763. [CrossRef] [PubMed]
84. Puxeddu, E.; Susta, F.; Orvietani, P.L.; Chiasserini, D.; Barbi, F.; Moretti, S.; Cavaliere, A.; Santeusanio, F.; Avenia, N.; Binaglia, L. Identification of differentially expressed proteins in papillary thyroid carcinomas with V600E mutation of BRAF. *Proteom. Clin. Appl.* **2007**, *1*, 672–680. [CrossRef] [PubMed]
85. Netea-Maier, R.T.; Hunsucker, S.W.; Hoevenaars, B.M.; Helmke, S.M.; Slootweg, P.J.; Hermus, A.R.; Haugen, B.R.; Duncan, M.W. Discovery and validation of protein abundance differences between follicular thyroid neoplasms. *Cancer Res.* **2008**, *68*, 1572–1580. [CrossRef] [PubMed]
86. Musso, R.; di Cara, G.; Albanese, N.N.; Marabeti, M.R.; Cancemi, P.; Martini, D.; Orsini, E.; Giordano, C.; Pucci-Minafra, I. Differential proteomic and phenotypic behaviour of papillary and anaplastic thyroid cell lines. *J. Proteom.* **2013**, *90*, 115–125. [CrossRef] [PubMed]
87. Chaker, S.; Kashat, L.; Voisin, S.; Kaur, J.; Kak, I.; MacMillan, C.; Ozcelik, H.; Siu, K.W.; Ralhan, R.; Walfish, P.G. Secretome proteins as candidate biomarkers for aggressive thyroid carcinomas. *Proteomics* **2013**, *13*, 771–787. [CrossRef] [PubMed]
88. Pagni, F.; L'Imperio, V.; Bono, F.; Garancini, M.; Roversi, G.; de Sio, G.; Galli, M.; Smith, A.J.; Chinello, C.; Magni, F. Proteome analysis in thyroid pathology. *Expert Rev. Proteom.* **2015**, *12*, 375–390. [CrossRef] [PubMed]
89. Galli, M.; Pagni, F.; de Sio, G.; Smith, A.; Chinello, C.; Stella, M.; L'Imperio, V.; Manzoni, M.; Garancini, M.; Massimini, D.; et al. Proteomic profiles of thyroid tumors by mass spectrometry-imaging on tissue microarrays. *Biochim. Biophys. Acta* **2016**. [CrossRef] [PubMed]
90. Giusti, L.; Iacconi, P.; Ciregia, F.; Giannaccini, G.; Donatini, G.L.; Basolo, F.; Miccoli, P.; Pinchera, A.; Lucacchini, A. Fine-needle aspiration of thyroid nodules: Proteomic analysis to identify cancer biomarkers. *J. Proteome Res.* **2008**, *7*, 4079–4088. [CrossRef] [PubMed]
91. Giusti, L.; Iacconi, P.; Ciregia, F.; Giannaccini, G.; Basolo, F.; Donatini, G.; Miccoli, P.; Lucacchini, A. Proteomic analysis of human thyroid fine needle aspiration fluid I. *J. Endocrinol. Nvestig.* **2007**, *30*, 865–869. [CrossRef] [PubMed]
92. Ciregia, F.; Giusti, L.; Molinaro, A.; Niccolai, F.; Agretti, P.; Rago, T.; Di Coscio, G.; Vitti, P.; Basolo, F.; Iacconi, P.; et al. Presence in the pre-surgical fine-needle aspiration of potential thyroid biomarkers previously identified in the post-surgical one. *PLoS ONE* **2013**, *8*, e72911. [CrossRef] [PubMed]
93. Mainini, V.; Pagni, F.; Garancini, M.; Giardini, V.; de Sio, G.; Cusi, C.; Arosio, C.; Roversi, G.; Chinello, C.; Caria, P.; et al. An alternative approach in endocrine pathology research: MALDI-IMS in papillary thyroid carcinoma. *Endocr. Pathol.* **2013**, *24*, 250–253. [CrossRef] [PubMed]
94. Pagni, F.; Mainini, V.; Garancini, M.; Bono, F.; Vanzati, A.; Giardini, V.; Scardilli, M.; Goffredo, P.; Smith, A.J.; Galli, M.; et al. Proteomics for the diagnosis of thyroid lesions: Preliminary report. *Cytopathology* **2015**, *26*, 318–324. [CrossRef] [PubMed]
95. Pagni, F.; de Sio, G.; Garancini, M.; Scardilli, M.; Chinello, C.; Smith, A.J.; Bono, F.; Leni, D.; Magni, F. Proteomics in thyroid cytopathology: Relevance of MALDI-imaging in distinguishing malignant from benign lesions. *Proteomics* **2016**, *16*, 1775–1784. [CrossRef] [PubMed]
96. Ferris, R.L.; Baloch, Z.; Bernet, V.; Chen, A.; Fahey, T.J., 3rd; Ganly, I.; Hodak, S.P.; Kebebew, E.; Patel, K.N.; Shaha, A.; et al. American thyroid association statement on surgical application of molecular profiling for thyroid nodules: Current impact on perioperative decision making. *Thyroid* **2015**, *25*, 760–768. [CrossRef] [PubMed]

6

VEGFA and *NFE2L2* Gene Expression and Regulation by MicroRNAs in Thyroid Papillary Cancer and Colloid Goiter

Leonardo P. Stuchi [1], Márcia Maria U. Castanhole-Nunes [1], Nathália Maniezzo-Stuchi [2], Patrícia M. Biselli-Chicote [1], Tiago Henrique [3], João Armando Padovani Neto [4], Dalisio de-Santi Neto [5], Ana Paula Girol [2], Erika C. Pavarino [1] and Eny Maria Goloni-Bertollo [1,*]

1 Research Unit in Genetics and Molecular Biology—UPGEM, Faculty of Medicine of São José do Rio Preto—FAMERP, São José do Rio Preto 15090-000, Brazil; prado_leonardo@yahoo.com.br (L.P.S.); mcastanhole@gmail.com (M.M.U.C.-N.); patriciabiselli@yahoo.com.br (P.M.B.-C.); erika@famerp.br (E.C.P.)

2 Padre Albino University Center—UNIFIPA, Catanduva, São Paulo 15809-144, Brazil; nmmbiomedica@hotmail.com (N.M.-S.); anapaula.girol@unifipa.com.br (A.P.G.)

3 Laboratory of Molecular Markers and Bioinformatics, Department of Molecular Biology, Faculty of Medicine of São José do Rio Preto —FAMERP, São José do Rio Preto 15090-000, Brazil; henrique@famerp.br

4 Department of Otolaryngology and Head and Neck Surgery, Faculty of Medicine of São José do Rio Preto —FAMERP, São José do Rio Preto 15090-000, Brazil; padovani.ja@gmail.com

5 Pathological Anatomy Service, Hospital de Base, Foundation Regional Faculty of Medicine of São José do Rio Preto—FUNFARME, São José do Rio Preto 15090-000, Brazil; dalisius@gmail.com

* Correspondence: eny.goloni@famerp.br

Abstract: Deregulation of VEGFA (Vascular Endothelial Growth Factor A) and NFE2L2 (Nuclear Factor (Erythroid-derived 2)-Like 2), involved in angiogenesis and oxidative stress, can lead to thyroid cancer progression. MiR-17-5p and miR-612 are possible regulators of these genes and may promote thyroid disorders. In order to evaluate the involvement of VEGFA, NFE2L2, hsa-miR-17-5p, and hsa-miR-612 in thyroid pathology, we examined tissue samples from colloid goiter, papillary thyroid cancer (PTC), and a normal thyroid. We found higher levels of VEGFA and NFE2L2 transcripts and the VEGFA protein in goiter and PTC samples than in normal tissue. In the goiter, miR-612 and miR-17-5p levels were lower than those in PTC. Tumors, despite showing lower *VEGFA* mRNA expression, presented higher VEGFA protein levels compared to goiter tissue. In addition, NRF2 (Nuclear Related Transcription Factor 2) protein levels in tumors were higher than those in goiter and normal tissues. Inhibition of miR-17-5p resulted in reduced NFE2L2 expression. Overall, both transcript and protein levels of NFE2L2 and VEGFA were elevated in PTC and colloid goiter. Hsa-miR-612 showed differential expression in PTC and colloid goiter, while hsa-miR-17-5p showed differential expression only in colloid goiter, suggesting that hsa-miR-17-5p may be a positive regulator of NFE2L2 expression in PTC.

Keywords: thyroid neoplasms; goiter; vascular endothelial growth factor A; NF-E2-related factor 2; microRNAs

---

1. Introduction

Colloid goiter is the most common disorder of the thyroid gland, even in non-endemic regions, and it is clinically detected in about 4% of individuals older than 30 years [1]. The presence of colloid goiter can indicate the beginning of malignant transformation of the thyroid leading to thyroid cancer [2,3].

Thyroid cancer is the most common endocrine neoplasia, accounting for about 1.7% of all cancer diagnoses worldwide [4], and it is the fifth most common type of cancer in women [5]. Papillary thyroid cancer (PTC) is the most common thyroid cancer, accounting for about 80% of diagnoses [6].

Angiogenesis plays a key role in the progression of cancer and the onset of metastases, as the newly formed blood vessels supply the nutrients and oxygen necessary for the maintenance of tumor growth [7]. VEGFA (Vascular Endothelial Growth Factor A) is the first angiogenic factor induced by hypoxia and promotes proliferation, budding, migration, and formation of the endothelial matrix [8]. Another important factor for angiogenesis is nuclear related transcription factor 2 (NRF2), encoded by the *NFE2L2* gene (*nuclear factor (erythroid-derived 2)-like 2*). NRF2 regulates the expression of antioxidant proteins in response to oxidative stress in various tissues [9]. Therefore, *VEGFA* and *NFE2L2* have been considered potential targets for new antiangiogenic therapies.

Gene expression can be regulated by microRNAs (miRNAs, miR), which control many cellular processes, including cell growth, differentiation, proliferation, and apoptosis [10]. Identification of the possible roles of miR-17-5p and miR-612 in the regulation of *NFE2L2* and *VEGFA* expression in PTC and colloid goiter can provide valuable insights for the development of strategies and drugs to inhibit tumor growth and also to restore sensitivity of tumors to chemotherapy.

In this study, we aimed to evaluate mRNA and protein levels of VEGFA and NFE2L2, as well as the expression patterns of miR-17-5p and miR-612 in human papillary thyroid cancer, colloid goiter, and normal thyroid tissues, and also to investigate the involvement of miR-17-5p and miR-612 in the regulation of *VEGFA* and *NFE2L2* expression in the thyroid papillary cancer cell line (TPC-1 line).

2. Materials and Methods

2.1. Specimens

Tumor and goiter tissue samples, along with adjacent tissues, as well as normal thyroid tissue samples were collected from 66 patients, as follows: 15 thyroid papillary cancer patients (13 females and 2 males), 15 goiter colloid patients (14 females and 1 male), and 6 patients with normal thyroid (4 females and 2 males). Tumor and goiter samples, along with adjacent tissue samples, were sent to the Pathology Service of Hospital de Base de São José do Rio Preto—SP for diagnosis and microdissection. The tumors were classified according to the parameters of "American Joint Committee for Cancer" (AJCC) [11]: tumor size (T), presence of nodal metastasis (N), and presence of distant metastasis (M). This study was approved by the Research Ethics Committee of the Medical School of São José do Rio Preto, FAMERP (No. 468.393).

2.2. Computer Prediction of miRs

miRs were selected in the DIANA-TarBase v7.0 database (http://diana.imis.athena-innovation.gr/DianaTools/index.php?r=tarbase/index), TargetScan (http://www.targetscan.org/vert_71) and mirDIP (http://ophid.utoronto.ca/mirDIP/). Two miRs with the highest score for regulation of *NFE2L2* and *VEGFA* were selected.

2.3. Expression of NFE2L2, VEGFA, miR-17-5p, and miR-612

RNA was extracted using the mirVana PARIS Kit (Applied Biosystems, Carlsbad, CA, USA). Complementary DNA (cDNA) from total RNA was synthesized using the High Capacity cDNA Archive Kit (Life Technologies, Carlsbad, CA, USA). The conversion of the miRs into cDNA was performed using the TaqMan-Micro RNA Reverse Transcription kit (Applied Biosystems).

Expression analyses of *NFE2L2* (Hs00975961_g1) and *VEGFA* (Hs00900055_m1), miR-17-5p (002308), and miR-612 (001579) were performed by quantitative real-time PCR (qPCR) using specific TaqMan probes (Thermo Fisher Scientific, Waltham, MA, USA) on the CFX 96 Real Time System

(Bio-Rad, Hercules, CA, USA). All reactions were performed in duplicates and included a contamination control. The genes *β-actin* (Hs01060665_g1) and *GAPDH* (Hs03929097_g1) were used as reference genes for normalization of *NFE2L2* and *VEGFA* expression data. The genes *RNU6B* (001093) and *RNU48B* (001006) were used for normalization of miR-17-5p and miR-612 expression data (Thermo Fisher Scientific). Relative quantification (RQ) of genes and miR expression in PTC and colloid goiter was calculated using the $2^{-\Delta\Delta Ct}$ method in relation to the normal tissues [12].

2.4. Quantification of Protein Expression in Tissue Samples

The proteins were extracted using the mirVana Paris Kit and Trizol Reagent (Applied Biosystems) and quantified using the BCA Protein Assay Kit (Abcam, Cambridge, United Kingdom).

Quantification of VEGFA protein in fresh tissue samples was performed using VEGFA Duo Set ELISA Kit (R&D Systems, Minneapolis, MN, USA) following the manufacturer's instruction. Immunohistochemistry was performed for analysis of NRF2 protein quantification. Briefly, after deparaffinization, the sections were rehydrated in a graded series of ethanol. The polyclonal rabbit anti-Nrf2 primary antibody (PA5-27882, Thermo Fisher Scientific) was used at a dilution of 1:100. After incubation, a biotinylated secondary antibody (Histostain-Plus IHC Kit, DAB, broad spectrum, 95-9943B, Invitrogen, Carlsbad, CA, USA) was used. The slides were incubated with streptavidin complex conjugated to peroxidase and 3,3'-diaminobenzidine (DAB 750118, Invitrogen) in the dark. For analysis of densitometry, the sections were photographed under a 40x objective (three fields per slide). For each sample, the cytoplasm and nucleus of epithelial cells were evaluated at 20 points equally distributed in the cytoplasm and 10 points in the nucleus.

2.5. Cell Line TPC-1 Culture

The TPC-1 cell line [13] derived from female papillary cancer was cultured in DMEM (Dulbecco's modified Eagle's medium, Cultilab, Campinas, Brazil), supplemented with 10% fetal bovine serum (Cultilab), 100 U/mL sodium penicillin, 100 mg/mL streptomycin (Cultilab), and 1% L-glutamine (Cultilab) at 37 °C in a 5% CO_2 incubator. The TPC-1 cell line authentication was performed by STR (Short Tandem Repeat) DNA typing profile using Gene Print 10 (Promega, Madison, WI, USA), ID 142738.

2.6. Transfection in the TPC-1 Cell Line

Transfection assays were conducted using mirVana™ inhibitor for miR-17-5p (MH12412, Thermo Scientific) and the mirVana™ miR-612 mimic (MC11461, Thermo Scientific) with Lipofectamine RNAiMAX (Invitrogen) following the manufacturer's instructions. Cells were cultured for 48 h in 100 μL of Opti-MEM serum-free medium (Invitrogen), 1 μL of Lipofectamine RNAiMAX (Invitrogen), and 10 mM of the inhibitor for miR-17-5p or the miR-612 mimic. RNA was extracted to verify the efficiency of transfection, using the respective positive and negative controls by qPCR.

2.7. Statistical Analyses

Statistical analyses were performed using GraphPad Prism software, version 6. The continuous data distribution was evaluated using D'Agostino and Pearson's normality test. The Wilcoxon signed rank test and the Mann–Whitney test were used to evaluate the gene expression data. The correlation between the expression of miRNAs and the genes was analyzed by Spearman's correlation. The Mann–Whitney test was used to evaluate the protein expression data. Values of $p < 0.05$ were considered significant.

3. Results

3.1. Characteristics of the Samples

The characteristics of the samples are summarized in Table 1.

Table 1. Characteristics of the collected samples.

Characteristics	Tumor	Goiter
Gender		
Female (F)	13 (86.7%)	14 (93.4%)
Male (M)	2 (13.3%)	1 (6.6%)
Age		
<45	F: 7 (46.6%); M: 1 (6.7%)	F: 6 (40%); M: 1 (6.7%)
≥45	F: 6 (40%); M: 1 (6.7%)	F: 8 (53.3%); M: 0 (-)
Tumor extent		
I	8 (53.4%)	
II-III	7 (46.6%)	
Nodal metastasis	2 (13.3%)	
Distant metastasis	2 (13.3%)	

3.2. Expression of VEGFA, NFE2L2, miR-17-5p, and miR-612 in Fresh Tissue Samples

Expression levels of *VEGFA*, *NFE2L2*, miR-17-5p, and miR-612 in the tumor tissues, colloid goiter, and their respective adjacent tissues were compared to those observed in the normal tissues. *VEGFA* and *NFE2L2* showed high expression levels in the tumor and goiter. MiR-17-5p and miR-612 did not exhibit differential expression in the tumor, but the expression levels of both miRs were reduced in the goiter (Table 2).

Table 2. Genes and miR expression in thyroid tumor and goiter in relation to normal thyroid tissue.

	Tumor				Goiter			
Gene	**RQ Median**	**Min**	**Max**	***P***	**RQ Median**	**Min**	**Max**	***P***
VEGFA	1.516	0.059	6.605	0.0125 *	20.010	8.595	32.260	<0.0001 *
NFE2L2	5.446	0.045	40.76	0.0061 *	23.380	0.278	68.780	0.0009 *
MicroRNAs								
miR-17-5p	0.206	0.007	3.305	0.094	0.099	0.006	0.879	<0.0001 *
miR-612	0.181	0.002	7.097	0.135	0.044	0.003	0.238	0.015 *

RQ, relative quantification; *P*, *p* value; *, Wilcoxon signed rank test.

VEGFA and *NFE2L2* also showed elevated expression in the tumor- and goiter-adjacent tissues. MiR-612 showed reduced expression in the tumor-adjacent tissue and in the goiter-adjacent tissue, whereas miR-17-5p showed reduced expression only in the goiter-adjacent tissue (Table 3).

Table 3. Gene and miR expression in tumor- and goiter-adjacent tissues in relation to normal thyroid tissue.

	Tumor-Adjacent Tissue				Goiter -Adjacent Tissue			
Gene	**RQ Median**	**Min**	**Max**	***P***	**RQ Median**	**Min**	**Max**	***P***
VEGFA	3.405	0.010	8.190	0.0023 *	20.720	13.820	55.970	<0.0001 *
NFE2L2	23.990	0.039	76.920	0.0149 *	15.870	2.417	83.740	<0.0001 *
MicroRNAs								
miR-17-5p	0.256	0.059	11.020	0.118	0.209	0.043	10.930	0.0448 *
miR-612	0.128	0.003	20.790	0.016 *	0.092	0.001	4.413	0.0131 *

RQ, relative quantification; *P*, *p* value; *, Spearman correlation.

Comparisons between the groups revealed that *VEGFA* gene expression was higher in the goiter than in the tumor (RQ median = 20.28 vs. 1.5; $p < 0.0001$) and also in the goiter-adjacent tissue than in the tumor-adjacent tissue (RQ median = 20.72 vs. 3.40, $p < 0.0001$) (Figure 1). No significant difference was detected in *NFE2L2* expression between the groups.

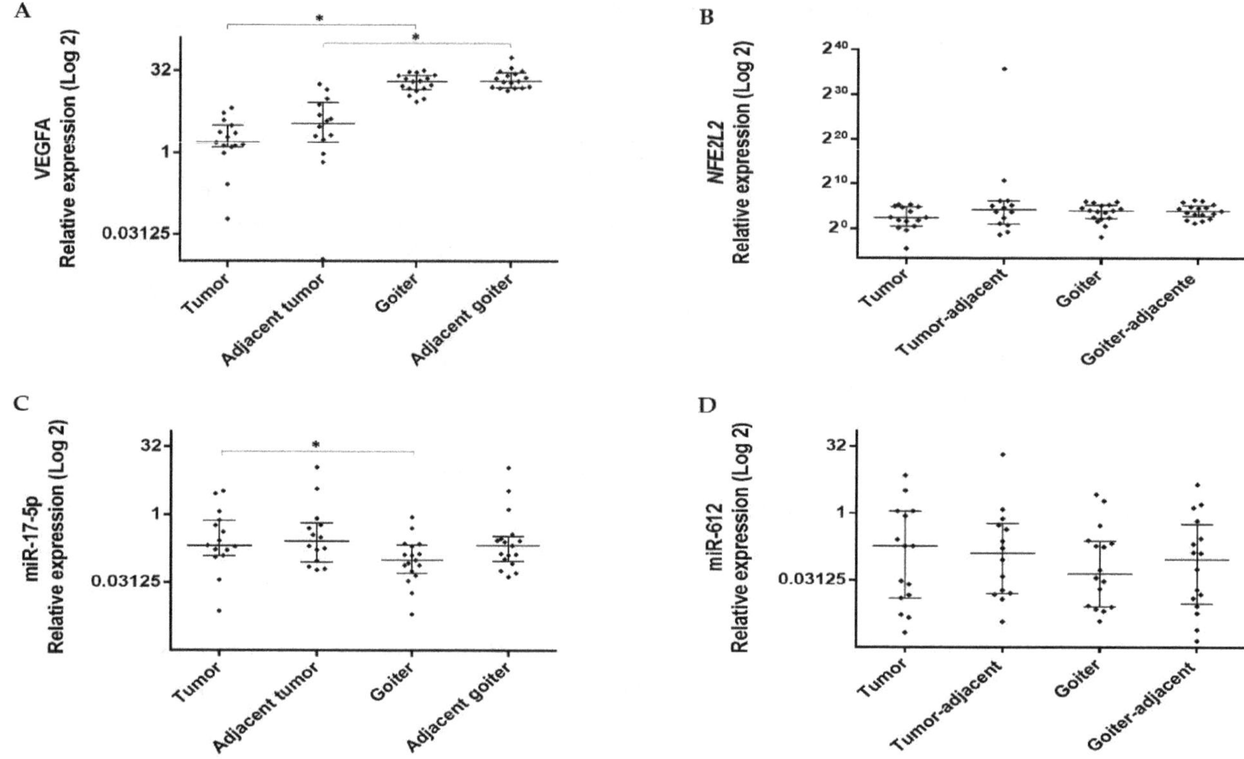

Figure 1. Expression levels of (**A**) *VEGFA* (*Vascular Endothelial Growth Factor A*), (**B**) *NFE2L2 (Nuclear Factor (Erythroid-derived 2)-Like 2)*, (**C**) miR-17-5p, and (**D**) miR-612 in tumor and goiter tissues and their respective adjacent tissues. Data are presented as median with interquartile range (25% percentile and 75% percentile). The relative expression value was Log2 transformed (*y*-axis). Calibrator (normal tissue) log RQ = 1. *, Statistically significant (panel A, Mann–Whitney, $p < 0.0001$; panel C, Mann–Whitney, $p = 0.033$).

Regarding miR expression, miR-17-5p expression was higher in the tumor than in the goiter (RQ median = 0.20 vs. 0.09; $p = 0.033$) (Figure 1). Expression of miR-612 did not differ significantly between the groups.

3.3. Correlation between Expression Levels of VEGFA, NFE2L2, miR-17-5p, and miR-612

There was a negative correlation in the tumor tissue between miR-612 and *VEGFA* expression, and between miR-612 and miR-17-5p and *NFE2L2* expression. In relation to the goiter, only miR-612 expression presented a negative correlation with *NFE2L2* expression (Table 4; Figure 2).

Table 4. Correlation between expression levels of *VEGFA* and *NFE2L2* and the miR-17-5p and miR-612 miRs in thyroid tumors and colloid goiter.

	Tumor				Goiter			
	VEGFA		*NFE2L2*		*VEGFA*		*NFE2L2*	
	R^2	*P*	R^2	*P*	R^2	*P*	R^2	*P*
miR17-5p	−0.411	0.130	−0.067	0.019 *	−0.118	0.653	−0.174	0.503
miR-612	−0.546	0.038 *	−0.679	0.007 *	-0.479	0.062	−0.724	0.002 *

R^2, correlation coefficient; *P*, *p* value; *, Spearman correlation.

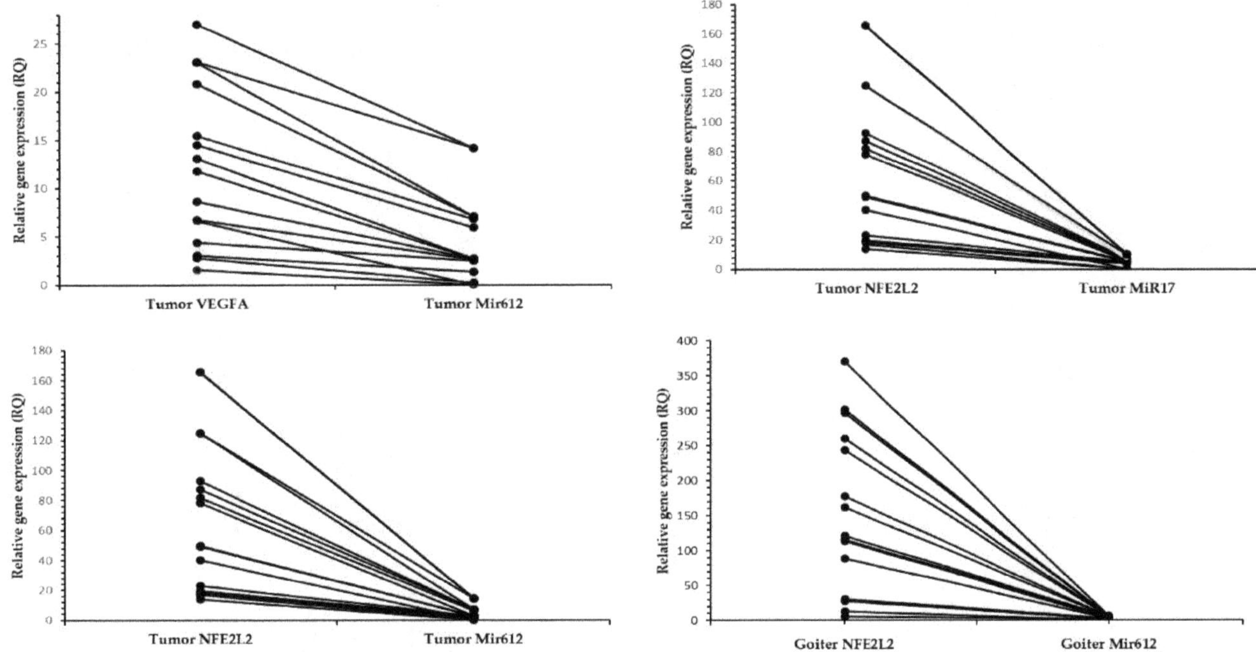

Figure 2. Relationship between relative expression levels of miRs and genes, showing high expression levels of genes and low expression levels of miRs. Each point represents an individual sample, for which the two gene expression levels are correspondingly connected. RQ, relative quantification.

3.4. Expression of VEGFA and NRF2 Proteins in Tissues

The protein levels of VEGFA were higher in the tumor compared to those in normal tissue ($p = 0.0009$), the goiter ($p = 0.0222$), and goiter-adjacent tissue ($p = 0.0003$). Tumor-adjacent tissue also presented elevated VEGFA protein levels compared to the normal tissues ($p = 0.0138$). The expression of VEGFA was upregulated in the goiter compared to the normal tissues ($p = 0.0397$) (Figure 3).

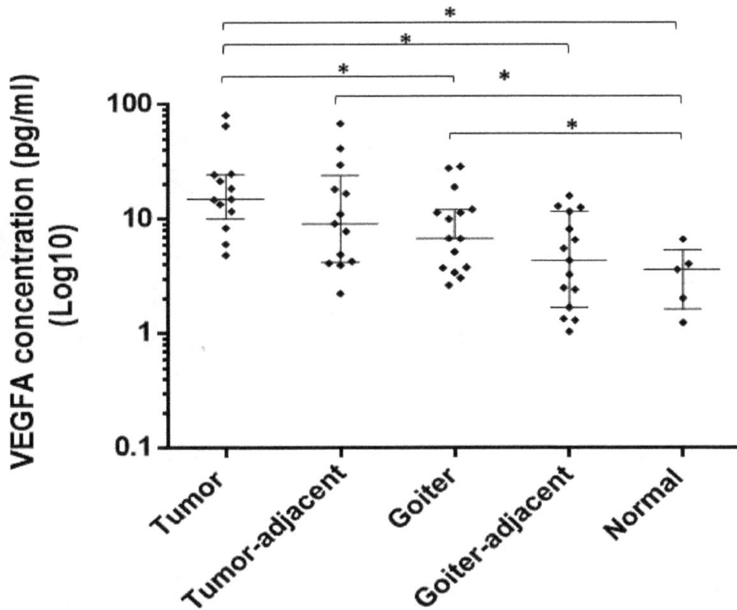

Figure 3. Protein expression of VEGFA in tumor, goiter, and normal tissue samples. VEGFA concentration was Log10 transformed (y-axis). Mann–Whitney test (* p value).

Expression of NRF2 protein in tumor tissues, colloid goiter, and normal tissues is shown in Figure 4. The cytoplasmic expression of NRF2 was higher in the tumor tissues compared to the normal tissues ($p < 0.0001$) and the goiter ($p < 0.0001$). In the nucleus, there was a stronger staining in the tumor tissue compared to the goiter tissue ($p < 0.0001$); no nuclear staining was observed in the normal thyroid tissues.

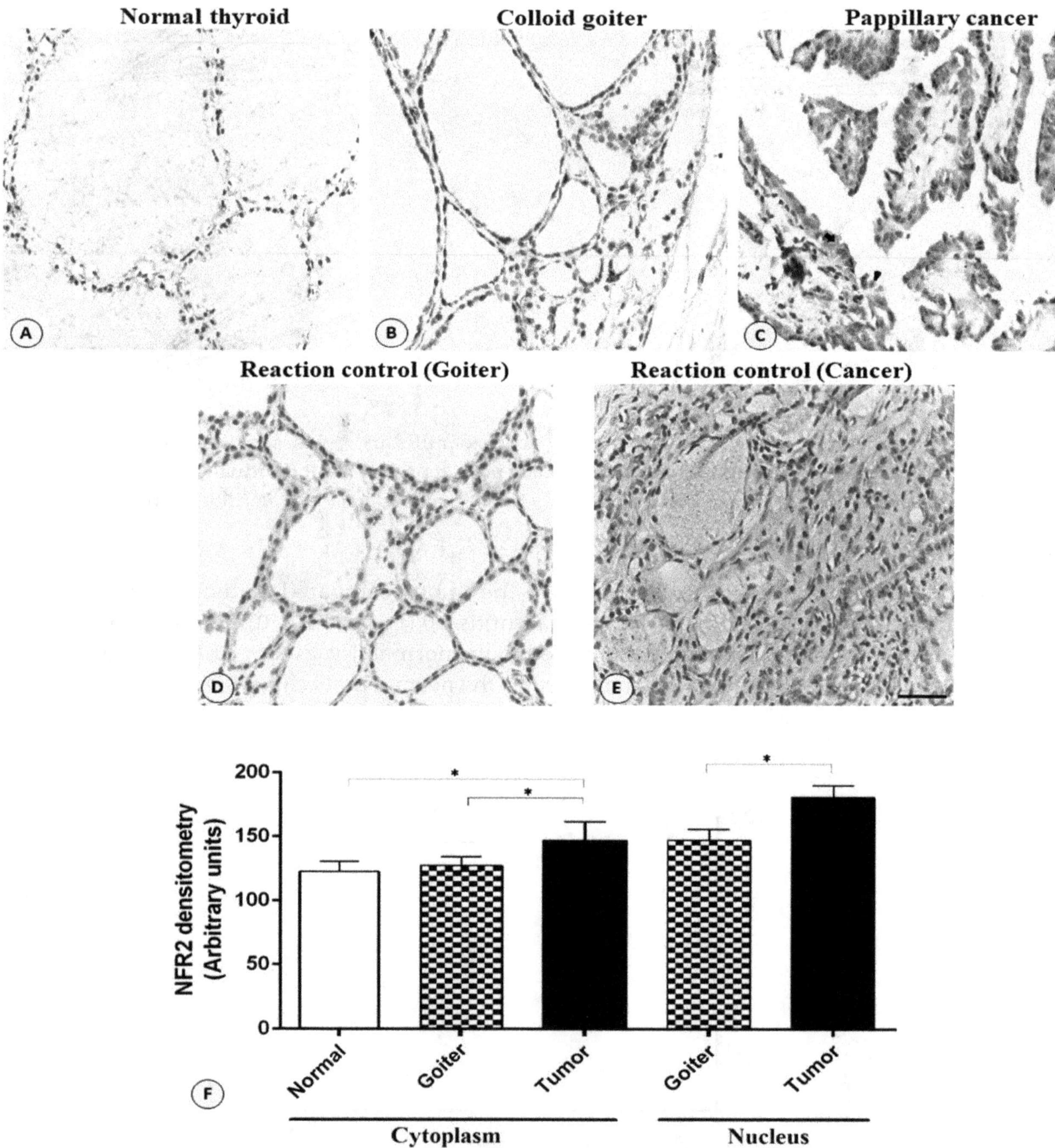

Figure 4. Expression of the NRF2 protein in the thyroid gland. Increased expression in the cytoplasm and nucleus in different tissues. (**A**) Normal thyroid tissue. (**B**) Colloid goiter. (**C**) Papillary thyroid cancer. (**D**) Negative controls of the goiter and (**E**) tumor. Section thickness, 5 μm; contra-staining, hematoxylin; scale bars, 20 μm. (**F**) Densitometric analysis of NRF2 quantification. The data represent the mean ± SEM of the densitometric index. *, $p < 0.0001$; bar size, 20 μm; arrows, cytoplasm; arrowhead, nucleus.

3.5. Superexpression Assay of miR-612 in the TPC-1 Cell Line

The transfection efficiency was checked on TPC-1 cells using the positive (mirVana™ miRNA Mimic miR-1 Positive Control, Life Technologies) and negative controls (mirVana ™ miRNA Mimic, Negative Control # 1, Life Technologies). Relative quantification ($2^{-\Delta\Delta Ct}$ method) of *TWF1* in cells treated with mirVana ™ miRNA Mimic miR-1 Positive Control revealed a 60% reduction in *TWF1* expression. The transfection with miR-612 did not show any significant difference in the expression of *VEGFA* and *NFE2L2* in the treated cells.

3.6. Inhibition Assay of miR-17-5p in the TPC-1 Cell Line

The transfection efficiency test for the inhibition assay using the positive control mirVana™ miRNA Inhibitor, let-7c positive control (Life Technologies) showed a 60% reduction in *HMGA2* expression. Transfection of miR-17-5p inhibitor into TPC-1 cells showed no difference in *VEGFA* expression, however, an approximately 73% inhibition in *NFE2L2* expression was noted (Figure 5).

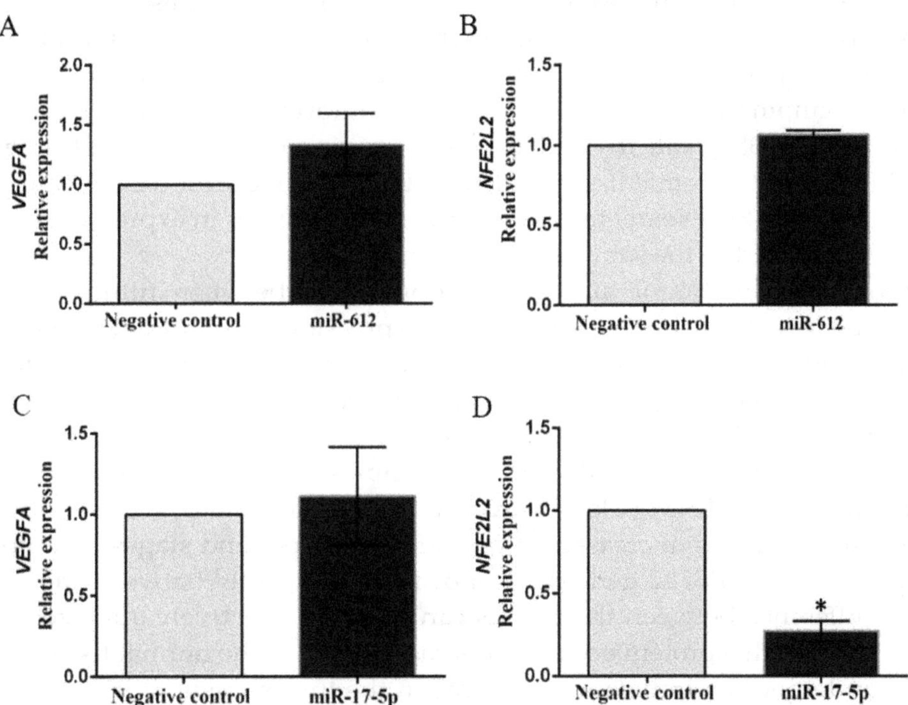

Figure 5. Results of the transfection assay on the TPC-1 cell line using mirVana™ miRNA Inhibitor for miR-17-5p, and mirVana™ miRNA Mimic for miR-612. *VEGFA* expression did not differ between cells transfected and non-transfected with miR-612 (**A**) and the inhibitor for miR-17-5p (**C**). *NFE2L2* expression did not differ between cells transfected and non-transfected with miR-612 (**B**); the inhibition of miR-17-5p resulted in approximately 73% inhibition of *NFE2L2* expression (**D**). *, approximately 73% inhibition of gene expression in relation to the negative control. Calibrator (negative control) log RQ = 1.

4. Discussion

We noted higher prevalence of cancer and goiter in females, which may be related to sex-differences. Porc et al. reported the first meta-analysis and revealed genetic factors that differentially affect thyroid function in males and females [14]. The present study shows that tissues affected by papillary thyroid cancer or colloid goiter, and their respective adjacent tissues present increased expression of *VEGFA* and *NFE2L2*, thereby providing evidence that vascularization and oxidative stress are imbalanced in these tissues. Corroborating with our results, earlier studies have shown that the expression of the *VEGFA* is higher in thyroid cancer, and may be crucial for the development of goiter, since the proliferation of endothelial cells precedes that of thyroid cells [15–18]. Studies have reported functional defects and increased expression of *NFE2L2* in the thyroid. Since this gene is involved in the maintenance of homeostasis against the physiologically generated oxidative stress during thyroid hormone synthesis, its dysregulation may contribute to the development of goiter as well as tumorigenesis of thyroid [19–21]. It is noteworthy that the expression levels of these genes increase according to the type and degree of thyroid cancer progression [15,22].

We also observed the elevated expression of these genes in the tissues adjacent to the tumor tissues in relation to the normal tissues. This indicates that the organ affected by cancer and goiter present altered physiology. This result highlights the importance of the normal tissue as a normalizer of the expression data in gene expression studies, since the tissue adjacent to tumor may not represent the normality of the tissue in true sense and, in fact, may present some of cellular alterations that precede these diseases. To the best of our knowledge, this is the first study to analyze the expression of *VEGFA* and *NFE2L2* in normal thyroid tissue for comparison with tumor tissue and goiter, as other studies have used adjacent non-malignant tissues for comparison.

The TCGA (The Cancer Genome Atlas Program) thyroid cancer dataset showed that VEGFA and NFE2L2 were highly expressed in normal tissue (n = 59) when compared with the primary tumor (n = 505). When analyzing the histology of thyroid tumors, it was found that, for VEGFA, the follicular thyroid papillary carcinoma (n = 102) was the closest to normal tissue, while the classical thyroid papillary carcinoma (n = 358), tall thyroid papillary carcinoma (n = 36) and others (n = 9) were down-regulated in relation to normal tissue. All NFE2L2 levels in cancer tissues were down-regulated in relation to normal tissue (Supplementary Material). These changes in expression levels in relation to normal tissue may be related to the sample number analyzed.

A comparison between tumor and colloid goiter and between tumor-adjacent tissue and goiter-adjacent tissue revealed a significantly higher expression of the *VEGFA* gene in the samples of colloid goiter and its adjacent tissue. This increase in the expression of the *VEGFA* gene in goiter may be due to several factors. Increasing endothelial cells is the first step in goiter formation, which exhibits levels of *VEGFA* expression similar to those observed in some types of thyroid cancer [23–25]. It is also worth mentioning that most of the papillary cancer samples analyzed in the present study presented early stages according to the TNM (Classification of Malignant Tumors) classification and that the levels of *VEGFA* gene expression increased according to the types and stages of tumor [15].

The expression of the *NFE2L2* gene did not differ significantly between the tissues. Evidence suggests that the difference between the tissues can be more effectively analyzed with the protein analysis of NRF2, because this protein occurs in degraded form in the normal tissue. In benign lesions, this degradation undergoes an imbalance, whereas in the tumor tissue it is possible to observe the migration of NRF2 to the nucleus, where this factor acts in response to oxidative stress, thus activating antioxidant enzymes [20,22].

In addition, the expression of miR-17-5p and miR-612 in PTC and colloid goiter samples and their respective adjacent tissues was also verified in comparison to the normal tissues, since these miRs may be related to the regulation of the genes investigated in this study. The results showed that miR-17-5p and miR-612 were not differentially expressed in tumor samples, and only miR-612 expression was reduced in tumor-adjacent tissue. In colloid goiter samples and goiter-adjacent tissue, the expression of these miRs was reduced.

MiR-17-5p has been studied in several cancers types, including thyroid cancer, and the results point to an elevated expression in tumor tissues [26–28]. However, the data available for PTC are not consistent with our findings. Zhao and Li (2015) observed significantly reduced miR-17-5p expression in thyroid papillary cancer samples in comparison to tumor-adjacent tissues [29]. The present study, however, did not find significant differences between the expression levels of miR-17-5p in tumor and non-tumor adjacent tissues, but a slight decrease in expression was observed; a larger sample size is required to reach a conclusion. Expression levels of miR-17-5p, on the other hand, were significantly reduced in the colloid goiter samples compared to those in normal tissues. No reports were found in the literature that corroborate or contrast with the findings of the present study. In the comparison between the tumor and goiter samples, we detected a significant increase in miR-17-5p expression in the tumor samples, indicating that even in initial stages the malignant tissue presents alteration of expression in comparison to the benign tissue.

Expression of miR-612 showed no significant difference in the tumor tissues, although its relative expression was low in these samples. However, in the tumor-adjacent tissues, colloid goiter and goiter-adjacent tissues, the expression of miR-612 was significantly reduced compared to that in the normal tissues. It was previously shown that this miR-612 exhibits reduced expression in colorectal cancer [30] and hepatocellular carcinoma (HCC), and that its expression is inversely proportional to tumor progression and aggressiveness in HCC [31]. Our results, deviating from the observations in HCC and colorectal cancer, suggest that the expression of this miR could increase with the degree of cellular alterations that lead to tumor formation, since the tumor-adjacent tissues and the goiter samples have significantly reduced expression of miR-612. As no data on miR-612 expression in PTC are available, further investigations are needed to clarify the role of miR-612 in this and other types of thyroid disorders.

The protein quantification results of VEGFA showed that the papillary cancer samples, the tumor-adjacent tissues, and the colloid goiter samples had increased expression of this protein in comparison to the normal tissues. In the comparisons between goiter and tissues adjacent to the goiter as well as between tumor tissues and tumor-adjacent tissues, no difference in VEGFA protein or transcript levels was observed. A comparison of VEGFA levels between tumor and goiter samples showed significantly higher expression in the tumor, a result suggesting a relation at the protein level opposite to that we observed in mRNA levels. This contradictory result between protein and transcript levels suggests that tumor tissue and goiter may present different mechanisms of post-transcriptional or post-translational regulation that could result in lower amounts of protein present in goiter.

In addition, VEGFA also participates in angiogenic stimulation through inhibition of PTEN (phosphatase and tensin homolog) expression. VEGFA triggers a cascade of signaling events, including activation of mitogen-activated protein kinase (MAPK) and phosphorylation of the Elk-1 transcription factor. These events promote an increase in the expression of members of the miR-17-92 group, repressing PTEN expression. It is known that the reduced expression of PTEN protein is associated with the development of thyroid cancer through the proliferation of endothelial cells. On the contrary, the genetic inactivation of miR-17-92 in endothelial cells results in peripheral vascular impairment in vivo [32,33]. These findings reinforce the importance of increased VEGFA protein in tumors and may explain the higher protein quantification observed in the tumor samples in comparison to the goiter.

Using the immunohistochemistry technique, it was possible to observe the presence of NRF2 protein, which is activated by oxidative stress, migrating from the cell cytoplasm to the nucleus where it exerts the function of transcription factor. The results observed in the present study showed that the labeling of this protein in the normal tissue is very weak (almost undetectable), and is observed only in the cytoplasm. In goiter, the labeling is intensified and it is already possible, in some cases, to observe the protein in the nucleus. Finally, in the tumor tissue, it is possible to see a strong labeling in the cytoplasm and nucleus. These data indicate that NRF2 protein is activated in PTC. Consistent with our data, Ziros et al. (2013) also observed the same labeling pattern in normal thyroid tissue, benign lesions and papillary cancer [20]. A recent study by Geng et al. (2017) indicates that the Nrf2 pathway is commonly activated in PTC and occasionally is activated in benign thyroid lesions, suggesting that prolonged activation of NRF2 and its elevated expression may contribute to the occurrence of nodular goiter and PTC [22]. The presence of strong labeling of the NRF2 protein in the nucleus of tumor cells reinforces its role in the regulation of antioxidant response related genes [34].

To obtain information about the possible miRs involved in the regulation of the *NFE2L2* and *VEGFA* genes, a database search was performed. Bioinformatic analysis revealed that miR-17-5p targets both *VEGFA* and *NFE2L2* genes. Previous studies have shown the interaction between miR-17 and *VEGFA* in the skin [35] and kidney [36,37]. The interaction of this miR with the *NFE2L2* gene was observed in the mammary gland [38]. The miR-612 showed regular expression of the *VEGFA* gene in the bone marrow [39]. To date, there are no studies that prove the interaction of miR-612 with *NFE2L2;* however, according to the databases consulted, miR-612 is predicted to regulate the *NFE2L2* gene.

After bioinformatic analysis, the inhibitor for miR-17-5p and the miR-612 mimic were selected for transfection into the TPC-1 cell line. The present study showed that inhibition of miR-17-5p resulted in reduced expression of the *NFE2L2* gene in the TPC-1 cells. The miR-17 cluster is known to reduce the expression of the *PTEN* gene. The *PTEN* gene is important for angiogenesis as it regulates genes such as *NFE2L2*. Rojo et al. (2014) showed that the inhibition of miR-17 increased *PTEN* expression, which in turn has a role in Nrf2 degradation pathway [40]. In the present study inhibition of miR-17-5p resulted in a decrease in *NFE2L2* expression, corroborating previous findings; however, the tissue expression data showed a negative correlation between the expression of this miR-17-5p and the *NFE2L2* gene. These contrasting results may reflect the participation of other active pathways in thyroid cancer that could influence *NFE2L2* expression. It is also worth mentioning the differences found between the findings of fresh tumor tissue samples and cell culture. Although in vitro studies are extremely important for functional studies, they cannot reproduce the complexity of the tumor microenvironment, nor can they mimic the different pathways involved in the disease progression.

The genes and miRs evaluated in this study present great potential for the diagnosis of colloid goiter and papillary cancer since they presented differential expression in these tissues. VEGFA and NRF2 proteins have been shown to be efficient in differentiating normal tissues from PTC. The negative regulation of miR-17-5p and miR-612 in colloid goiter also suggest the performance of these miRs as biomarkers for this thyroid condition.

Angiogenesis, oxidative stress, and deregulation of miRs are crucial for the development of thyroid disorders and cancer. The two genes evaluated in the present study can be possible therapeutic targets in the angiogenesis of thyroid disorders since the feedback between these genes and their regulation via miRs is of great importance for tumor development.

5. Conclusions

NFE2L2 and *VEGFA* genes and their protein products are widely expressed in PTC and colloid goiter. miR-612 has differential expression in the thyroid tumor and colloid goiter, while miR-17 is expressed only in the goiter. Hsa-miR-17-5p positively regulates the expression of the *NFE2L2* gene in PTC. This study showed the important relationship between miR-17-5p and *NFE2L2*, evidenced by the functional experiments. However, further studies regarding the influence of miR17-5p on *NFE2L2* and *VEGFA* and on the formation of new vessels in the colloid goiter and in PTC are needed.

Author Contributions: Conceptualization, L.P.S.; data curation, L.P.S. and P.M.B.-C.; formal analysis, L.P.S. and M.M.U.C.-N.; methodology, L.P.S., M.M.U.C.-N., N.M.-S., J.A.P.N., D.d.-S.N. and A.P.G.; resources, E.C.P. and E.M.G.-B.; supervision, E.M.G.-B.; bioinformatics analysis, T.H.; validation, L.P.S.; writing—original draft, L.P.S. and N.M.-S.; writing—review and editing, L.P.S. All authors have read and agreed to the published version of the manuscript.

Acknowledgments: TPC-1 cells were provided by Janete Cerutti, Federal University of São Paulo (UNIFESP).

References

1. Medeiros-Neto, G. Multinodular Goiter. In *Endotext*; De Groot, L.J., Chrousos, G., Dungan, K., Feingold, K.R., Grossman, A., Hershman, J.M., Koch, C., Korbonits, M., McLachlan, R., New, M., et al., Eds.; MDText.com, Inc.: Dartmouth, MA, USA, 2016.
2. Gandolfi, P.P.; Frisina, A.; Raffa, M.; Renda, F.; Rocchetti, O.; Ruggeri, C.; Tombolini, A. The incidence of thyroid carcinoma in multinodular goiter: Retrospective analysis. *Acta Bio Med. Atenei Parm.* **2004**, *75*, 114–117.
3. Campbell, M.J.; Seib, C.D.; Candell, L.; Gosnell, J.E.; Duh, Q.Y.; Clark, O.H.; Shen, W.T. The underestimated risk of cancer in patients with multinodular goiters after a benign fine needle aspiration. *World J. Surg.* **2015**, *39*, 695–700. [CrossRef]
4. Ferlay, J.; Shin, H.-R.; Bray, F.; Forman, D.; Mathers, C.; Parkin, D.M. Estimates of worldwide burden of cancer in 2008: GLOBOCAN 2008. *Int. J. Cancer* **2010**, *127*, 2893–2917. [CrossRef]
5. Jemal, A. Cancer Statistics, 2010. *CA Cancer J. Clin.* **2011**, *61*, 133. [CrossRef]
6. DeLellis, R.A. *Pathology and Genetics of Tumours of Endocrine Organs*; IARC Press: Lyon, France, 2004; p. 320.
7. Biselli-Chicote, P.M.; Oliveira, A.R.; Pavarino, E.C.; Goloni-Bertollo, E.M. VEGF gene alternative splicing: Pro- and anti-angiogenic isoforms in cancer. *J. Cancer Res. Clin. Oncol.* **2012**, *138*, 363–370. [CrossRef]
8. Ferrara, N.; Gerber, H.P.; LeCouter, J. The biology of VEGF and its receptors. *Nat. Med.* **2003**, *9*, 669–676. [CrossRef]
9. Sporn, M.B.; Liby, K.T. NRF2 and cancer: The good, the bad and the importance of context. *Nat. Rev. Cancer* **2012**, *12*, 564–571. [CrossRef]
10. Bartel, D.P. MicroRNAs: Genomics, biogenesis, mechanism, and function. *Cell* **2004**, *116*, 281–297. [CrossRef]
11. Greene, F.L. The American Joint Committee on Cancer: Updating the strategies in cancer staging. *Bull. Am. Coll. Surg.* **2002**, *87*, 13–15. [PubMed]
12. Pfaffl, M.W. A new mathematical model for relative quantification in real-time RT-PCR. *Nucleic Acids Res.* **2001**, *29*, e45. [CrossRef] [PubMed]
13. Tanaka, J.; Ogura, T.; Sato, H.; Hatano, M. Establishment and biological characterization of an in vitro human cytomegalovirus latency model. *Virology* **1987**, *161*, 62–72. [CrossRef]
14. Porcu, E.; Medici, M.; Pistis, G.; Volpato, C.B.; Wilson, S.G.; Cappola, A.R.; Bos, S.D.; Deelen, J.; den Heijer, M.; Freathy, R.M.; et al. A meta-analysis of thyroid-related traits reveals novel loci and gender-specific differences in the regulation of thyroid function. *PLoS Genet.* **2013**, *9*, e1003266. [CrossRef] [PubMed]
15. Salajegheh, A.; Pakneshan, S.; Rahman, A.; Dolan-Evans, E.; Zhang, S.; Kwong, E.; Gopalan, V.; Lo, C.Y.; Smith, R.A.; Lam, A.K. Co-regulatory potential of vascular endothelial growth factor-A and vascular endothelial growth factor-C in thyroid carcinoma. *Hum. Pathol.* **2013**, *44*, 2204–2212. [CrossRef] [PubMed]
16. Salajegheh, A.; Vosgha, H.; Rahman, M.A.; Amin, M.; Smith, R.A.; Lam, A.K. Interactive role of miR-126 on VEGF-A and progression of papillary and undifferentiated thyroid carcinoma. *Hum. Pathol.* **2016**, *51*, 75–85. [CrossRef] [PubMed]
17. Malkomes, P.; Oppermann, E.; Bechstein, W.O.; Holzer, K. Vascular endothelial growth factor–marker for proliferation in thyroid diseases? *Exp. Clin. Endocrinol. Diabetes* **2013**, *121*, 6–13. [CrossRef]
18. Mohamad Pakarul Razy, N.H.; Wan Abdul Rahman, W.F.; Win, T.T. Expression of Vascular Endothelial Growth Factor and Its Receptors in Thyroid Nodular Hyperplasia and Papillary Thyroid Carcinoma: A Tertiary Health Care Centre Based Study. *Asian Pac. J. Cancer Prev. APJCP* **2019**, *20*, 277–282. [CrossRef] [PubMed]
19. Martinez, V.D.; Vucic, E.A.; Pikor, L.A.; Thu, K.L.; Hubaux, R.; Lam, W.L. Frequent concerted genetic mechanisms disrupt multiple components of the NRF2 inhibitor KEAP1/CUL3/RBX1 E3-ubiquitin ligase complex in thyroid cancer. *Mol. Cancer* **2013**, *12*, 124. [CrossRef]
20. Ziros, P.G.; Manolakou, S.D.; Habeos, I.G.; Lilis, I.; Chartoumpekis, D.V.; Koika, V.; Soares, P.; Kyriazopoulou, V.E.; Scopa, C.D.; Papachristou, D.J.; et al. Nrf2 is commonly activated in papillary thyroid carcinoma, and it controls antioxidant transcriptional responses and viability of cancer cells. *J. Clin. Endocrinol. Metab.* **2013**, *98*, E1422–E1427. [CrossRef]
21. Teshiba, R.; Tajiri, T.; Sumitomo, K.; Masumoto, K.; Taguchi, T.; Yamamoto, K. Identification of a KEAP1 germline mutation in a family with multinodular goitre. *PLoS ONE* **2013**, *8*, e65141. [CrossRef]
22. Geng, W.J.; Shan, L.B.; Wang, J.S.; Li, N.; Wu, Y.M. Expression and significance of Nrf2 in papillary thyroid carcinoma and thyroid goiter. *Zhonghua Zhong Liu Za Zhi [Chin. J. Oncol.]* **2017**, *39*, 367–368. [CrossRef]

23. Ramsden, J.D. Angiogenesis in the thyroid gland. *J. Endocrinol.* **2000**, *166*, 475–480. [CrossRef] [PubMed]
24. Klein, M.; Catargi, B. VEGF in physiological process and thyroid disease. *Annales d Endocrinologie* **2007**, *68*, 438–448. [CrossRef] [PubMed]
25. Wolinski, K.; Stangierski, A.; Szczepanek-Parulska, E.; Gurgul, E.; Budny, B.; Wrotkowska, E.; Biczysko, M.; Ruchala, M. VEGF-C Is a Thyroid Marker of Malignancy Superior to VEGF-A in the Differential Diagnostics of Thyroid Lesions. *PLoS ONE* **2016**, *11*, e0150124. [CrossRef] [PubMed]
26. Gu, R.; Huang, S.; Huang, W.; Li, Y.; Liu, H.; Yang, L.; Huang, Z. MicroRNA-17 family as novel biomarkers for cancer diagnosis: A meta-analysis based on 19 articles. *Tumour Biol. J. Int. Soc. Oncodevelopmental Biol. Med.* **2016**, *37*, 6403–6411. [CrossRef] [PubMed]
27. Yuan, Z.M.; Yang, Z.L.; Zheng, Q. Deregulation of microRNA expression in thyroid tumors. *J. Zhejiang Univ. Sci. B* **2014**, *15*, 212–224. [CrossRef]
28. Yang, Z.; Yuan, Z.; Fan, Y.; Deng, X.; Zheng, Q. Integrated analyses of microRNA and mRNA expression profiles in aggressive papillary thyroid carcinoma. *Mol. Med. Rep.* **2013**, *8*, 1353–1358. [CrossRef]
29. Zhao, S.; Li, J. Sphingosine-1-phosphate induces the migration of thyroid follicular carcinoma cells through the microRNA-17/PTK6/ERK1/2 pathway. *PLoS ONE* **2015**, *10*, e0119148. [CrossRef]
30. Sheng, L.; He, P.; Yang, X.; Zhou, M.; Feng, Q. miR-612 negatively regulates colorectal cancer growth and metastasis by targeting AKT2. *Cell Death Dis.* **2015**, *6*, e1808. [CrossRef]
31. Tao, Z.H.; Wan, J.L.; Zeng, L.Y.; Xie, L.; Sun, H.C.; Qin, L.X.; Wang, L.; Zhou, J.; Ren, Z.G.; Li, Y.X.; et al. miR-612 suppresses the invasive-metastatic cascade in hepatocellular carcinoma. *J. Exp. Med.* **2013**, *210*, 789–803. [CrossRef]
32. Fiedler, J.; Thum, T. New Insights Into miR-17-92 Cluster Regulation and Angiogenesis. *Circ. Res.* **2016**, *118*, 9–11. [CrossRef]
33. Chamorro-Jorganes, A.; Lee, M.Y.; Araldi, E.; Landskroner-Eiger, S.; Fernandez-Fuertes, M.; Sahraei, M.; Quiles Del Rey, M.; van Solingen, C.; Yu, J.; Fernandez-Hernando, C.; et al. VEGF-Induced Expression of miR-17-92 Cluster in Endothelial Cells Is Mediated by ERK/ELK1 Activation and Regulates Angiogenesis. *Circ. Res.* **2016**, *118*, 38–47. [CrossRef] [PubMed]
34. Zhou, S.; Ye, W.; Zhang, M.; Liang, J. The effects of nrf2 on tumor angiogenesis: A review of the possible mechanisms of action. *Crit. Rev. Eukaryot. Gene Expr.* **2012**, *22*, 149–160. [CrossRef] [PubMed]
35. Greenberg, E.; Hajdu, S.; Nemlich, Y.; Cohen, R.; Itzhaki, O.; Jacob-Hirsch, J.; Besser, M.J.; Schachter, J.; Markel, G. Differential regulation of aggressive features in melanoma cells by members of the miR-17-92 complex. *Open Biol.* **2014**, *4*, 140030. [CrossRef] [PubMed]
36. Ye, W.; Lv, Q.; Wong, C.K.; Hu, S.; Fu, C.; Hua, Z.; Cai, G.; Li, G.; Yang, B.B.; Zhang, Y. The effect of central loops in miRNA:MRE duplexes on the efficiency of miRNA-mediated gene regulation. *PLoS ONE* **2008**, *3*, e1719. [CrossRef]
37. Karginov, F.V.; Hannon, G.J. Remodeling of Ago2-mRNA interactions upon cellular stress reflects miRNA complementarity and correlates with altered translation rates. *Genes Dev.* **2013**, *27*, 1624–1632. [CrossRef]
38. Pillai, M.M.; Gillen, A.E.; Yamamoto, T.M.; Kline, E.; Brown, J.; Flory, K.; Hesselberth, J.R.; Kabos, P. HITS-CLIP reveals key regulators of nuclear receptor signaling in breast cancer. *Breast Cancer Res. Treat.* **2014**, *146*, 85–97. [CrossRef]
39. Baraniskin, A.; Kuhnhenn, J.; Schlegel, U.; Chan, A.; Deckert, M.; Gold, R.; Maghnouj, A.; Zollner, H.; Reinacher-Schick, A.; Schmiegel, W.; et al. Identification of microRNAs in the cerebrospinal fluid as marker for primary diffuse large B-cell lymphoma of the central nervous system. *Blood* **2011**, *117*, 3140–3146. [CrossRef]
40. Rojo, A.I.; Rada, P.; Mendiola, M.; Ortega-Molina, A.; Wojdyla, K.; Rogowska-Wrzesinska, A.; Hardisson, D.; Serrano, M.; Cuadrado, A. The PTEN/NRF2 axis promotes human carcinogenesis. *Antioxid. Redox Signal.* **2014**, *21*, 2498–2514. [CrossRef]

7

The Adverse Effect of Hypertension in the Treatment of Thyroid Cancer with Multi-Kinase Inhibitors

Ole Vincent Ancker [1], Markus Wehland [2], Johann Bauer [3], Manfred Infanger [2] and Daniela Grimm [1,2,*]

1 Department of Biomedicine, Aarhus University, Wilhelm Meyers Allé 4, 8000 Aarhus C, Denmark; ole.vincent.ancker@post.au.dk
2 Clinic and Policlinic for Plastic, Aesthetic and Hand Surgery, Otto von Guericke University, Leipziger Str. 44, 39120 Magdeburg, Germany; markus.wehland@med.ovgu.de (M.W.); manfred.infanger@med.ovgu.de (M.I.)
3 Max-Planck-Institute for Biochemistry, Am Klopferspitz 18, 82152 Martinsried, Germany; jbauer@biochem.mpg.de
* Correspondence: dgg@biomed.au.dk

Academic Editor: Harry A. J. Struijker-Boudier

Abstract: The treatment of thyroid cancer has promising prospects, mostly through the use of surgical or radioactive iodine therapy. However, some thyroid cancers, such as progressive radioactive iodine-refractory differentiated thyroid carcinoma, are not remediable with conventional types of treatment. In these cases, a treatment regimen with multi-kinase inhibitors is advisable. Unfortunately, clinical trials have shown a large number of patients, treated with multi-kinase inhibitors, being adversely affected by hypertension. This means that treatment of thyroid cancer with multi-kinase inhibitors prolongs progression-free and overall survival of patients, but a large number of patients experience hypertension as an adverse effect of the treatment. Whether the prolonged lifetime is sufficient to develop sequelae from hypertension is unclear, but late-stage cancer patients often have additional diseases, which can be complicated by the presence of hypertension. Since the exact mechanisms of the rise of hypertension in these patients are still unknown, the only available strategy is treating the symptoms. More studies determining the pathogenesis of hypertension as a side effect to cancer treatment as well as outcomes of dose management of cancer drugs are necessary to improve future therapy options for hypertension as an adverse effect to cancer therapy with multi-kinase inhibitors.

Keywords: thyroid cancer; hypertension; vascular endothelial growth factor; multi-kinase inhibitors; lenvatinib; sorafenib; sunitinib

1. Introduction

The most common and effective strategies to treat thyroid cancer are surgery, radioactive iodine (RAI) therapy and thyroid-stimulating hormone (TSH) suppression treatment. This therapy regimen shows good results in patients affected by differentiated thyroid carcinoma (DTC) as well as a long-term survival rate of up to 90% [1]. The therapy options for de-differentiated thyroid cancers or for recurrent thyroid cancer are extremely limited. Poorly differentiated thyroid cancer types (PDTC) do not respond to RAI treatment and have a remarkably reduced survival rate. Under these circumstances, multi-kinase inhibitors, such as lenvatinib, sorafenib and sunitinib, may be useful. The multi-kinase inhibitors target an important step in the development of tumors. When a tumor reaches a critical level in its development, oxygen must be delivered through blood vessels and not simply by diffusion. At this point, the tumor produces new blood vessels and thereby obtains the required oxygen and nutrition to grow. The multi-kinase inhibitors work anti-angiogenically by preventing the transmission of signals from multiple tyrosine kinases, which are essential for the development of a new vasculature [2].

Along with their effects as cancer drugs, multi-kinase inhibitors have been shown to cause several unwanted side effects; examples are proteinuria, stomatitis, diarrhea and hypertension, the latter of which had been observed in up to half of the treated patients [3].

Hypertension, or elevated blood pressure, is a physical condition in which the pressure in the blood vessels is persistently raised and the heart must labor against higher systolic and/or higher diastolic pressure. Hypertension exists per definition when the systolic blood pressure (SBP) equals or exceeds 140 mmHg and/or the diastolic pressure (DBP) equals or exceeds 90 mmHg, whereas normal blood pressure is defined as 120 mmHg systolic and 80 mmHg diastolic [4].

Hypertension can physically be described by Ohm's law:

$$\text{blood pressure} = \text{cardiac output} \times \text{total periphery resistance}$$

Isolated hypertension, when not extremely elevated, is not dangerous and many people live with raised blood pressure without even being aware of it. However, hypertension can have severe impacts on overall health, numerous studies have shown that patients with hypertension have a higher risk of cardiovascular and renal diseases [5].

The aim of this review is to create an overview of hypertension as an adverse effect (AE) of multi-kinase inhibitors when treating metastatic RAI-refractory thyroid cancer. In addition, this review will focus on the function of multi-kinase inhibitors, and on the mechanisms of the development of hypertension. It will reflect the importance of hypertension as an AE.

This review will consider and address the following questions: (1) How do multi-kinase inhibitors cause hypertension? (2) How can we manage hypertension induced by tyrosine kinase inhibitor (TKI)-treatment? (3) Is the relationship between the efficacy of cancer treatment and the AE of hypertension favorable? (4) Is hypertension as a side effect of the multi-kinase inhibitors a severe concern?

2. Background

2.1. Thyroid Cancer

The thyroid gland is located in front of the tracheal tube. The function of the thyroid gland is to produce the thyroid hormones T3 and T4, which stimulate a great number of processes in the human body, such as metabolic rate, protein synthesis, development, and they also influence the cardiovascular system. Furthermore, the thyroid produces calcitonin, which plays a role in calcium homeostasis. The thyroid gland can be enlarged both by benign and malignant causes: it is often enlarged due to a dietary iodine deficiency that is not cancer associated (struma), but other tumors of the thyroid are caused by malignant alterations [6]. Thyroid cancer can be classified into several categories: differentiated (DTC), covering papillary (PTC) and follicular (FTC), medullary (MTC) and anaplastic thyroid cancer (ATC). The cancer cells in DTC appear similar to normal thyroid cells, whereas poorly differentiated thyroid cancer (PDTC) is comprised of cancer cells that do not share the same characteristics or abilities as normal thyroid cells [7].

PDTC is accountable for up to 10% of thyroid cancer forms and is more aggressive than DTC. Unfortunately, the prognosis for PDTC is not encouraging: the 5-, 10- and 15-year survival rates are 50%, 34% and 0%, respectively [8]. MTC has a 10-year survival rate of 75%–80% [9], whereas the 5-year survival rate for DTC is as high as 98% due to successful treatment, such as surgery, RAI ablation and treatment with thyroid stimulating hormone [10]. Regrettably, about 20% of patients experience recurrence of the disease. The recurrent form of thyroid cancer is poorly differentiated and thereby more malignant; this makes it for example resistant to RAI ablation because due to an inability to take up iodine [11].

The incidence of thyroid cancer in Denmark in 2012 was estimated to be 220 new cases, both sexes included, which places it in the intermediary group below the most common cancer types as colorectal, breast and prostate cancer [12]. In 2012, the incidence worldwide was 298,102 new cases for both sexes representing 2.1% of all cancers [13].

2.2. Multi-Kinase Inhibitors

Most thyroid cancer types have promising prospects as a result of surgical treatment and radioactive iodine ablation. PDTC, RAI-refractory carcinomas and tumors showing resistance to various forms of available treatment must be treated with alternatives in the hope of a good result [14].

Angiogenesis is the formation of new blood vessels from pre-existing vasculature and is a normal physiological process that starts during fetal development and persists in adults during inflammation and vascular or wound healing [15]. Angiogenesis is utilized by tumors to create new blood supply, so forming a path for the delivery of oxygen and nutrients, and in turn supporting tumor growth. Several factors play a role in the creation of new blood vessels, both in normal physiology and in pathophysiology. The growth of a tumor is determined by its nutrient supply. By diffusion alone, only very limited amounts can reach the tumor, and especially its core, so that for continued expansion, an increased internal blood supply is necessary. The central hypothesis is that an increase in tumor size must be preceded by expansion of tumor vasculature, which is stimulated by the tumor. Tumor cells take advantage of the normal physiological process involving the secretion of vascular endothelial growth factor (VEGF). VEGF is of high importance in the induction of new vessel formation and in the survival of endothelial cells [16–18]. Therefore, angiogenesis is a critical process for the development and subsequent growth of tumors.

The superfamily of VEGF comprises VEGF-A, VEGF-B, VEGF-C, VEGF-D and placental growth factor (PGF). Their corresponding tyrosine kinase receptors, the vascular endothelial growth factor receptors (VEGFRs) VEGFR-1, -2 and -3, are distinguished according to their affinities to different VEGFs. VEGFR-1 and -2 are found in endothelial cells, while VEGFR-3 is expressed in lymphatic endothelial cells. VEGFR-1 binds VEGF-A, VEGF-B and PGF, whereas VEGFR-2 binds VEGF-A and proteolytically modified VEGF-C and VEGF-D. Finally, VEGFR-3 is activated by VEGF-C and VEGF-D [19–21].

In addition, growth factors platelet derived growth factor (PDGF), epidermal growth factor (EGF), and fibroblast growth factor (FGF) also play a significant role in angiogenesis [19,20]. The ligand FGF and its receptor FGFR play an important role in cell growth, proliferation, differentiation and survival of thyroid cancer cells, where FGFR-1, -3 and -4 are overexpressed and expression of FGFR-2 is reduced. Binding of a growth factor to one of the receptors leads to a tyrosine kinase activation of either the mitogen activated protein kinase (MAPK) or the phosphatidylinositol-3-kinase (PI3K) pathway that eventually affect oncogenic gene expression [22].

There are two main pathways by which VEGF signaling can be interfered pharmacologically. Direct inhibition of VEGF is one possibility: an immunoglobulin designed specifically for VEGF targets and binds before the interaction with the corresponding receptor [23]. Another pathway focuses on inhibition of the phosphorylation cascade triggered after the binding of ligand and receptor by blocking the signal from the tyrosine receptor and thereby preventing the oncogenic features such as angiogenesis, proliferation and growth. Lenvatinib, sorafenib and sunitinib (Table 1) are drugs used in cancer therapy that inhibit multiple tyrosine kinases in thyroid cancer treatment [22].

Table 1. Characteristics of lenvatinib, sorafenib, and sunitinib.

Drug	Targets	Half-Life	Bioavailability	Metabolism
Lenvatinib	VEGF-R1-3, FGFR1-4, PDGF-RA, c-KIT, RET	28 h	85%	Hepatic CYP3A4
Sorafenib	VEGF-R1-3, PDGF-RA-D, C-RAF, B-RAF	25–48 h	38%–49%	Hepatic CYP3A4
Sunitinib	VEGF-R1-3, PDGF-RA-D, c-KIT, RET, CD114, CD135	40–60 h	50%	Hepatic CYP3A4

Lenvatinib is an orally taken TKI that targets VEGF-R1/-3, FGFR1-4, ret proto-oncogene (RET), and platelet derived growth factor receptor (PDGFRβ). By blocking these receptors, lenvatinib disturbs angiogenesis of the tumor, invasion of tissue and metastasis. By inhibiting VEGF-R1/-3, lenvatinib disrupts angiogenic processes in the tumor. Furthermore, lenvatinib inhibits RET, which is important for controlling tumor growth and, by hitting FGFR and PDGFRβ, it also influences the tumor's microenvironment, as presented in Figure 1 [22].

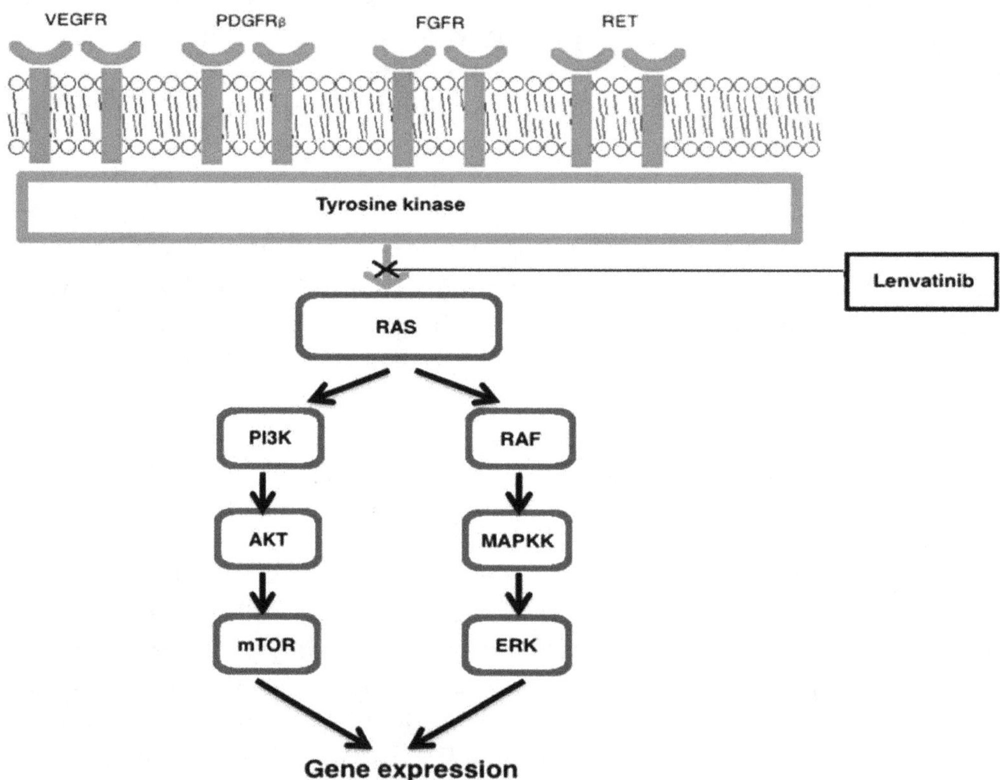

Figure 1. Lenvatinib inhibits signaling from VEGFR, PDGFRβ, FGFR and RET. It decreases angiogenesis and lymphogenesis, stunts tumor growth and damages the tumor's microenvironment [11,22]. VEGFR (vascular endothelial growth factor receptor), PDGFR (platelet derived growth factor receptor), FGFR (fibroblast growth factor receptor), RET (rearranged during transfection), RAS (rat sarcoma), PI3K (phosphatidylinositol-3-kinase), AKT (protein kinase B), mTOR (mammalian target of rapamycin), RAF (rapidly accelerated fibrosarcoma kinase), MAPKK (mitogen activated protein kinase kinase), ERK (extracellular signal regulated kinase).

Sunitinib (Sunitinib malate; Sutent; Pfizer, New York, USA) is a multi-targeted TKI used in the treatment of metastatic renal cell carcinomas (RCC) and gastrointestinal stromal tumors, and is under evaluation for other malignancies [11]. It inhibits VEGFR-1 and -2, platelet-derived growth factor receptors, stem cell factor receptor (c-KIT), FLT3 as well as RET kinases. Sunitinib acts on VEGF receptors and on RET and is therefore a suitable drug to treat RAI-refractory thyroid cancer. Sunitinib is still not approved for thyroid cancer therapy by the FDA, and therefore therapy approaches applying sunitinib are still off-label [11].

Sorafenib (NEXAVAR®) is widely used in cancer therapy and is an oral serine-threonine TKI that targets VEGFR-1/–3, PDGFR, BRAF, RET/PTC, and c-kit. The agent has an anti-proliferative effect and an anti-angiogenic activity by blocking the intracellular signal transduction of VEGFR2 in endothelial cells [11]. Sorafenib is a FDA-approved drug for patients with RAI-refractory metastatic thyroid cancer. The approval of sorafenib is based on the results of the randomized DECISION (stuDy of sorafEnib in loCally advanced or metastatIc patientS with radioactive Iodine refractory thyrOid caNcer) trial.

This was an international, multi-center, placebo-controlled study involving 417 thyroid cancer patients. The patients (400 mg oral sorafenib twice daily) lived on average nearly 11 months longer without disease progression compared to the placebo group [24–26].

2.3. Hypertension

The effects of VEGF are not only present in cancer cells: healthy endothelial cells also express VEGFRs and, because of this property, unwanted consequences may appear [20,27,28]. Hypertension is the most common adverse effect in the treatment of the tyrosine kinase inhibitors. VEGF is known to regulate the vasomotor tonus and maintains blood pressure by dilating small arterioles and venules. In case of an anti-VEGF therapy the result is a reduced density of microvessels (Figure 2). Hypertension has been reported to occur at a higher incidence in patients with DTC and treated with sorafenib [29]. Hypertension usually occurs in the first six weeks of treatment with sorafenib; therefore, blood pressure (BP) should be monitored regularly (at least once a week) at the start of sorafenib therapy [30].

In the SELECT trial (ClinicalTrials.gov number, NCT01321554), lenvatinib, compared to placebo, revealed significant improvements in progression-free survival and the response rate in patients with RAI-refractory thyroid cancer, but it also induced more adverse effects [31]. Treatment-related adverse effects (TEAE) of any grade, occurring in more than 40% of lenvatinib-treated patients were hypertension (in 67.8% of the patients), diarrhea (in 59.4%), fatigue or asthenia (in 59.0%), decreased appetite (in 50.2%), decreased weight (in 46.4%), and nausea (in 41.0%) [31]. Cabanillas et al. [32] investigated 58 patients with advanced, progressive, RAI-refractory DTC, receiving lenvatinib 24 mg once daily in 28-day cycles until disease progression, unmanageable toxicity, withdrawal, or death. TEAE were evaluated: 44 patients had hypertension (all grades 76%) and six patients had grade 3 TEAE (10%). Most patients with hypertension and proteinuria were managed successfully without lenvatinib dose adjustments [32].

There is no unanimous agreement on how these cancer drugs result in hypertension, but some hypotheses have gained a footing in explaining why. One explanation depends on reduced production of the vasodilator, nitric oxide (NO). Blockage of VEGF induces vasoconstriction. VEGFR-2 signaling generates nitric oxide (NO) and prostaglandin I2, which induces endothelial cell-dependent vasodilatation in arterioles and venules. Inhibition of VEGFR-2 signaling reduces NO synthase expression and NO synthesis. Normally, activation of VEGFR-2, by VEGF or shear stress in the vessel walls, induces the PI3K pathway, resulting in an increased production of the vasodilator NO and hence a reduction of peripheral resistance and blood pressure. VEGF inhibition results in an increase in vascular resistance, followed by hypertension. The multi-kinase inhibitors prevent the phosphorylation cascade and thus the formation of NO, leading to a rise in blood pressure [33]. In addition, an increase in blood pressure may also result from the VEGF/VEGFR inhibition in the kidney. VEGF and VEGFR are also expressed in podocytes. Electron microscopy images revealed glomerular lesions associated with VEGF-targeted therapies [34]. The reduced VEGF activity influences renal endothelial cells and podocytes and results in a dysregulation of VEGF expression and a downregulation of tight junction proteins with the consequence of proteinuria. As an alternative explanation to the theory of the lack of NO, an increased amount of the vasoconstrictor endothelin-1 (ET-1) has been suggested. ET-1 binds to its receptors in endothelial cells causing the smooth muscle cells to contract and thus increase resistance in the vessels and raise the blood pressure [35,36].

A study has considered a third theory that suggests hypertension is due to a decrease in the number of small arterioles and capillaries, leading to higher peripheral resistance and thereby to increased blood pressure. The authors found that patients treated with anti-angiogenic medicaments showed fewer mucosal capillaries. However, the study was not able to determine whether the observed effects were a consequence of a direct lack of small arterioles or simply a hypo-perfusion of these, since the technique used for recording the numbers of vessels depended on perfusion. Both a decreased number of arterioles or a stopping of perfusion of existing ones could explain a rise in blood pressure, since the blood is distributed in fewer vessels, increasing resistance inside them [37].

Some studies have shown a rapid increase in blood pressure, which challenges the understanding of the mechanisms giving rise to hypertension, and argues against a structural or anatomical explanation of acute induced hypertension. However, rapid rises of hypertension make a theory of active vasomodulators more likely [38]. Risk factors for hypertension occurring upon TKI therapy are of older age, obesity, high sodium intake, alcohol abuse, smoking or reduced physical activity. A pre-existing high blood pressure or certain VEGF polymorphisms might be associated with a lower risk of grade 3 or 4 hypertension.

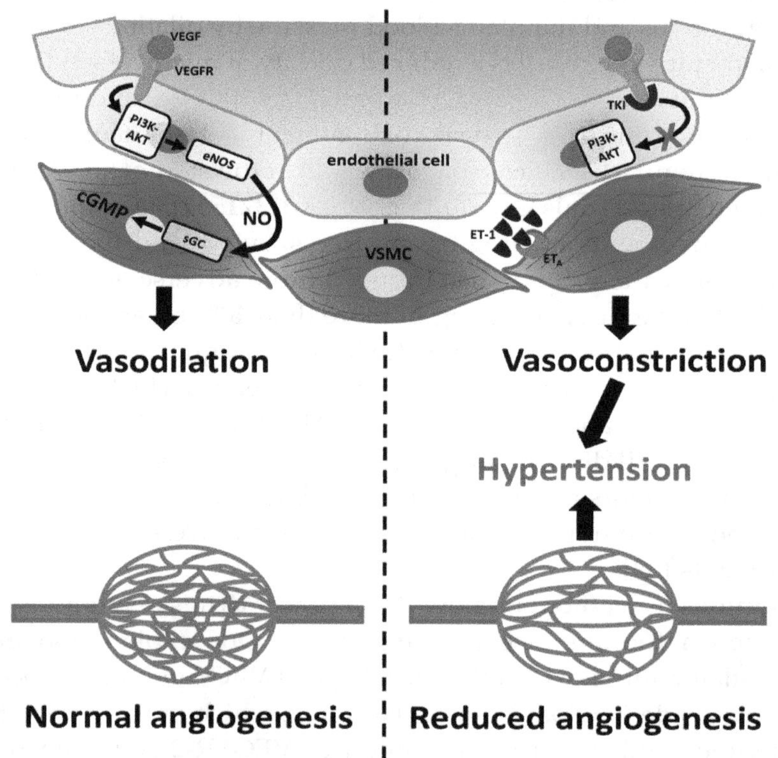

Figure 2. The effects of VEGF on blood pressure and capillary vascularization under: physiological conditions (**left**); and TKI therapy (**right**) (adapted from [39]). VEGF (vascular endothelial growth factor), VEGFR (vascular endothelial growth factor receptor), PI3K (phosphatidylinositol-3-kinase), AKT (protein kinase B), eNOS (endothelial nitric oxide synthase), sGC (soluble guanylyl cyclase), ET-1 (endothelin-1), ET_A (endothelin receptor type A), NO (nitric oxide), cGMP (cyclic guanosine monophosphate).

2.4. *Efficacy of Cancer Drug Treatment*

A recent study [31] has monitored the efficacy of lenvatinib, compared with placebo, in adults with DTC, RAI-refractory cancer and without prior treatment with a multi-kinase inhibitor. The primary endpoints were either progression of the cancer disease or death. Patients treated with lenvatinib had a median progression-free survival of 18.3 months, whereas placebo-treated patients had a progression-free survival of only 3.6 months. The six month progression-free survival rate for the patients treated with lenvatinib was 77.5%, while the rate for placebo-treated patients was 25.4%. Patients receiving lenvatinib also had more AE. Treatment-related AE of any grade occurred in more than 40% of patients in the lenvatinib group; for example, hypertension (in 67.8% of the patients), diarrhea (in 59.4%), and others [31].

Another study published in December 2015 showed similar results: Japanese patients with DTC, RAI-refractory disease and a progression in disease in the last 13 months were eligible. Patients treated with lenvatinib experienced a median progression-free survival of 16.5 months, while the placebo group had a progression-free survival of 3.7 months. The six-month progression-free survival rate was 70.0% for lenvatinib-treated patients and 31.7% for placebo-treated patients [40]. The most common AE (any grade) in Japanese patients from the SELECT trial was hypertension (86.7%).

Taken together, the findings of the SELECT trial provided the basis for the FDA approval of lenvatinib for the treatment of progressive RAI-refractory thyroid cancer. Another study investigated 59 patients with unresectable progressive MTC [41]. They received lenvatinib (24 mg daily, 28-day cycles) until disease progression, unmanageable toxicity, withdrawal, or death. Lenvatinib had a high objective response rate, a high disease control rate, and a short median time to response. Toxicities were managed with dose modifications and medications. Most hypertension and proteinuria events were grade 1 or 2 and managed with standard drug therapy. The median duration of treatment was 264 days (range, 13–547 days). Withdrawal from therapy due to hypertension: one patient (2%).

Hypertension is a condition that affects the cardiovascular system in the body. It is an abstract condition because not all patients have the same tolerance of raised pressure. Some may experience serious cardiovascular outcomes, while others can live their whole life with hypertension without showing any symptoms. Studies show that hypertension is associated with many different cardiovascular diseases, where almost all have a high mortality rate, such as intracerebral hemorrhage, subarachnoid hemorrhage, stable angina pectoris, myocardial infarction, aorta aneurysm and heart failure [42].

Most patients with hypertension as an adverse effect continue the treatment of cancer. In a lenvatinib-versus-placebo study, only 1.1% of patients had to stop the treatment because of hypertensive effects and 19.9% were given a lower dose because of a rise in BP [31]. Nearly all patients with this form of hypertension manage the symptoms with normal anti-hypertensive drugs. Patients with unmanageable hypertension and signs of organ damage, renal dysfunction or cardiovascular diseases need intervention in the form of either a lower dose or a total stop of treatment [38]. Hypertension, and other AE from TKI-treatment are currently under investigation. Several clinical trials are investigating this concern, both examining the direct AE of lenvatinib, but also whether lower doses of the drug can show the same effect while giving fewer unwanted effects. An overview of recent studies is given in Table 2.

Table 2. Overview of recent clinical trials studying lenvatinib, sunitinib, and sorafenib, website used on 7 March 2017 [43].

Title	Design	Objective	Status
A phase I trial of lenvatinib (multi-kinase inhibitor) and capecitabine (Antimetabolite) in patients with advanced malignancies. NCT02915172	Interventional open label	This phase I study aims to find the highest tolerable dose of lenvatinib and Capecitabine that can be given to patients with advanced cancer.	Not yet recruiting
Post-marketing surveillance of lenvatinib mesylate in patients with unresectable thyroid cancer. NCT02430714	Observational cohort prospective	The objective of this study is to find unknown adverse reactions, adverse drug reactions, efficacy, safety and effectiveness factors, incidence of hypertension, hemorrhagic, and thromboembolic effects and liver disorder.	Recruiting
A multi center, randomized, double-blind phase II trial of lenvatinib (E7080) in subjects with iodine-131 refractory differentiated thyroid cancer (RR-DTC) to evaluate whether an oral starting dose of 20 mg or 14 mg daily will provide comparable efficacy to a 24 mg starting dose, but have a better safety profile. NCT02702388	Interventional double blind randomized	This randomized double-blinded study aims to investigate whether a lower starting dose of lenvatinib can provide comparable efficacy whilst showing a better safety profile for the patients.	Active Not recruiting

Table 2. *Cont.*

Title	Design	Objective	Status
An open label phase I dose escalation study of E7080 administered to patients with solid tumors. NCT00280397	Interventional open label	This study investigates the maximum tolerable dose and the related effects of E7080 (lenvatinib) given to patients with solid tumors with no successful treatment.	Completed
A phase II study of E7080 in subjects with advanced thyroid cancer. NCT01728623	Interventional open label	This study was performed to evaluate the safety, efficacy and pharmacokinetics of E7080 (lenvatinib), taken orally daily in patients with advanced thyroid cancer.	Completed
An open label phase I dose escalation study of E7080. NCT00121719	Interventional open label	This study aims to find the maximum tolerated dose of lenvatinib in patients with solid tumors or lymphomas.	Active Not recruiting
Phase II, multi-center, open-label, single arm trial to evaluate the safety and efficacy of oral E7080 in medullary and iodine-131 refractory, unresectable differentiated thyroid cancers, stratified by histology. NCT00784303	Interventional open label non-randomized	This is a phase II study that aimed to investigate the safety and efficacy of oral E7080 (lenvatinib) in medullary and iodine-131 refractory, unresectable differentiated thyroid cancer.	Completed
Phase II study assessing the efficacy and safety of lenvatinib for anaplastic thyroid cancer (HOPE). NCT02726503	Interventional open label	This phase II study aims to investigate the efficacy and safety of lenvatinib for unresectable anaplastic thyroid cancer.	Recruiting
A multi-center, randomised, double-blind, placebo-controlled, phase III trial of lenvatinib (E7080) in I-131-refractory differentiated thyroid cancer in China. NCT02966093	Interventional double blind randomized	This phase III study primarily aims to compare progression-free survival of participants with radioiodine refractory differentiated thyroid cancer treated with lenvatinib or placebo, and secondarily to investigate adverse events.	Not yet recruiting
Post-marketing surveillance of Lenvima in Korean patients. NCT02764554	Observational prospective	This study aims to observe the safety profile of lenvatinib (Lenvima) in normal clinical practice.	Recruiting
Prospective, non-interventional, post-authorization safety study that includes all patients diagnosed as unresectable differentiated thyroid carcinoma and treated with sorafenib (JPMS-DTC). NCT02185560	Observational	Safety study that includes all patients diagnosed as unresectable differentiated thyroid carcinoma (DTC) and treated with sorafenib within a certain period.	Recruiting
Safety and efficacy of sorafenib in patients with advanced thyroid cancer: a Phase II clinical study. NCT02084732	Interventional	Describe the clinical activity and safety profile of sorafenib in the treatment of patients with advanced thyroid cancer (metastatic or recurrent) among a selected group of patients refractory to or ineligible to radioactive iodine (RAI) therapy.	Recruiting
Prospective, non-interventional, post-authorization safety study that includes all patients diagnosed as unresectable differentiated thyroid carcinoma and treated with sorafenib (JPMS-DTC). NCT02185560	Observational	This is a non-interventional, multi center post-authorization safety study that includes all patients diagnosed as unresectable differentiated thyroid carcinoma (DTC) and treated with sorafenib within a certain period.	Recruiting

Table 2. *Cont.*

Title	Design	Objective	Status
Thyroid cancer and sunitinib (THYSU). NCT00510640	Interventional	The objective of the trial is to determine the objective tumor response rate (efficacy) in patients with locally advanced or metastatic anaplastic, differentiated or medullary thyroid carcinoma treated with sunitinib; a secondary objective is to evaluate the safety of sunitinib in these patients	Completed
Sutent adjunctive treatment of differentiated thyroid cancer (IIT Sutent). NCT00668811	Interventional	The primary objective is to assess clinical benefit rate, defined as complete response, partial response, or stable disease per RECIST criteria. The secondary objective will be to assess the safety of Sutent in this patient population.	Completed

The study NCT02915172 includes both a phase I and a phase II study. The phase I study aims to decide the highest tolerable dose of lenvatinib and capecitabine in patients with advanced cancer. The initial dose for the first included group is 10 mg orally taken lenvatinib in a 21-day cycle. The phase II study wishes to determine whether the maximal tolerated dose found in the phase I study can be used for treating patients with advanced cancer including thyroid cancer. NCT02915172 takes place at the MD Anderson Cancer Center, Texas, USA, which is also the responsible party. The study will include 46 participants over the age of 18. The study was set to start December 2016 and the final data collection date is set to December 2022.

NCT02430714 and NCT02764554 are post-marketing surveillance studies of lenvatinib in patients with unresectable thyroid cancer. In NCT02430714, a dose of 24 mg orally taken once daily is administered to the patients and, in NCT02764554, the participants are in groups with 4 mg and 10 mg orally taken lenvatinib. The primary outcome is to decide the number of AE in the following year. NCT02430714 is conducted by the Japanese pharmaceutical company Eisai Co., Ltd., Japan, recruiting 400 participants including children, adults and seniors from centers in Osaka and Tokyo, Japan. The study was set to start May 2015 and the final data collection date is March 2025. NCT02764554 is performed by the Korean pharmaceutical company Eisai Korea Inc. The estimated number of enrolled patients is 3000 including children, adults and seniors recruiting from Seoul, Republic of Korea. The start date of the surveillance study was September 2016 with a final data collection date of July 2021.

The study NCT02702388 investigates whether a lower dose, than the currently approved dose of 24 mg orally taken lenvatinib once daily, shows a comparable effect but a better safety profile in patients with RAI-refractory DTC. The two experimental starting doses are 20 mg and 14 mg reducing down to a dose of 4 mg. NCT02702388 includes 41 participants over the age of 18. The start date was set to March 2016 and the final data collection date is May 2019. The 78 centers of the study are located in Australia, Austria, Belgium, Denmark, France, Germany, Italy, Philippines, Poland, Portugal, Romania, Spain, Sweden, United Kingdom and United States of America. The responsible party of the study is Eisai Inc.

The aim of the studies NCT00280397 (solid tumors) and NCT00121719 (solid tumors) is to investigate the maximal tolerated dose of lenvatinib and furthermore, to provide a summary of AE and the pharmacokinetic properties of lenvatinib. NCT00280397 started in January 2006 and had its final data collection date in September 2008. The study consisted of 27 participants with an age span from 20 to 75 years. The study was performed by Eisai Inc. with a center in Tokyo, Japan. The study found the maximal tolerated dose of lenvatinib to be 13 mg, when orally taken two times daily two-weeks-on/one-week-off [44]. NCT00121719 began in July 2005 with a final data collection date in June 2009. Eighty-seven participants over the age of 18 were enrolled in the study. The study was conducted by Eisai Inc. with centers in Amsterdam, Netherlands and Glasgow, United Kingdom. The study found the maximal tolerated dose of lenvatinib to be 25 mg orally taken once daily.

The studies NCT01728623, NCT02726503, NCT00784303, and NCT02966093 intend to determine the overall- and progression-free survival rates of participants treated with 24 mg lenvatinib orally taken once daily, moreover the studies aim to investigate the AE of the drug. NCT02726503 also studies the efficacy on ATC (Phase II) and NCT00784303 furthermore investigates the tumor response rate and the pharmacokinetic profile of lenvatinib. NCT01728623 started September 2012 and had its last data collection date in July 2015. In this study 37 participants over the age of 20 years were enrolled from three centers in Japan. The responsible party of the study was Eisai Inc. NCT02726503 started in January 2016 and has its last data collection date in July 2018. The study consists of 39 participants over the age of 20 years recruiting from 12 Japanese hospitals. The responsible party of this study is the Translational Research Informatics Center, Kobe, Hyogo, Japan. NCT00784303 started in August 2009 and had its last data collection date in April 2011. One hundred sixteen participants over the age of 18 were enrolled from 51 centers in the United States, Australia, France, Germany, Italy, Poland and the United Kingdom. The responsible party is Eisai Inc. NCT02966093 is set to start in January 2017 and has its final data collection date in January 2020. The estimated number of participants is 150 over the age of 18. Recruiting from 13 centers in China. Eisai Co., Ltd. is the responsible party of this study.

Study NCT02185560 aims to analyze patients of all ages and sexes, suffering from unresectable differentiated thyroid carcinoma and receiving sorafenib treatment. Standard follow-up length will be 9 months (or until lost to follow-up). For patients with a possible follow-up of 24 months, additional data, such as survival status and keratoacanthoma and/or squamous cell cancer development will be collected. Primary end points are the number of participants with adverse and serious adverse drug reactions as well as the number of participants with serious AE as a measure of safety and tolerability. This study is conducted by Bayer Clinical Trials.

The Phase 2 study NCT02084732, conducted by the Instituto Nacional de Cancerologia, Columbia, is also directed towards an assessment of the safety and efficacy of sorafenib in the treatment of patients with advanced thyroid cancer. It is currently in the recruiting stage and is open for adult patients of both sexes. The follow-up period is 24 months, and besides its primary objective of determining the clinical activity and safety profile of sorafenib in the treatment of patients with advanced thyroid cancer, its secondary aims are the measurement of PFS and the description of AE associated with sorafenib used in advanced thyroid cancer.

Study NCT02185560 is similar in design and scope to NCT02185560 discussed above, just substituting sorafenib with sunitinib. Bayer Clinical Trials is the responsible party.

Study NCT00510640 has been conducted by the University Hospital Bordeaux, France under collaboration with Pfizer. Patients suffering from locally advanced or metastatic anaplastic, differentiated or medullary thyroid carcinoma receive 50 mg/day sunitinib for four weeks followed by a rest-period of two weeks. Cycles are repeated until disease progression or severe toxicity. Based on tolerability, doses can be reduced to 12.5 mg/day. Adult patients of both sexes are eligible. The primary outcome measure of this study is the objective response rate (ORR) (the proportion of patients with confirmed complete (CR) or partial response (PR) according to the RECIST), secondary outcome measures are the safety of sunitinib in patients with thyroid carcinoma and time to disease progression, response, and duration of response. The study is completed, and no results are published so far.

In the study NCT00668811 a total of 23 patients with advanced differentiated thyroid cancer received 37.5 mg/day sunitinib for treatment cycles of 28 days. Adult patients with advanced DTC were eligible and of the 23 subjects, 74% (17) were male. The primary objective is to assess clinical benefit rate, defined as complete response, partial response, or stable disease and the secondary objective is to assess the safety of sunitinib in this patient population. Overall, this study found, that sunitinib was relatively well tolerated and had good anti-tumor activity for this kind of thyroid cancer [45]. The responsible party for this study was the Washington Hospital Center in collaboration with the company Pfizer.

For an overview of adverse effects observed in larger clinical trials with lenvatinib, sofrafenib, and sunitinib, see Table 3.

Table 3. Overview of serious AE observed in clinical trials investigating TKI treatment; website used on 7 March 2017 [43].

Clinical Trial Title ID	Dose (mg/day)	# of Patients	Most Frequent Serious Adverse Effects	
SELECT: A multi center, randomized, double-blind, placebo-controlled, phase 3 trial of Lenvatinib (E7080) in ^{131}I-refractory differentiated thyroid cancer. NCT01321554 [31,40]	24 Per os (PO)	261	4% 3% 3% 2% 2% 2% 2%	Pneumonia Hypertension Dehydration Physical health deterioration Renal failure Pulmonary embolism Sepsis
An open label phase I dose escalation study of E7080 (solid tumors). NCT00121719	0.1–32 PO	93	5% 5% 4% 3% 3%	Abdominal pain Vomiting Hypertension Physical health deterioration Pyrexia
Sorafenib in treating patients with advanced anaplastic thyroid cancer. NCT00126568 [46]	2 × 400 PO	20	15% 10% 10% 5% 5%	Disease progression Death Dyspnea Thrombosis Pulmonary disorders
Nexavar® versus placebo in locally advanced/metastatic RAI-refractory differentiated thyroid cancer. NCT00984282 [24–26]	2 × 400 PO	207	5% 4% 4% 3% 2%	Secondary malignancy Dyspnea Musculoskeletal disorders Pleural effusion Fever
A continuation study using sunitinib malate for patients leaving treatment on a previous sunitinib study. NCT00428220	37.5 PO	223	5% 4% 3% 3% 2% 2% 2%	Disease progression Abdominal pain Vomiting Diarrhea Physical health deterioration Pyrexia Anemia
Sutent adjunctive treatment of differentiated thyroid cancer (IIT Sutent). NCT00668811 [45]	37.5 PO	23	13% 13% 9% 9% 4% 4% 4% 4% 4%	Hypertension Leukopenia Hand-foot syndrome Anorexia Neutropenia Lymphopenia Thrombocytopenia Nausea Gastrointestinal bleeding

2.5. Management of Multi-Kinase Inhibitor-Caused Hypertension

It is important to measure baseline BP in order to better determine cardiovascular risk factors after administering treatment. If the BP < 120/80 mmHg, TKI therapy can begin [47]. BP monitoring under TKI therapy should be performed every week for the first eight weeks, and before any infusion or cycle.

When patients show prehypertension values (120 < SBP < 140 mmHg and 80 < DBP < 90 mmHg), it is important to search for cardiovascular risk factors. If no risk factors are present, TKI treatment can begin and BP should be controlled accordingly. In cases when cardiovascular risk factors are detectable, an antihypertensive therapy, for example, calcium channel blockers (CCB), should be started 3–7 days before the start of TKI therapy.

Nebivolol is a β-adrenoceptor antagonist (BAA) whose antihypertensive effect is mainly related to a reduction in peripheral resistance; therefore, this is a good candidate for treating the TKI-induced rise in BP [48]. However, it is important to consider each patient individually, as there is no golden standard for treatment of TKI-induced hypertension and because every patient is diverse in his or her anamnesis. Some patients may take medicine that affects the metabolism of the antihypertensive or the anti-angiogenic drug and an individual plan must be made for each patient. For example, the multi-kinase inhibitor sunitinib affects the CYP3A4 enzyme, which is of high importance in metabolizing many drugs. This property of sunitinib is important to keep in mind when planning an antihypertensive strategy [49].

Hypertension should be monitored and treated according to standard medical practice, i.e., it should be managed as in patients without cancer. For a patient without comorbidities, the target blood pressure should be <140/90 mmHg. For patients with chronic kidney disease, the target BP is <135/85 mmHg, and for patients with proteinuria, drugs inhibiting the renin-angiotensin system should be applied. The anti-angiogenic therapy should be continued without dose reduction unless severe or persistent hypertension is present [47].

It is difficult to determine which is the best antihypertensive drug because there has been a lack of controlled clinical studies until now. In general, there are several classes of antihypertensive drugs, which can be applied. When a patient exerts signs of proteinuria, angiotensin converting enzyme inhibitors (ACEi) or angiotensin 2 receptor antagonists can be given. In addition, calcium channel blockers such as amlodipine can be considered. Non-dihydropyridine drugs such as verapamil or diltiazem should be avoided because of CYP3A4 metabolism. They are contraindicated in combination with oral angiogenesis inhibitors. In addition, medicaments increasing NO, like nitrates, or the BAA nebivolol can be applied. Common treatments of hypertension involve BAA, CCB, diuretics, ACEi, angiotensin-II receptor antagonists (AIIA), and NO donors [49]. The current treatment of TKI-induced hypertension uses therapeutic options that are already established and is summarized in Table 4. Studies have shown that dihydropyridine CCBs, such as amlodipine, have a great effect on relaxing smooth muscle cells and thereby lowering the total periphery resistance and hence the blood pressure. ACEi and AIIA have also shown good results in the antihypertensive treatment and concurrent renal-protecting effects in these treated cancer patients [39,50].

Finally, based on the proposed mechanisms regarding the lack of NO production, therapeutic considerations may include NO derivatives. Agents that increase NO bioavailability, such as long-acting nitrates are interesting. By giving long lasting precursors of NO, the desired effect is to neutralize or minimize the multi-kinase inhibitor-induced hypertension. In general, NO donors are known to be well tolerated and cause relatively harmless adverse effects such as headache, flushing, nausea and hypotension. Therefore, long lasting NO donors are suggested as a first line treatment [51].

An alternative and newer way to manage TKI-induced hypertension is the application of endothelin receptor antagonists, because it is assumed that ET-1 concentration increases in patients treated with multi-kinase inhibitors. This kind of hypertensive treatment is a novel regimen to handle the AE. Studies have shown that the combination of two or three of the suggested treatments may have a beneficial effect on TKI-induced hypertension [39,52].

Table 4. Different antihypertensive drugs for the management of TKI-induced hypertension.

Class	Drug	Dose	Recommendation
CCB Dihydropyridines	Amlodipine	2.5–10 mg/day	Great potency for reducing arterial smooth muscle cell contractility [39], effective therapy [49].
ACEi	Enalapril	Start with 5–20 mg/12–24 h, then max 40 mg/12–24 h	Particularly indicated in the setting of proteinuria [39], effective [49].
	Ramipril	Start with 2.5 mg/day, then 5 mg/day after 2 weeks, after another 2 weeks max 10 mg/day	
ARB	Losartan	50–100 mg/day	Particularly indicated in the setting of proteinuria [39], effective [49].
	Valsartan	80–320 mg/day	
	Irbesartan	150–300 mg/day	
BBA	Nebivolol	2.5–5 mg/day	Indicated for DTC; begin therapy of hypertension with a BBA [53].
Diuretics/Thiazides	Hydrochlorothiazide	Start with 12.5–25 mg/day, then 12.5 mg/day	Less-effective than CCB, ACEi or ARB [39], but often used [54].
Nitrate derivates	Long-acting nitrates: Isosorbide dinitrate (ISDN) or Isosorbide mononitrate (ISMN)	40–60 mg/day	Adequate response in hypertension refractory to ACEi and CCB [51].
α-blockers	Prazosin	2–20 mg/day	Used as additional therapy if BP is not sufficiently controlled.

CCB, calcium channel blockers; ACEi, Angiotensin converting enzyme inhibitors; ARB, angiotensin II receptor blockers; BBA, β-adrenoceptor antagonists; d, day.

2.6. Discussion

Hypertension as an AE of multi-kinase inhibitor treatment is an important and frequent concern over TKI treatment. As summarized in the previous sections, numerous AE are occurring with multi-kinase inhibitor treatment of cancer. Grade 1 and grade 2 hypertension, experienced by patients treated with TKI, can frequently be managed without the need for dose reduction or discontinuation of treatment. Hypertension is linked with several cardiovascular and renal diseases, and higher mortality, which make it crucial to investigate [54–59].

Not all patients who meet the requirements of the definition of hypertension are affected. Some will never feel any change in their state of health or experience any pathogenic outcomes as a result of hypertension. Meanwhile, other groups of patients suffer from the impact of hypertension consisting of either cardiovascular events or even death. In particular, patients already suffering from risk factors, such as diabetes mellitus, cardiovascular conditions, chronic renal disease or are weakened in other ways are affected [60].

The patients treated with multi-kinase inhibitors, such as lenvatinib and sorafenib, are already in a late stage of their cancer illness and it must be assumed that this group of patients is, in some way, weakened or have sequelae from either the illness itself or from previous treatment. When considering whether hypertension as an AE is critical, it is important to be aware of the individual patient's anamnesis and general state of health. If the patient shows no previous signs of, for example, cardiovascular events, hypertension usually takes some time to affect the well-being of the patient or to induce life-threatening conditions.

Currently, treatment with multi-kinase inhibitors prolongs progression-free survival by about 12 to 16 months, from a starting point of a couple of months to half a year. Whether this time is enough to develop life-threatening conditions arising from unwanted effects such as hypertension is questionable, but must be considered when evaluating AE. Some above-mentioned studies [31,32] showed that patients either had to stop treatment entirely or lower the dose because of an alarming rise in BP. Other studies suggested the presence of hypertension as a biomarker for a good response to the anti-angiogenic treatment and therefore that hypertension may be necessary, but must also be treated [1,20,32,61]. Similarly, the sunitinib-associated rise in BP, as well as neutropenia, is discussed as biomarkers in metastatic renal cell carcinoma patients: both side effects were associated with longer progression-free survival and a higher overall-survival rate [20]. At the moment, various possible anti-angiogenic biomarkers are under examination, such as hypertension, altered VEGF plasma levels, interleukin (IL)-8 polymorphisms, or a change in tumor microvessel density. Today, promising candidates are detected, but important challenges limit their translation into practice.

Since there is still no generally accepted explanation for the cause of hypertension as an AE in multi-kinase inhibition, a specific therapy to manage this form of hypertension is not given. Various strategies of treating hypertension are suggested, some with good results, but these treatments are only symptomatic and also have accompanying side effects. Therefore, it is important to perform more studies investigating the mechanisms of hypertension induced by TKI, as well as to know the risk factors and the frequency of hypertension induced by anti-angiogenic drugs in different cancer types.

3. Conclusions

The multi-kinase inhibition by targeted therapy offers new strategies of treating cancer diseases that otherwise are considered untreatable. Unfortunately, many AE follow this kind of treatment, especially hypertension.

Hypertension is a well-known systemic AE of treatment with VEGF-inhibitors. Treatment induced-hypertension has been associated with sunitinib therapy for different forms of cancer. The TKIs are included in international clinical guidelines as first-line and second-line therapy in metastatic renal cell carcinoma (mRCC). Hypertension is an adverse effect of these drugs and the degree of hypertension associates with the anti-tumor effect in mRCC [62]. More recent phase II trials have shown a significant risk of treatment-induced hypertension with sunitinib in patients suffering from pancreatic neuroendocrine tumors [63] and endometrial carcinoma [64].

In addition, the incidence of treatment-associated hypertension with sorafenib was increased in patients with hepatocellular carcinoma [65] and non-small cell lung cancer [50]. Besides to locally recurrent or metastatic, progressive, RAI-refractory differentiated thyroid cancer, lenvatinib is indicated for the treatment of patients with advanced renal cell carcinoma in combination with everolimus following prior anti-angiogenic therapy. The frequency of hypertension, which is a known class effect of VEGF-targeting agents, was increased in both treatment groups in which lenvatinib was administered [66].

Therapy with multi-kinase inhibitors leads to a relatively large increase in the progression-free survival of patients with late stage metastatic thyroid cancer and not all patients are directly affected by the rise in BP. For some groups of patients with diseases other than thyroid cancer, either simultaneously or previously, hypertension is a great concern that can be dangerous for the individual. Currently, biomarkers for the prediction of the effectiveness of anti-angiogenic therapy are being investigated [67] and in this course, it might be helpful to analyze possible predictors of AE such as hypertension, too. Management of hypertension is somewhat possible, but not with a curative result, and is thereby only symptomatic with the antihypertensive drugs listed in Table 4. Hence, it is important to focus on different regimens for managing high blood pressure, or even to use other strategies to specifically target the cancer cells without causing systemic adverse events.

In summary, the relationship between angiogenic inhibitors and a rise in BP has now been established: angiogenic inhibitors used to treat cancer may exacerbate cardiac risk factors. Introduction or even prophylactic use of antihypertensive drugs can allow maintenance of therapy despite the onset of hypertension. In addition to cancer therapy, the reduction of hypertension risk factors should be addressed.

4. Outlook

Several studies have already shown hypertension and other unwanted events in response to multi-kinase inhibition treatment. Future and on-going studies have adjusted their aims to consider the AE of this type of treatment, since many studies with these aims are now registered. It is of great interest and import to examine how to reduce or eliminate AE by dose-finding studies or by determining the mechanisms inducing hypertension and thus being able to properly treat this effect.

5. Materials and Methods

Literature and information used for this review can be found using online databases, such as Pubmed, Scopus and clinicaltrials.gov by using the search terms "multi-kinase inhibitors", "antiangiogenesis", "multi-kinase inhibitors and hypertension", "thyroid cancer" and others.

Acknowledgments: This review was the bachelor thesis of Ole Vincent Ancker. The authors would like to thank Petra Wise, USC, Los Angeles, CA, USA and Proof-Reading-Service.com, Devonshire Business Center, Works Road, Letchworth Garden City, SG6 1GJ, Hertfordshire, United Kingdom for reviewing the article for language and grammatical errors.

Author Contributions: Ole Vincent Ancker, Markus Wehland and Daniela Grimm wrote the review; Johann Bauer searched and checked the references; Manfred Infanger and Johann Bauer supported the paper; and Markus Wehland, and Ole Vincent Ancker contributed with drafting the figures and tables.

Abbreviations

AIIA	angiotensin II receptor antagonists
ACEi	angiotensin converting enzyme inhibitors
AE	adverse effects
AKT	protein kinase B
ATC	anaplastic thyroid cancer
CCB	calcium channel blockers
cGMP	cyclic guanosine monophosphate
DTC	differentiated thyroid cancer
EGF	endothelial growth factor
eNOS	endothelial nitric oxide synthase
ERK	extracellular signal regulated kinase
ET-1	endothelin-1
ET_A	endothelin receptor type A
FGF	fibroblast growth factor
FGFR	fibroblast growth factor receptor
FTC	follicular thyroid cancer
MAPKK	mitogen activated protein kinase kinase
MTC	medullary thyroid cancer
NO	nitric oxide
PDGF	platelet derived growth factor
PDGFR	platelet derived growth factor receptor
PI3K	phosphatidylinositol-3-kinase
PDTC	poorly differentiated thyroid cancer
PO	per os
PTC	papillary thyroid cancer
RAI	radioactive iodine
RAS	rat sarcoma
RET	ret proto-oncogene

sGC	soluble guanylyl cyclase
TKI	tyrosine kinase inhibitor
VEGF	vascular endothelial growth factor
VEGFR	vascular endothelial growth factor receptor

References

1. Costa, R.; Carneiro, B.A.; Chandra, S.; Pai, S.G.; Chae, Y.K.; Kaplan, J.B.; Garrett, H.B.; Agulnik, M.; Kopp, P.A.; Giles1, F.J. Spotlight on lenvatinib in the treatment of thyroid cancer: Patient selection and perspectives. *Drug Des. Dev. Ther.* **2016**, *10*, 873–884. [CrossRef] [PubMed]
2. O'Neill, C.J.; Oucharek, J.; Learoyd, D.; Sidhu, S.B. Standard and emerging therapies for metastatic differentiated thyroid cancer. *Oncologist* **2010**, *15*, 146–156. [CrossRef] [PubMed]
3. Cabanillas, M.E.; Habra, M.A. Lenvatinib: Role in thyroid cancer and other solid tumors. *Cancer Treat. Rev.* **2016**, *42*, 47–55. [CrossRef] [PubMed]
4. Mancia, G.; Fagard, R.; Narkiewicz, K.; Redon, J.; Zanchetti, A.; Bohm, M.; Christiaens, T.; Cifkova, R.; De Backer, G.; Dominiczak, A.; et al. 2013 ESH/ESC guidelines for the management of arterial hypertension: The Task Force for the Management of Arterial Hypertension of the European Society of Hypertension (ESH) and of the European Society of Cardiology (ESC). *Eur. Heart J.* **2013**, *34*, 2159–2219. [CrossRef] [PubMed]
5. He, J.; Whelton, P.K. Elevated systolic blood pressure and risk of cardiovascular and renal disease: Overview of evidence from observational epidemiologic studies and randomized controlled trials. *Am. Heart J.* **1999**, *138*, 211–219. [CrossRef]
6. Thyroid Cancer 2016 Updated 31 March 2016. Available online: http://www.cancer.org/cancer/thyroidcancer/detailedguide/thyroid-cancer-what-is-thyroid-cancer (accessed on 27 December 2016).
7. Tiedje, V.; Schmid, K.W.; Weber, F.; Bockisch, A.; Fuhrer, D. Differentiated thyroid cancer. *Internist* **2015**, *56*, 153–166. [CrossRef] [PubMed]
8. Patel, K.N.; Shaha, A.R. Poorly differentiated thyroid cancer. *Curr. Opin. Otolaryngol. Head Neck Surg.* **2014**, *22*, 121–126. [CrossRef] [PubMed]
9. Roy, M.; Chen, H.; Sippel, R.S. Current understanding and management of medullary thyroid cancer. *Oncologist* **2013**, *18*, 1093–1100. [CrossRef] [PubMed]
10. Krook, K.A.; Fedewa, S.A.; Chen, A.Y. Prognostic indicators in well-differentiated thyroid carcinoma when controlling for stage and treatment. *Laryngoscope* **2015**, *125*, 1021–1027. [CrossRef] [PubMed]
11. Laursen, R.; Wehland, M.; Kopp, S.; Pietsch, J.; Infanger, M.; Grosse, J.; Grimm, D. Effects and Role of Multi-kinase Inhibitors in Thyroid Cancer. *Curr. Pharm. Des.* **2016**, *22*, 5915–5926. [CrossRef] [PubMed]
12. Ferlay, J.; Steliarova-Foucher, E.; Lortet-Tieulent, J.; Rosso, S.; Coebergh, J.W.; Comber, H.; Forman, D.; Bray, F. Cancer incidence and mortality patterns in Europe: Estimates for 40 countries in 2012. *Eur. J. Cancer* **2013**, *49*, 1374–1403. [CrossRef] [PubMed]
13. GLOBOCAN 2012: Estimated Cancer Incidence, Mortality and Prevalence Worldwide in 2012. Available online: http://globocan.iarc.fr/Pages/fact_sheets_population.aspx (accessed on 31 December 2016).
14. Anderson, R.T.; Linnehan, J.E.; Tongbram, V.; Keating, K.; Wirth, L.J. Clinical, safety, and economic evidence in radioactive iodine-refractory differentiated thyroid cancer: A systematic literature review. *Thyroid* **2013**, *23*, 392–407. [CrossRef] [PubMed]
15. Dvorak, H.F. Angiogenesis: Update 2005. *J. Thromb. Haemost.* **2005**, *3*, 1835–1842. [CrossRef] [PubMed]
16. Infanger, M.; Shakibaei, M.; Kossmehl, P.; Hollenberg, S.M.; Grosse, J.; Faramarzi, S.; Schulze-Tanzil, G.; Paul, M.; Grimm, D. Intraluminal application of vascular endothelial growth factor enhances healing of microvascular anastomosis in a rat model. *J. Vasc. Res.* **2005**, *42*, 202–213. [CrossRef] [PubMed]
17. Infanger, M.; Kossmehl, P.; Shakibaei, M.; Baatout, S.; Witzing, A.; Grosse, J.; Bauer, J.; Cogoli, A.; Faramarzi, S.; Derradji, H.; et al. Induction of three-dimensional assembly and increase in apoptosis of human endothelial cells by simulated microgravity: Impact of vascular endothelial growth factor. *Apoptosis* **2006**, *11*, 749–764. [CrossRef] [PubMed]
18. Infanger, M.; Grosse, J.; Westphal, K.; Leder, A.; Ulbrich, C.; Paul, M.; Grimm, D. Vascular endothelial growth factor induces extracellular matrix proteins and osteopontin in the umbilical artery. *Ann. Vasc. Surg.* **2008**, *22*, 273–284. [CrossRef] [PubMed]

19. Ferrara, N. Vascular endothelial growth factor: Basic science and clinical progress. *Endocr. Rev.* **2004**, *25*, 581–611. [CrossRef] [PubMed]
20. Frandsen, S.; Kopp, S.; Wehland, M.; Pietsch, J.; Infanger, M.; Grimm, D. Latest Results for Anti-Angiogenic Drugs in Cancer Treatment. *Curr. Pharm. Des.* **2016**, *22*, 5927–5942. [CrossRef] [PubMed]
21. Kowanetz, M.; Ferrara, N. Vascular endothelial growth factor signaling pathways: Therapeutic perspective. *Clin. Cancer Res.* **2006**, *12*, 5018–5022. [CrossRef] [PubMed]
22. Stjepanovic, N.; Capdevila, J. Multi-kinase inhibitors in the treatment of thyroid cancer: Specific role of lenvatinib. *Biologics* **2014**, *8*, 129–139. [PubMed]
23. Hayman, S.R.; Leung, N.; Grande, J.P.; Garovic, V.D. VEGF inhibition, hypertension, and renal toxicity. *Curr. Oncol. Rep.* **2012**, *14*, 285–294. [CrossRef] [PubMed]
24. Worden, F.; Fassnacht, M.; Shi, Y.; Hadjieva, T.; Bonichon, F.; Gao, M.; Fugazzola, L.; Ando, Y.; Hasegawa, Y.; Park do, J.; et al. Safety and tolerability of sorafenib in patients with radioiodine-refractory thyroid cancer. *Endocr. Relat. Cancer* **2015**, *22*, 877–887. [CrossRef] [PubMed]
25. Brose, M.S.; Nutting, C.M.; Jarzab, B.; Elisei, R.; Siena, S.; Bastholt, L.; de la Fouchardiere, C.; Pacini, F.; Paschke, R.; Shong, Y.K.; et al. Sorafenib in radioactive iodine-refractory, locally advanced or metastatic differentiated thyroid cancer: A randomised, double-blind, phase 3 trial. *Lancet* **2014**, *384*, 319–328. [CrossRef]
26. Brose, M.S.; Nutting, C.M.; Sherman, S.I.; Shong, Y.K.; Smit, J.W.; Reike, G.; Chung, J.; Kalmus, J.; Kappeler, C.; Schlumberger, M. Rationale and design of decision: A double-blind, randomized, placebo-controlled phase III trial evaluating the efficacy and safety of sorafenib in patients with locally advanced or metastatic radioactive iodine (RAI)-refractory, differentiated thyroid cancer. *BMC Cancer* **2011**, *11*, 349.
27. Ma, X.; Wehland, M.; Schulz, H.; Saar, K.; Hübner, N.; Infanger, M.; Bauer, J.; Grimm, D. Genomic approach to identify factors that drive the formation of three-dimensional structures by EA.hy926 endothelial cells. *PLoS ONE* **2013**, *8*, e64402. [CrossRef] [PubMed]
28. Kristensen, T.B.; Knutsson, M.L.; Wehland, M.; Laursen, B.E.; Grimm, D.; Warnke, E.; Magnusson, N.E. Anti-vascular endothelial growth factor therapy in breast cancer. *Int. J. Mol. Sci.* **2014**, *15*, 23024–23041. [CrossRef] [PubMed]
29. Gupta-Abramson, V.; Troxel, A.B.; Nellore, A.; Puttaswamy, K.; Redlinger, M.; Ransone, K.; Mandel, S.J.; Flaherty, K.T.; Loevner, L.A.; O'Dwyer, P.J.; et al. Phase II trial of sorafenib in advanced thyroid cancer. *J. Clin. Oncol.* **2008**, *26*, 4714–4719. [CrossRef] [PubMed]
30. Nexavar (Sorafenib). *Tablets Prescribing Information*; Bayer Health Care Pharmaceuticals, Inc.: Wayne, NJ, USA, 2012.
31. Schlumberger, M.; Tahara, M.; Wirth, L.J.; Robinson, B.; Brose, M.S.; Elisei, R.; Habra, M.A.; Newbold, K.; Shah, M.H.; Hoff, A.O.; et al. Lenvatinib versus placebo in radioiodine-refractory thyroid cancer. *N. Engl. J. Med.* **2015**, *372*, 621–630. [CrossRef] [PubMed]
32. Cabanillas, M.E.; Schlumberger, M.; Jarzab, B.; Martins, R.G.; Pacini, F.; Robinson, B.; McCaffrey, J.C.; Shah, M.H.; Bodenner, D.L.; Topliss, D.; et al. A phase 2 trial of lenvatinib (E7080) in advanced, progressive, radioiodine-refractory, differentiated thyroid cancer: A clinical outcomes and biomarker assessment. *Cancer* **2015**, *121*, 2749–2756. [CrossRef] [PubMed]
33. Bair, S.M.; Choueiri, T.K.; Moslehi, J. Cardiovascular complications associated with novel angiogenesis inhibitors: Emerging evidence and evolving pers Phase I dose-escalation study and biomarker analysis of E7080 in patients with advanced solid tumors pectives. *Trends. Cardiovasc. Med.* **2013**, *23*, 104–113. [CrossRef] [PubMed]
34. Ollero, M.; Sahali, D. Inhibition of the VEGF signalling pathway and glomerular disorders. *Nephrol. Dial. Transplant.* **2015**, *30*, 1449–1455. [CrossRef] [PubMed]
35. Kappers, M.H.; de Beer, V.J.; Zhou, Z.; Danser, A.H.; Sleijfer, S.; Duncker, D.J.; van den Meiracker, A.H.; Merkus, D. Sunitinib-induced systemic vasoconstriction in swine is endothelin mediated and does not involve nitric oxide or oxidative stress. *Hypertension* **2012**, *59*, 151–157. [CrossRef] [PubMed]
36. Kappers, M.H.; van Esch, J.H.; Sluiter, W.; Sleijfer, S.; Danser, A.H.; van den Meiracker, A.H. Hypertension induced by the tyrosine kinase inhibitor sunitinib is associated with increased circulating endothelin-1 levels. *Hypertension* **2010**, *56*, 675–681. [CrossRef] [PubMed]
37. Steeghs, N.; Gelderblom, H.; Roodt, J.O.; Christensen, O.; Rajagopalan, P.; Hovens, M.; Putter, H.; Rabelink, T.J.; de Koning, E. Hypertension and rarefaction during treatment with telatinib, a small molecule angiogenesis inhibitor. *Clin. Cancer Res.* **2008**, *14*, 3470–3476. [CrossRef] [PubMed]

38. Eskens, F.A.; Verweij, J. The clinical toxicity profile of vascular endothelial growth factor (VEGF) and vascular endothelial growth factor receptor (VEGFR) targeting angiogenesis inhibitors: A review. *Eur. J. Cancer* **2006**, *42*, 3127–3139. [CrossRef] [PubMed]
39. De Jesus-Gonzalez, N.; Robinson, E.; Moslehi, J.; Humphreys, B.D. Management of antiangiogenic therapy-induced hypertension. *Hypertension* **2012**, *60*, 607–615. [CrossRef] [PubMed]
40. Kiyota, N.; Schlumberger, M.; Muro, K.; Ando, Y.; Takahashi, S.; Kawai, Y.; Wirth, L.; Robinson, B.; Sherman, S.; Suzuki, T.; et al. Subgroup analysis of Japanese patients in a phase 3 study of lenvatinib in radioiodine-refractory differentiated thyroid cancer. *Cancer Sci.* **2015**, *106*, 1714–1721. [CrossRef] [PubMed]
41. Schlumberger, M.; Jarzab, B.; Cabanillas, M.E.; Robinson, B.; Pacini, F.; Ball, D.W.; McCaffrey, J.; Newbold, K.; Allison, R.; Martins, R.G.; et al. A Phase II Trial of the Multitargeted Tyrosine Kinase Inhibitor Lenvatinib (E7080) in Advanced Medullary Thyroid Cancer. *Clin Cancer Res.* **2016**, *22*, 44–53. [CrossRef] [PubMed]
42. Rapsomaniki, E.; Timmis, A.; George, J.; Pujades-Rodriguez, M.; Shah, A.D.; Denaxas, S.; White, I.R.; Caulfield, M.J.; Deanfield, J.E.; et al. Blood pressure and incidence of twelve cardiovascular diseases: Lifetime risks, healthy life-years lost, and age-specific associations in 1.25 million people. *Lancet* **2014**, *383*, 1899–1911. [CrossRef]
43. ClinicalTrials.gov. Available online: http://www.clinicaltrials.gov (accessed on 7 March 2017).
44. Yamada, K.; Yamamoto, N.; Yamada, Y.; Nokihara, H.; Fujiwara, Y.; Hirata, T.; Koizumi, F.; Nishio, K.; Koyama, N.; Tamura, T. Phase I dose-escalation study and biomarker analysis of E7080 in patients with advanced solid tumors. *Clin. Cancer Res.* **2011**, *17*, 2528–2537. [CrossRef] [PubMed]
45. Bikas, A.; Kundra, P.; Desale, S.; Mete, M.; O'Keefe, K.; Clark, B.G.; Gandhi, R.; Barett, C.; Jelinek, J.S.; Wexler, J.A.; et al. Phase 2 clinical trial of sunitinib as adjunctive treatment in patients with advanced differentiated thyroid cancer. *Eur. J. Endocrinol.* **2016**, *174*, 373–380. [CrossRef] [PubMed]
46. Savvides, P.; Nagaiah, G.; Lavertu, P.; Fu, P.; Wright, J.J.; Chapman, R.; Wasman, J.; Dowlati, A.; Remick, S.C. Phase II trial of sorafenib in patients with advanced anaplastic carcinoma of the thyroid. *Thyroid* **2013**, *23*, 600–604. [CrossRef] [PubMed]
47. Izzedine, H.; Ederhy, S.; Goldwasser, F.; Soria, J.C.; Milano, G.; Cohen, A.; Khayat, D.; Spano, J.P. Management of hypertension in angiogenesis inhibitor-treated patients. *Ann. Oncol.* **2009**, *20*, 807–815. [CrossRef] [PubMed]
48. Porta, C.; Paglino, C.; Imarisio, I.; Bonomi, L. Uncovering Pandora's vase: The growing problem of new toxicities from novel anticancer agents. The case of sorafenib and sunitinib. *Clin. Exp. Med.* **2007**, *7*, 127–134. [CrossRef] [PubMed]
49. Leon-Mateos, L.; Mosquera, J.; Anton Aparicio, L. Treatment of sunitinib-induced hypertension in solid tumor by nitric oxide donors. *Redox. Biol.* **2015**, *6*, 421–425. [CrossRef] [PubMed]
50. Wasserstrum, Y.; Kornowski, R.; Raanani, P.; Leader, A.; Pasvolsky, O.; Iakobishvili, Z. Hypertension in cancer patients treated with anti-angiogenic based regimens. *Cardio-Oncology* **2015**, *1*, 6. [CrossRef]
51. Kruzliak, P.; Novak, J.; Novak, M. Vascular endothelial growth factor inhibitor-induced hypertension: From pathophysiology to prevention and treatment based on long-acting nitric oxide donors. *Am. J. Hypertens* **2014**, *27*, 3–13. [CrossRef] [PubMed]
52. Laffin, L.J.; Bakris, G.L. Endothelin Antagonism and Hypertension: An Evolving Target. *Semin. Nephrol.* **2015**, *35*, 168–175. [CrossRef] [PubMed]
53. Brose, M.S.; Frenette, C.T.; Keefe, S.M.; Stein, S.M. Management of sorafenib-related adverse events: A clinician's perspective. *Semin. Oncol.* **2014**, *41*, S1–S16. [CrossRef] [PubMed]
54. Walko, C.M.; Grande, C. Management of common adverse events in patients treated with sorafenib: Nurse and pharmacist perspective. *Semin. Oncol.* **2014**, *41*, S17–S28. [CrossRef] [PubMed]
55. Sim, J.J.; Bhandari, S.K.; Shi, J.; Reynolds, K.; Calhoun, D.A.; Kalantar-Zadeh, K.; Jacobsen, S.J. Comparative risk of renal, cardiovascular, and mortality outcomes in controlled, uncontrolled resistant, and nonresistant hypertension. *Kidney Int.* **2015**, *88*, 622–632. [CrossRef] [PubMed]
56. Wehland, M.; Grosse, J.; Simonsen, U.; Infanger, M.; Bauer, J.; Grimm, D. The Effects of Newer β-Adrenoceptor Antagonists on Vascular Function in Cardiovascular Disease. *Curr. Vasc. Pharmacol.* **2012**, *10*, 378–390. [CrossRef] [PubMed]
57. Fisker, F.Y.; Grimm, D.; Wehland, M. Third-generation β-adrenoceptor antagonists in the treatment of hypertension and heart failure. *Basic Clin. Pharmacol. Toxicol.* **2015**, *117*, 5–14. [CrossRef] [PubMed]

58. Andersen, M.B.; Simonsen, U.; Wehland, M.; Pietsch, J.; Grimm, D. LCZ696 (Valsartan/Sacubitril)—A possible new treatment for hypertension and heart failure. *Basic Clin. Pharmacol. Toxicol.* **2016**, *118*, 14–22. [CrossRef] [PubMed]
59. Semeniuk-Wojtaś, A.; Lubas, A.; Stec, R.; Szczylik, C.; Niemczyk, S. Influence of Tyrosine Kinase Inhibitors on Hypertension and Nephrotoxicity in Metastatic Renal Cell Cancer Patients. *Int. J. Mol. Sci.* **2016**, *17*, 2073. [CrossRef] [PubMed]
60. Sim, J.J.; Shi, J.; Kovesdy, C.P.; Kalantar-Zadeh, K.; Jacobsen, S.J. Impact of achieved blood pressures on mortality risk and end-stage renal disease among a large, diverse hypertension population. *J. Am. Coll. Cardiol.* **2014**, *64*, 588–597. [CrossRef] [PubMed]
61. Small, H.Y.; Montezano, A.C.; Rios, F.J.; Savoia, C.; Touyz, R.M. Hypertension due to antiangiogenic cancer therapy with vascular endothelial growth factor inhibitors: Understanding and managing a new syndrome. *Can. J. Cardiol.* **2014**, *30*, 534–543. [CrossRef] [PubMed]
62. Randrup Hansen, C.; Grimm, D.; Bauer, J.; Wehland, M.; Magnusson, N.E. Effects and side effects of using sorafenib and sunitinib in the treatment of metastatic renal cell carcinoma. *Int. J. Mol. Sci.* **2017**, *18*, 461. [CrossRef] [PubMed]
63. Raymond, E.; Dahan, L.; Raoul, J.L.; Bang, Y.J.; Borbath, I.; Lombard-Bohas, C.; Valle, J.; Metrakos, P.; Smith, D.; Vinik, A.; et al. Sunitinib malate for the treatment of pancreatic neuroendocrine tumors. *N. Engl. J. Med.* **2011**, *364*, 501–513. [CrossRef] [PubMed]
64. Castonguay, V.; Lheureux, S.; Welch, S.; Mackay, H.J.; Hirte, H.; Fleming, G.; Morgan, R.; Wang, L.; Blattler, C.; Ivy, P.S.; et al. A phase II trial of sunitinib in women with metastatic or recurrent endometrial carcinoma: A study of the Princess Margaret, Chicago and California Consortia. *Gynecol. Oncol.* **2014**, *134*, 274–280. [CrossRef] [PubMed]
65. Granito, A.; Marinelli, S.; Negrini, G.; Menetti, S.; Benevento, F.; Bolondi, L. Prognostic significance of adverse events in patients with hepatocellular carcinoma treated with sorafenib. *Therap. Adv. Gastroenterol.* **2016**, *9*, 240–249. [CrossRef] [PubMed]
66. Motzer, R.J.; Hutson, T.E.; Glen, H.; Michaelson, M.D.; Molina, A.; Eisen, T.; Jassem, J.; Zolnierek, J. Lenvatinib, everolimus, and the combination in patients with metastatic renal cell carcinoma: A randomised, phase 2, open-label, multicentre trial. *Lancet Oncol.* **2015**, *16*, 1473–1482. [CrossRef]
67. Wehland, M.; Bauer, J.; Magnusson, N.E.; Infanger, M.; Grimm, D. Biomarkers for anti-angiogenic therapy in cancer. *Int. J. Mol. Sci.* **2013**, *14*, 9338–9364. [CrossRef] [PubMed]

8

Biomarkers, Master Regulators and Genomic Fabric Remodeling in a Case of Papillary Thyroid Carcinoma

Dumitru A. Iacobas

Personalized Genomics Laboratory, CRI Center for Computational Systems Biology, Roy G Perry College of Engineering, Prairie View A&M University, Prairie View, TX 77446, USA; daiacobas@pvamu.edu

Abstract: Publicly available (own) transcriptomic data have been analyzed to quantify the alteration in functional pathways in thyroid cancer, establish the gene hierarchy, identify potential gene targets and predict the effects of their manipulation. The expression data have been generated by profiling one case of papillary thyroid carcinoma (PTC) and genetically manipulated BCPAP (papillary) and 8505C (anaplastic) human thyroid cancer cell lines. The study used the genomic fabric paradigm that considers the transcriptome as a multi-dimensional mathematical object based on the three independent characteristics that can be derived for each gene from the expression data. We found remarkable remodeling of the thyroid hormone synthesis, cell cycle, oxidative phosphorylation and apoptosis pathways. Serine peptidase inhibitor, Kunitz type, 2 (*SPINT2*) was identified as the Gene Master Regulator of the investigated PTC. The substantial increase in the expression synergism of *SPINT2* with apoptosis genes in the cancer nodule with respect to the surrounding normal tissue (NOR) suggests that *SPINT2* experimental overexpression may force the PTC cells into apoptosis with a negligible effect on the NOR cells. The predictive value of the expression coordination for the expression regulation was validated with data from 8505C and BCPAP cell lines before and after lentiviral transfection with *DDX19B*.

Keywords: 8505C cell line; apoptosis; BCPAP cell line; BRAF; CFLAR; IL6; oxidative phosphorylation; SPINT2; thyroid hormone synthesis; weighted pathway regulation

---

1. Introduction

Thyroid cancer (**TC**) has a lower incidence and mortality rate compared to other malignancies. Still, in 2020 in the USA, 52,440 new cases (12,270 men and 40,170 women) are expected to be added. Although TC affects over three times more women than men, the number of deaths (2180) is practically equally distributed between the two sexes (1040 men and 1140 women) [1]. There are four major types of thyroid cancers: papillary (hereafter denoted as **PTC**, 70–80% of total cases), follicular (**FTC**, 10–15%), medullary (**MTC**, ~2%) and anaplastic (**APC**, ~2%). PTC, FTC and MTC are composed of well-differentiated cells and are treatable, while APC is undifferentiated and has a poor prognosis [2].

Considerable effort has been invested in recent decades to identify DNA mutations and the oncogenes (which turn on) and tumor suppressor factors (which turn off) that are responsible for triggering TC. The 25.0 release (22 July 2020) of the Genomic Data Commons Data Portal [3] includes 11,128 confirmed mutations detected on 13,564 genes sequenced from 1440 (553 male and 887 female) TC cases. The most frequently mutated gene reported in the portal is *BRAF* (B-Raf proto-oncogene, serine/threonine kinase), with up to 10 mutations identified in 20.56% of cases. Further down in terms of mutation frequency are: *NRAS* (neuroblastoma RAS viral (v-ras) oncogene homolog) with two mutations in 2.71% of cases, *TTN* (titin), with a total of 40 mutations in 2.29% of cases, and *TG* (thyroglobulin), with a total of 26 mutations in 1.67% of cases [3]. For most genes, the portal [3] shows the specific types and locations of the mutations and the cancer form(s) where these mutations were found. However, there is no bi-univocal correspondence between cancer forms and mutated genes: each cancer was associated with numerous mutated genes and mutations of the same gene were identified in several forms of cancer. How many mutated genes does one need in order to decide upon the right form of cancer? Are there exclusive combinations of mutations for a particular form of cancer and only for that form? If present, the number of the affected genes should be large enough to avoid any overlap with other form of cancer. Although the incidence of each particular mutation in the explored cohort of patients is known, it is impossible to determine the predictive values of combinations of mutated genes because for more than three genes the number of possibilities ($\geq 2.3 \times 10^{11}$) exceeds the human population of the Earth. Even though one can determine via conditioned probabilities (actual conditioned frequencies) the chance of finding the same combination of mutations in other persons, the diagnostic value is very poor. Moreover, one should not forget that the mutations were identified with respect to a reference human genome obtained by averaging the DNA sequence results from a large number of healthy individuals regardless of race, sex, age, environmental conditions, etc. However, even among genomes of healthy individuals there are 0.1% (i.e., ~3mln nucleotides) differences (0.6% when considering indels) [4].

There are several commercially available gene assays used for the preoperative diagnostic and classification of TCs (e.g., [5,6]). Recently, Foundation Medicine [7] compiled a list of 310 genes with full coding exonic regions for the detection of substitutions, insertion–deletions and copy-number alterations. An additional list of the same Foundation contains 36 genes with intronic regions useful for the detection of gene rearrangements (one gene with a promoter region and one non-coding RNA gene) [7]. For all these assays, the question is how many and what genes should be mutated/regulated to assign an accurate diagnostic? Most importantly, how did the researchers determine the predictive values of each combination of genes? In [7], there are 346 combinations of one gene, 59,685 of two, 6,843,880 combinations of three, 587 million of four and over 40 billion of five and more. Therefore, for practical reasons, only the most relevant three biomarkers, at most, are currently used, which considerably limits the diagnostic accuracy.

While the diagnostic value of mutations and/or regulations is doubtful, what about their use for therapeutic purposes? Is restoring the normal sequence/expression level of one biomarker enough to cure the cancer? Considering that the "trusted" biomarkers were selected from the genes with the most frequently altered sequence and/or expression level in large populations, this means that they are less protected by the cellular homeostatic mechanisms. The cells are supposed to invest energy to protect the sequence and expression level of genes, critical for their survival, proliferation, and integration in multicellular structures. The low level of protection indicates that biomarkers are minor players, and therefore the restoration of their structure/expression level may be of little consequence to the cancer cells.

While we do not see a genomic solution for the cancer diagnostic at present, we believe that our Gene Master Regulator (**GMR**) approach [8,9] is a reasonable alternative to the actual biomarker-oriented gene therapy. The GMR of a particular cell phenotype is the gene whose highly protected sequence/expression by the cellular homeostatic mechanisms regulates major functional pathways through expression coordination with many of their genes. In our cancer genomic studies [8–10], we found that the GMR of the cancer nodule is very low in the gene hierarchy of the surrounding cancer-free tissue of the tumor. For this reason, manipulation of the GMR's expression is expected to selectively destroy cancer cells without affecting the normal ones much.

In this report, we analyze previously published transcriptomic data [8] to quantify the cancer-related remodeling of major functional pathways in the PTC nodule with respect to the normal tissue of the resection margins (**NOR**) of a surgically removed thyroid tumor. The Gene Commanding Height (**GCH**) hierarchy and the GMRs are determined in both PTC and NOR, and the potential regulations of the apoptosis genes in response to the cancer GMR expression manipulation are predicted. The GCH scores of the top genes are compared to those of the most mutated genes in TC as well as those of the usually considered cancer biomarkers. Transcriptomic profiles of two standard TC cell lines before and after stable transfection with a gene were used to determine the predictive value of the expression coordination with that gene in untreated cells for the regulation in treated ones. The analysis presented here was derived from the Genomic Fabric Paradigm (GFP) that assigns three independent measures to each gene and considers the transcriptome as a multi-dimensional mathematical object [11].

2. Materials and Methods

2.1. Gene Expression Data

We used gene expression data from one case of papillary thyroid carcinoma, pathological stage pT3NOMx, deposited in the Gene Expression Omnibus (GEO) of the National Center for Biotechnology Information (NCBI) [12] as GSE97001. In that study, the quarters of the most homogeneous 20-mm^3 part of the frozen unilateral, single, 32.0-mm PTC nodule and four small pieces from the NOR of the same gland from the same patient were profiled separately. Thus, we got data from four biological replicas of each region. Since each human is subjected to a unique set of transcriptome-regulating factors (race, sex, age, medical history, environmental conditions, exposure to stress and toxins, etc.), the normal tissue surrounding the cancer nodule is a far better reference than tissues from other healthy persons. Expression values were normalized iteratively to the median of all quantifiable genes in all samples and transcript abundances were presented as multiples of the expression level of the median gene in each region.

Transcriptomic data from the surgically removed tumor were compared to the gene expression profiles of two standard human thyroid cancer cell lines: BCPAP (papillary) and 8505C (anaplastic) deposited as GSE97002. We determined the predictive value of the coordination analysis in untreated cells for the expression regulation in treated ones by comparing the transcriptomic profiles of these cell lines before and after stable transfection with *DDX19B, NEMP1, PANK2* and *UBALD1*. The results of transfection with DEAD (Asp-Glu-Ala-Asp) box polypeptide 19B (*DDX17B*) were collected from GSE97028, those for nuclear envelope integral membrane protein 1 (*NEMP1*) from GSE97031, for pantothenate kinase 2 (*PANK2*) from GSE97030 and for UBA-like domain containing 1 (*UBALD1*) from GSE97427. Although alterations of *DDX19B* [13], *NEMP1* [14] and *PANK2* [15] were linked to some forms of cancer by other authors, these genes were selected only because their different GCH scores in the two cell lines made them suitable to validate the GMR approach [8,9].

2.2. Single-Gene Transcriptomic Quantifiers

2.2.1. Biological Replicas, Profiling Redundancy and Average Expression Level

The four biological replicas experimental design provided for every single gene in each region three independent measures: (i) average expression level, (ii) expression variation and (iii) expression coordination with each other gene [16]. We used these three measures and combinations of them to establish the gene hierarchies and characterize the contribution of each gene to the cancer-related reorganization of the thyroid transcriptome.

The Agilent two-color expression microarrays used in the analyzed experiment redundantly probed the genes with various number of spots from 1 to 20 (as for *MIEF1* = mitochondrial elongation factor 1) and *SRRT* = serrate, RNA effector molecule). Therefore, for each gene "*i*", we computed the average expression level over the group of R_i spots redundantly probing the same transcript of the average expression levels measured by spot "*k*" across the biological replicas.

$$\mu_i^{(NOR/PTC)} = \frac{1}{R_i}\sum_{k=1}^{R_i}\mu_{i,k}^{(NOR/PTC)} = \frac{1}{R_i}\sum_{k=1}^{R_i}\left(\frac{1}{4}\sum_{j=1}^{4}a_{i,k,j}^{(NOR/PTC)}\right), \quad where: \tag{1}$$
$$a_{i,k,j}^{(NOR/PTC)} = \text{expression level of gene "}i\text{" probed by spot "}k\text{" on biological replica "}j\text{"}$$

2.2.2. Expression Variation

Because of the probing redundancy, instead of the coefficient of variation (CV), we used the *Relative Expression Variability* (*REV*). *REV* is the Bonferroni-like corrected mid-interval of the chi-square estimate of the pooled CV for all quantifiable transcripts of the same gene [17]

$$REV_i^{(NOR/PTC)} = \underbrace{\frac{1}{2}\left(\sqrt{\frac{r_i}{\chi^2(r_i;0.975)}} + \sqrt{\frac{r_i}{\chi^2(r_i;0.025)}}\right)}_{\text{correction coefficient}} \underbrace{\sqrt{\frac{1}{R_i}\sum_{k=1}^{R_i}\left(\frac{s_{ik}^{(NOR/PTC)}}{\mu_{ik}^{(NOR/PTC)}}\right)^2}}_{\text{pooled CV}} \times 100\% \quad (2)$$

μ_{ik}= average expression level of gene i probed by spot k ($= 1, \ldots, R_i$) in the 4 biological replicas
s_{ik} = standard deviation of the expression level of gene i probed by spot k
$r_i = 4R_i - 1$ = number of degrees of freedom
R_i= number of microarray spots probing redundantly gene *i*

A lower *REV* indicates stronger control by the cellular homeostatic mechanisms to limit the expression fluctuations, expected for genes critical for survival, proliferation and phenotypic expression. Therefore, we also use the *Relative Expression Control* (*REC*)

$$REC_i^{(NOR,PTC)} \equiv \frac{\langle REV\rangle^{(NOR/PTC)}}{REV_i^{(NOR/PTC)}} - 1 \quad (3)$$

$\langle\rangle$= median for all genes profiled in that phenotype

As defined, positive *REC*s point to genes that are more controlled than the median while negative *REC*s identify less controlled genes in that phenotype. It is natural to assume that the cell invests more energy to control the expressions of more important genes for its survival, phenotypic expression and integration into a multi-cellular structure. As such, *REC* is a major factor to consider in establishing the gene hierarchy.

2.2.3. Expression Coordination

The expression coordination of two genes in the same region was quantified by their pair-wise momentum-product Pearson correlation coefficient between the two sets of expression levels across biological replicas, "$\rho_{ij}^{(NOR/PTC)}$". The statistical significance was evaluated with the two-tail *t*-test for the degrees of freedom df = 4(biological replicas)*R (number of spots probing redundantly each of the correlated transcripts) − 2. Two genes were considered as synergistically expressed (positive or in-phase coordination) if their expression levels fluctuated in phase across biological replicas. They are considered as antagonistically expressed (negative or anti-phase coordination) when their expression levels manifest opposite tendencies and are independently expressed (neutral coordination) when the expression fluctuations of one gene are not related to the fluctuations of the other [17]. Although not (yet) validated through molecular biology studies, the expression coordination was speculated to reflect the "transcriptomic stoichiometry" of the encoded proteins that are produced in certain proportions to optimize the cellular functional pathways [18].

We also computed the coordination power $CP_{i,\Gamma}^{(NOR/PTC)}$ [19] and the Overall Coordination $OC_{i,\Gamma}^{(NOR/PTC)}$ of a gene "*i*" with respect to the functional pathway "Γ" in each of the two profiled regions (NOR and PTC)

$$CP_{i,\Gamma}^{(NOR/PTC)} \equiv \left.\overline{\rho_{ij}^{(NOR/PTC)}}\right|_{\forall j\in\Gamma.j\neq i} \times 100\%, \quad OC_{i,\Gamma}^{(NOR/PTC)} \equiv \exp\left(\frac{4}{N}\sum_{j\in\Gamma,j\neq i}\rho_{ij}^2 - 1\right) \quad (4)$$

Both $CP_{i,\Gamma}^{(NOR/PTC)}$ and $OC_{i,\Gamma}^{(NOR/PTC)}$ are measures of the gene "*i*" influence on "Γ".

2.3. Gene Commanding Height (GCH) and Gene Master Regulator (GMR)

In previous papers [8–10], we introduced the Gene Commanding Height (GCH), a combination of the expression control and expression coordination with all (ALL) other genes, to establish the gene hierarchy in each phenotype

$$GCH_i^{(NOR,PTC)} \equiv \left(REC_i^{(NOR,PTC)}+1\right)OC_{i,ALL}^{(NOR/PTC)} \equiv \frac{\langle REV\rangle^{(NOR/PTC)}}{REV_i^{(NOR/PTC)}}\exp\left(\frac{4}{N}\sum_{j\in ALL,j\neq i}\rho_{ij}^2-1\right) \quad (5)$$

The top gene (highest GCH) in each phenotype was termed Gene Master Regulator (GMR) of that phenotype. The very strict control of the GMR expression suggests that this gene is utterly important for cell survival, while the very high overall coordination indicates how much its expression regulates the expression of many other genes.

2.4. Expression Regulation

A gene was considered as significantly regulated in the PTC with respect to the NOR if the absolute expression ratio exceeds the cut-off (CUT) value computed individually for each gene by considering the expression variabilities of that gene in both compared conditions [9].

$$\begin{gathered}\left|x_i^{(NOR\to PTC)}\right| > CUT_i = 1+\tfrac{1}{100}\sqrt{2\left(\left(REV_i^{(NOR)}\right)^2+\left(REV_i^{(PTC)}\right)^2\right)}, \quad where: \\ x_i \equiv \begin{cases} \frac{\mu_i^{(PTC)}}{\mu_i^{(NOR)}} \;, & \text{if } \mu_i^{(PTC)} > \mu_i^{(NOR)} \\ -\frac{\mu_i^{(NOR)}}{\mu_i^{(PTC)}} \;, & \text{if } \mu_i^{(PTC)} < \mu_i^{(NOR)} \end{cases} , \quad \mu_i^{(PTC/NOR)} = \tfrac{1}{R_i}\sum_{k=1}^{R_i}\mu_{ik}^{(PTC/NOR)}\end{gathered} \quad (6)$$

The "CUT" criterion for individual genes eliminates the false positives and the false negatives selected by considering uniform absolute fold-change cut-off (e.g., 1.5*x*). In addition to the percentage of up- and down-regulated genes (that considers all genes as equal contributors to the alteration of a pathway), or the expression ratios "*x*", we prefer the Weighted Individual (gene) Regulation [20], "*WIR*":

$$\begin{aligned}&WIR_i^{(NOR\to PTC)} \equiv \mu_i^{(NOR)}\tfrac{x_i}{|x_i|}(|x_i|-1)(1-p_i) \quad where: \\ &\mu_i^{(NOR)} = \text{average expression in the normal tissue,} \\ &p_i = \text{p-value of the regulation}\end{aligned} \quad (7)$$

Note that in Equation (7), WIR takes into account the normal expression of that gene (i.e., in NOR), its expression ratio (PTC vs. NOR) and the confidence interval (1-p) of the regulation.

2.5. Quantifiers of the Functional Genomic Fabrics

The Kyoto Encyclopedia of Genes and Genomes [21,22] was used to select the genes involved in the thyroid hormone synthesis (THS), cell cycle (CC) and oxidative phosphorylation (OPH), as well as how experimental manipulation of the PTC GMR might regulate the programmed cell death (apoptosis, APO). Although almost all functional pathways were perturbed in cancer, THS, CC, OPH and APO were selected because of their importance for the thyroid function and cancer development. There are reports of altered THS in cancer progression and apoptosis (e.g., [23]) and the role of the thyroid hormone in regulating the cell-cycle [24] and the oxidative phosphorylation [25].

Median REC over a gene selection (e.g., apoptosis pathway) was used to compare the expression controls of that selection in different regions or two different gene selections in the same region. Alteration of the genomic fabrics was quantified by the average "X" of the absolute expression ratios and by Weighted Pathway Regulation (WPR), the average of the absolute *WIR*s over a particular "selection" of genes

$$X_{selection}^{(NOR \to PTC)} \equiv \overline{\left| x_i^{(NOR \to PTC)} \right|_{\forall i \in selection}} \\ WPR_{selection}^{(NOR \to PTC)} \equiv \overline{\left| WIR_i^{(NOR \to PTC)} \right|_{\forall i \in selection}} \quad (8)$$

3. Results

3.1. Overall Results

A total of 14,903 well-quantified unigenes in all PTC and NOR samples, and in BCPAP and 8505C cells before and after transfection with one of the four targeted genes, were considered in the sequent analyses. The groups redundantly probing the same transcript were replaced by their averages in each biological replica. Eukaryotic translation elongation factor 1 α 1 (*EEF1A1*) had the largest expression (82.31 median gene expression units) in NOR (not significantly regulated in PTC). Niemann-Pick disease, type C2 (*NPC2*) had the largest expression in PTC (86.97 median gene expression units), up-regulated by 7.24x with respect to NOR. Notch 1 (*NOTCH1*) with 82.35 had the largest expression in the BCPAP cells and myelin protein zero-like 3 (*MPZL3*) with 107.60 tops the gene expression level in the 8505C cells.

Out of the quantified unigenes, 1225 (8.22%) were down-regulated and 1852 (12.42%) were up-regulated in PTC with respect to NOR. The average absolute PTC/NOR expression ratio for all genes was $X = 1.768$ (median $|x| = 1.309$) and the *WPR* was 1.071 (median WIR = 0.046). Chitinase 3-like 1 (*CHI3L1*) was the most up-regulated ($x = 219.38$) and trefoil factor 3 (intestinal) (*TFF3*) the most down-regulated (x-99.86) gene in PTC. Because expression coordination and average expression level are independent measures, the high regulation of these genes in PTC with respect to NOR has no relevance for their networking in either of the two profiled regions.

3.2. Three Independent Measures for Each Gene

Figure 1 illustrates the independence of the three measures for the first 50 alphabetically ordered genes involved in the KEGG-derived [22] human apoptosis pathway (hsa04210). We chose *IL6* (interleukin 6) to illustrate the expression coordination of apoptotic genes owing to the significant role of the encoded protein (IL6) in the PTC development [26]. However, coordination with any other gene supports the same conclusion. In addition to the clear independence of the three measures, transcriptomic differences between the two histo-pathologically distinct profiled regions from the thyroid are evident.

In this gene selection, FBJ murine osteosarcoma viral oncogene homolog (*FOS*) has the highest average expression level (45.37) in NOR (significantly down-regulated by −2.06x in PTC). Cathepsin H (*CTSH*) had the largest expression (35.23), up-regulated by 6.78x with respect to NOR. *FOS*, cathepsin K (*CTSK*) and inhibitor of kappa light polypeptide gene enhancer in B-cells kinase γ (*IKBKG*) were among the significantly down-regulated genes. In contrast, *BID* (H3 interacting domain death agonist), *CTSH* and *DIABLO* (diablo, IAP-binding mitochondrial protein), were among the up-regulated genes of the selection.

CASP8 and FADD-like apoptosis regulator (*CLFAR*) was the most variably expressed gene in the normal tissue and DNA fragmentation factor (*DFFB*), 40kDa, β polypeptide (caspase-activated DNase) the most variably expressed in PTC. Note that most of the selected genes have larger expression variability in the normal tissue than in the cancer nodule. This result confirms our previous reports (see Discussions) about diseases triggering increased control exerted by the cellular homeostatic mechanisms on the transcripts abundances as a way to protect against extensive damages.

Observe also that 20 (40%) of the illustrated apoptotic genes are synergistically expressed with *IL6* in the normal tissue and only two (4%) in the PTC nodule, suggesting the decoupling of the programmed cell death from the inflammatory response in cancer.

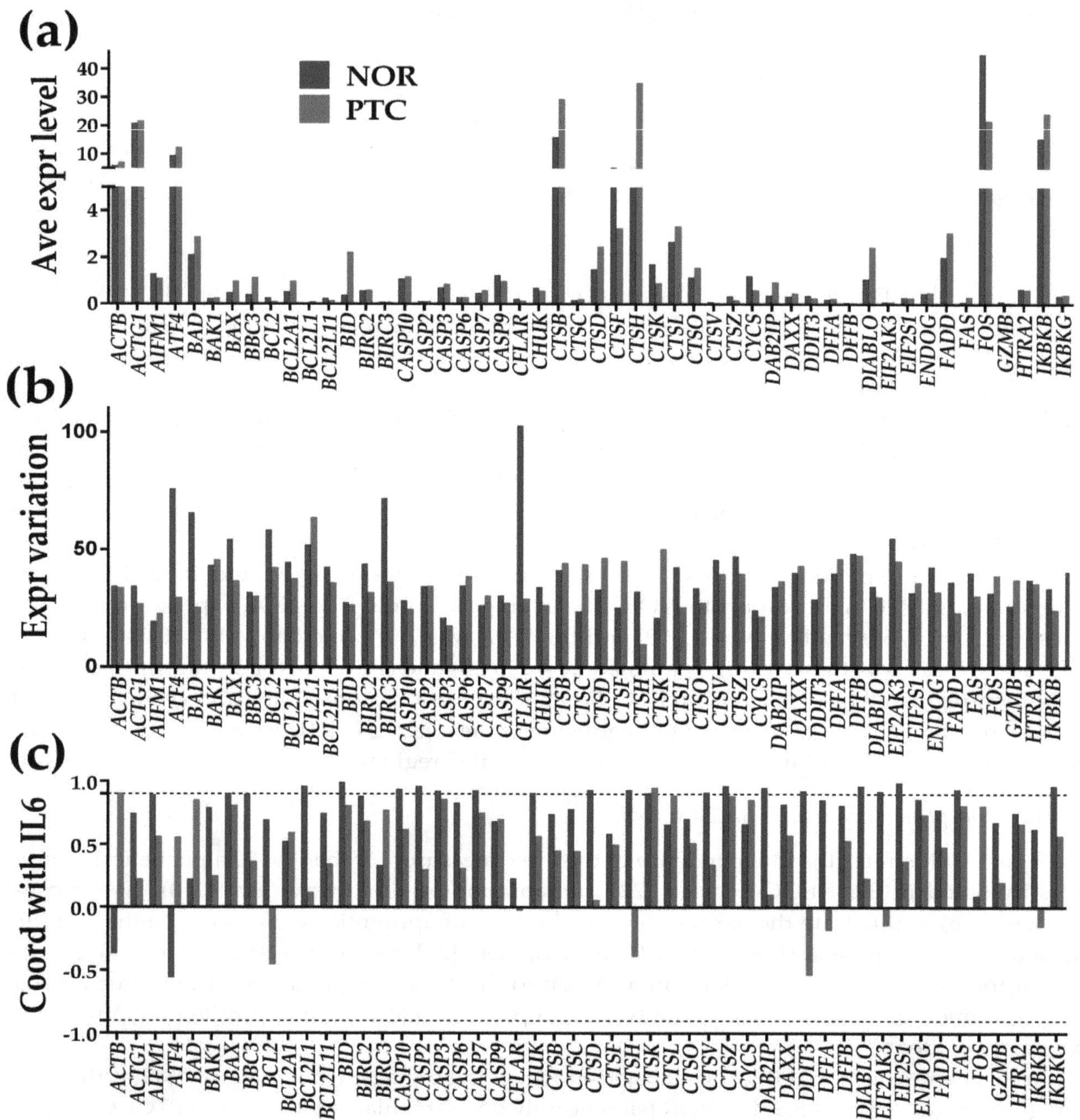

Figure 1. Three independent characteristics of every gene in each region. (**a**) average expression level, (**b**) expression variation and (**c**) expression coordination (here with IL6). The dashed black lines in panel (**c**) indicate the interval out of which the positive/negative coordination is considered as statistically significant.

3.3. Expression Regulation

Figure 2 illustrates the contributions of the first 50 alphabetically ordered quantified oncogenes to the overall regulation in PTC measured by the percentages of the up- and down-regulated genes, expression ratios and weighted individual (gene) regulations. The percentages are restricted to only the significantly regulated genes (considered as equal −1/+1 contributors). By contrast, both *X* and WIR take into account all (regulated and not regulated) genes and the contributions of these genes are no longer uniform. More informative than the expression ratio, WIR weights the contribution of each gene by its normal expression level (i.e., in NOR), fold-change in cancer and statistical significance of the regulation.

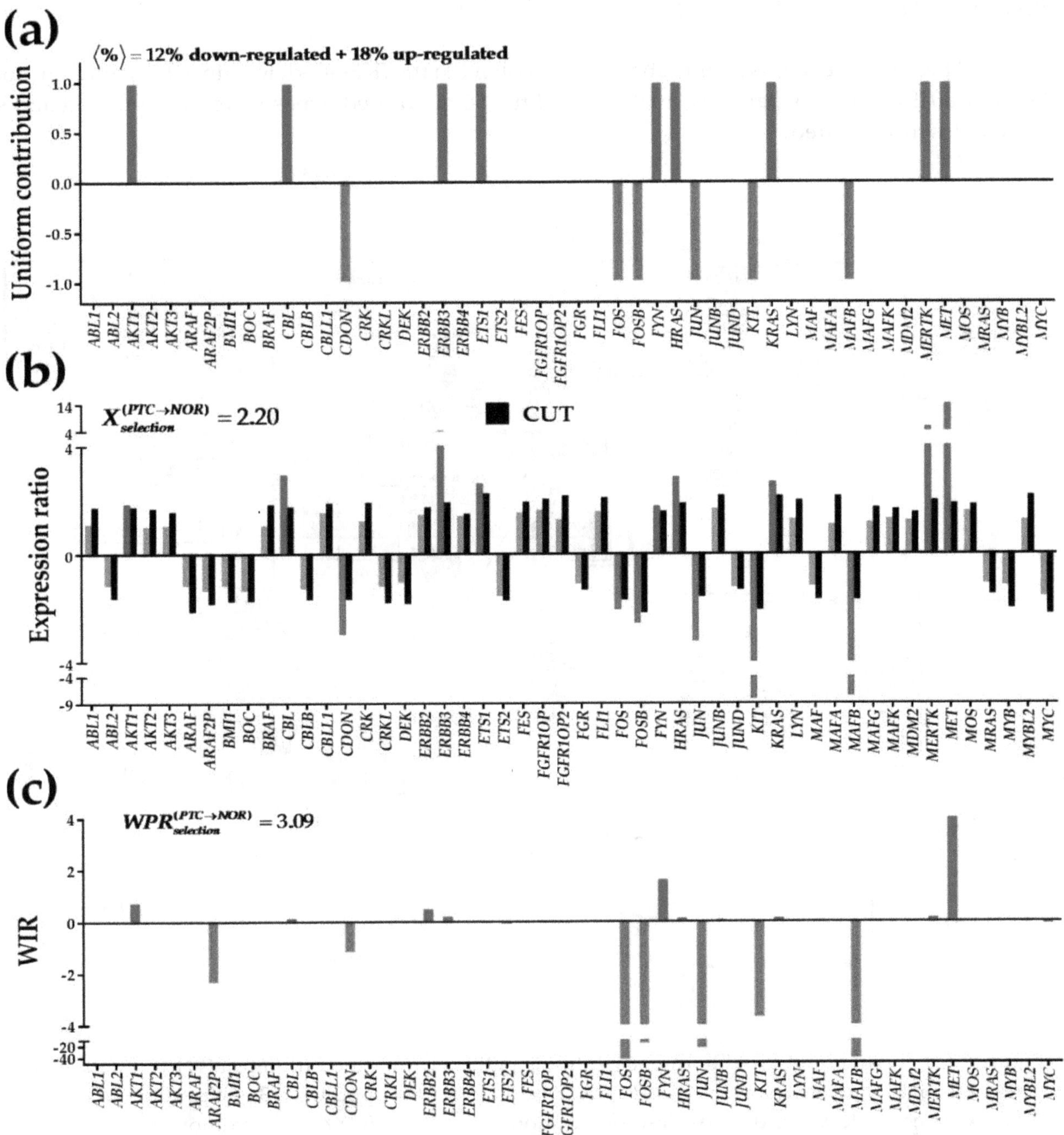

Figure 2. Three ways to consider the contribution of a gene to the pathway regulation. (**a**) uniform; (**b**) by expression ratio; (**c**) as Weighted Individual (gene) Regulation. Red/green/grey columns indicate up-/down-/not regulated genes. Black columns are the fold-change cut-offs (negative for down-regulation). Regulated genes: v-akt murine thymoma viral oncogene homolog 1 (*AKT1*), Cbl proto-oncogene, E3 ubiquitin protein ligase (*CBL*), cell adhesion associated, oncogene regulated (*CDON*), v-erb-b2 avian erythroblastic leukemia viral oncogene homolog 3 (*ERBB3*), v-ets avian erythroblastosis virus E26 oncogene homolog 1 (*ETS1*), homologs of FBJ murine osteosarcoma viral oncogene (*FOS/FOSB*), FYN proto-oncogene, Src family tyrosine kinase (*FYN*), Harvey rat sarcoma viral oncogene homolog (*HRAS*), jun proto-oncogene (*JUN*), Kirsten rat sarcoma viral oncogene homolog (*KRAS*), v-yes-1 Yamaguchi sarcoma viral related oncogene homolog (*LYN*), v-maf avian musculoaponeurotic fibrosarcoma oncogene homolog B (*MAFB*), c-mer proto-oncogene tyrosine kinase (*MERTK*) and met proto-oncogene (*MET*).

3.4. Regulation of the Thyroid Hormone Synthesis

Figure 3 presents the regulations of the genes involved in the (KEGG-determined) thyroid hormone synthesis (hsa04918). In this pathway, 10.0 (20%) of the 50 quantified genes were up-regulated and six (12%) were down-regulated.

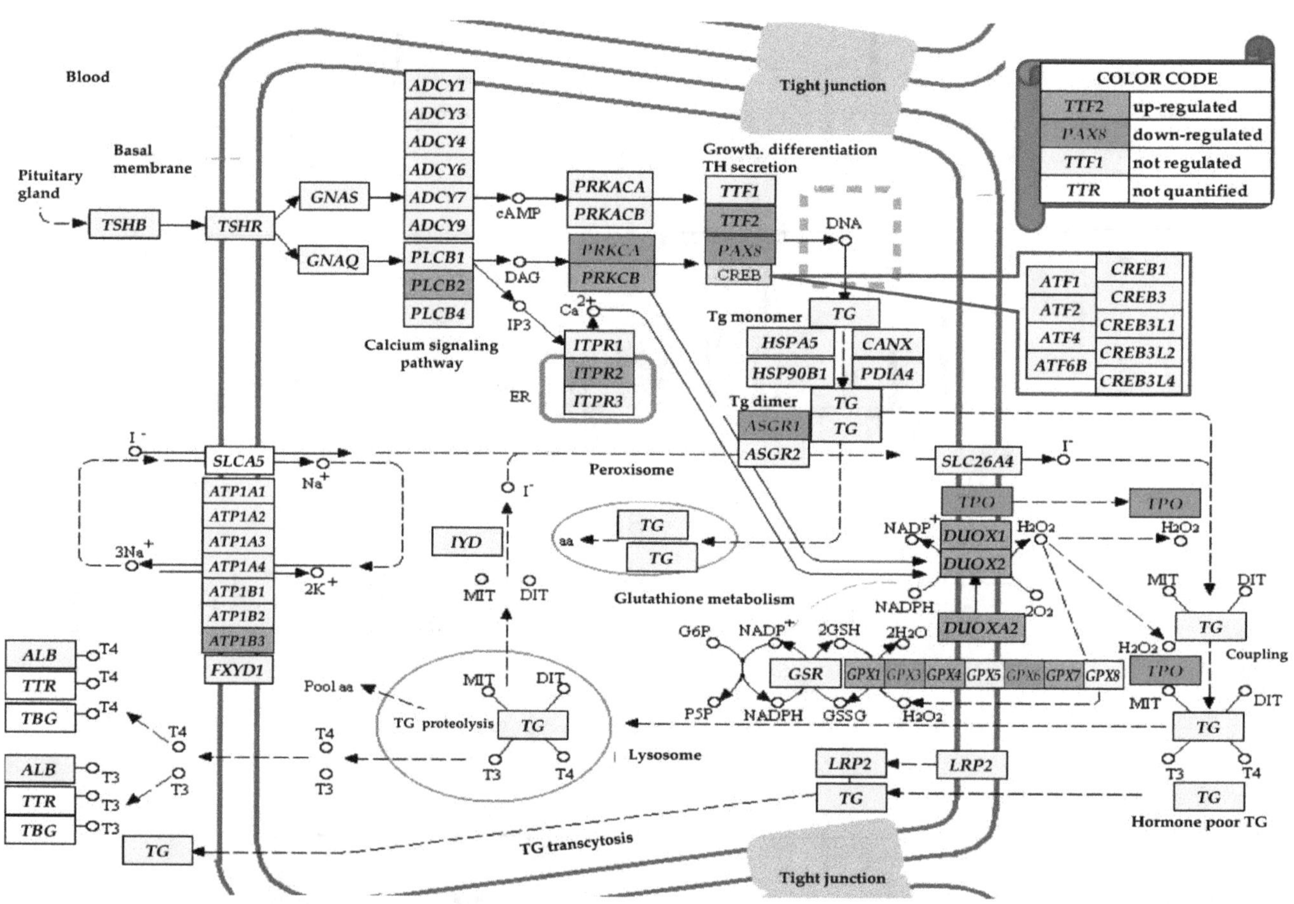

Figure 3. Regulation of thyroid hormone synthesis pathway (modified from hsa04918). Regulated genes: asialoglycoprotein receptor 1 (*ASGR1*), ATPase, Na+/K+ transporting, β 3 polypeptide (*ATP1B3*), dual oxidases (*DUOX1/2*), dual oxidase maturation factor 2 (*DUOXA2*), glutathione peroxidases (*GPX1/3/4/6/7*), inositol 1,4,5-trisphosphate receptor, type 2 (*ITPR2*), paired box 8 (*PAX8*), protein kinases C (*PRKCA/B*), thyroid peroxidase (*TPO*) and transcription termination factor, RNA polymerase II (*TTF2*).

3.5. Regulation of the Cell-Cycle Pathway

Figure 4 presents the regulation of the genes involved in the (KEGG-determined) cell cycle pathway (hsa04110), where, out of the 93 genes quantified, three (3.23%) were down-regulated and 14 (15.05%) were up-regulated. Except *PTTG2*, all other regulated genes are located in the DNA replication (S-phase) and the two temporal gaps, G1 and G2, separating the S phase from mitosis (M-phase), indicating faster replication but stationary differentiation.

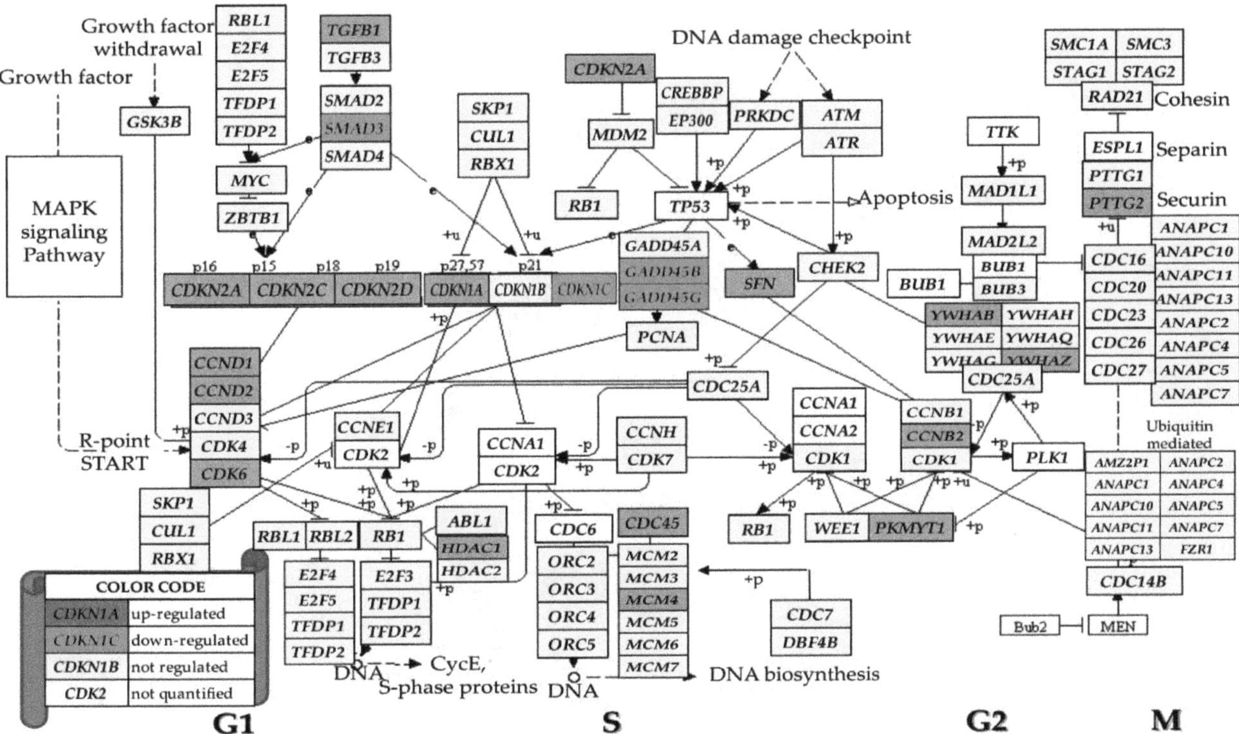

Figure 4. Regulation of the KEGG-determined cell cycle (hsa04110). Regulated genes: cyclins (*CCNB2/D1/D2*), cell division cycle 45 (*CDC45*), cyclin-dependent kinase inhibitors (*CDKN1A/1C/2A/2C/2D*), growth arrest and DNA-damage-inducibles (*GADD45B/D*), histone deacetylase 1 (*HDAC1*), minichromosome maintenance complex component 4 (*MCM4*), membrane associated tyrosine/threonine 1 (*PKMYT1*), pituitary tumor-transforming 2 (*PTTG2*), stratifin (*SFN*), SMAD family member 3 (*SMAD3*), transforming growth factor, β 1 (*TGFB1*) and tyrosine 3-monooxygenase/tryptophan 5-monooxygenase activation proteins (*YWHAB/Z*).

3.6. Remodeling of the Oxidative Phosphorylation Pathway

Figure 5 presents the remodeling of the coordination networks interlinking the five complexes ([C1], [C2], [C3], [C4], [C5]) of the oxidative phosphorylation in the PTC nodule with respect to NOR tissue. The genes were selected from the KEGG hsa 00190. Note the substantial increase in the synergistically expressed gene pairs in PTC (273) with respect of the NOR (155) and that there is no antagonistically expressed gene pair in PTC, while in NOR there are 105. When the coordination inside each complex is added, there are 781 synergistic and 0 antagonistic pairs in PTC versus 458 synergistic and 242 antagonistic pairs in NOR. In addition to the eight up-regulated and three down-regulated genes within the selection of the 92 oxidative-phosphorylation genes, these results indicate a significant increase in the coordination of the complexes involved in the OP activity.

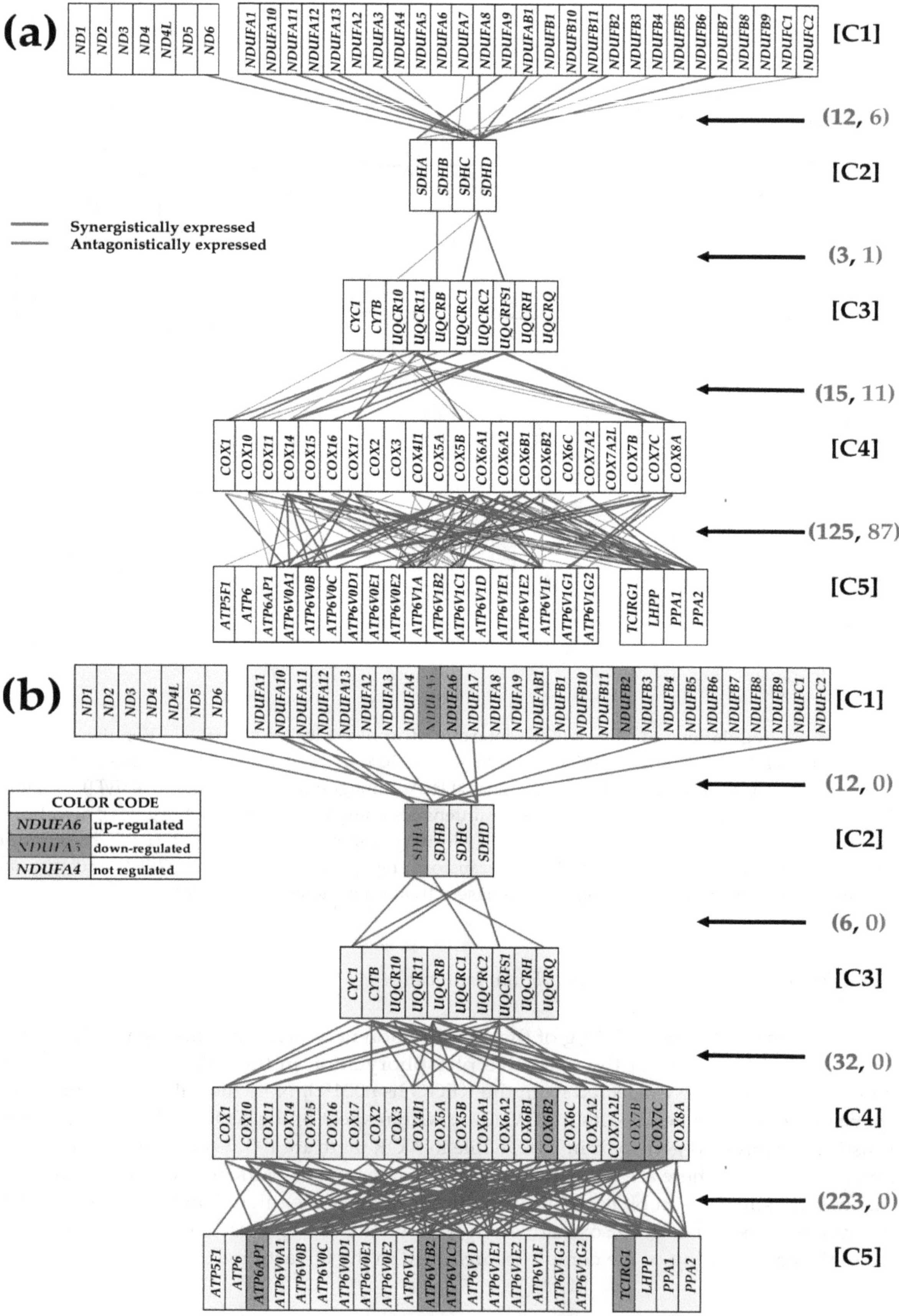

Figure 5. Remodeling of the coordination networks among the five complexes of the oxidative phosphorylation in the PTC nodule with respect to NOR tissue. The red/blue lines indicate that the

connected genes are synergistically/antagonistically expressed in that region. Red/blue numbers in parentheses indicate the number of synergistically/antagonistically expressed gene pairs between the two complexes. Regulated genes: ATPase, H+ transporting, lysosomal proteins (*ATP6AP1, ATP6V1B2, ATP6V1C1*), cytochrome c oxidase subunits (*COX6B2, COX7B, COX7C*), NADH dehydrogenase (ubiquinone) 1 α/β subcomplexes (*NDUFA5, NDUFA6, NDUFB2*), succinate dehydrogenase complex, subunit A, flavoprotein (Fp) (*SDHA*) and T-cell, immune regulator 1, ATPase, H+ transporting, lysosomal V0 subunit A3 (*TCIRG1*).

3.7. Gene Hierarchy

Figure 6 presents the GCH scores of the 12 most frequently mutated genes in TC (reported in [1]) and the top 12 genes in NOR and PTC. Mutated genes: B double prime 1, subunit of RNA polymerase III transcription initiation factor IIIB (*BDP1*), B-Raf proto-oncogene, serine/threonine kinase (*BRAF*), *DST* (dystonin), eukaryotic translation initiation factor 1A, X-linked (*EIF1AX*), Harvey rat sarcoma viral oncogene homolog (*HRAS*), lysine (K)-specific methyltransferase 2A (*KMT2A*), microtubule-actin crosslinking factor 1 (*MACR1*), metastasis associated lung adenocarcinoma transcript 1 (non-protein coding) (*MALAT1*), neuroblastoma RAS viral (v-ras) oncogene homolog (*NRAS*), thyroglobulin (*TG*), ubiquitin-specific peptidase 9, X-linked (*USP9X*), zinc finger homeobox 3 (*ZFHX3*). Note that none of the most frequently mutated genes are among the top 12 genes in either region. Even *BRAF*, mutated in 20.56% of the 1440 cases, has no competitive GCH to be a good candidate for the PTC gene therapy (GCH of *BRAF* in PTC is 11.79). However, *SPINT2*, the PTC's GMR ($GCH_{SPINT2}^{(PTC)}$ = 54.97), appears to be the most legitimate target for this case. While significant alteration of the expression of *SPINT2* would have lethal impact on the cancer cells, due to the very low GCH in NOR ($GCH_{SPINT2}^{(NOR)}$ = 1.93), it might have very little consequences on the normal cells. Importantly, the GCH scores of the top genes in PTC are substantially lower in NOR and vice-versa.

For comparison, we added the GCH scores of the top 23 genes in each of the standard TC cell lines BCPAP (papillary) and 8505C (anaplastic). Remarkably, 14 genes in the BCPAP cells and three genes in the 8505C cells have GCH scores higher than *SPINT2* in PTC. As an additional reference, Figure S1 shows the GCH scores of most of the genes from FoundationOne®CDx (Foundation Medicine, Cambridge, MA, U.S.A.) used by Foundation Medicine [7] for genomic testing of solid tumors, including "Non-Small Cell Lung (NSCLC), Colorectal, Breast, Ovarian, and Melanoma. The list contains genes with full coding exonic regions for the detection of substitutions, insertion-deletions (indels), and copy-number alterations (CNAs). It also includes genes with select intronic regions for the detection of gene rearrangements, one gene with a promoter region (telomerase reverse transcriptase (*TERT*)) and one non-coding RNA gene (*TERC*). These genes might be useful for diagnostic purposes. However, with their GCH score far below the GMR's and with not enough difference between PTC and NOR, they should have little therapeutic value for this particular case. Substantially lower than the PTC GMR were the biomarkers, oncogenes, apoptosis genes and the ncRNAs determined in the same specimens and presented in Figure 2 from [8].

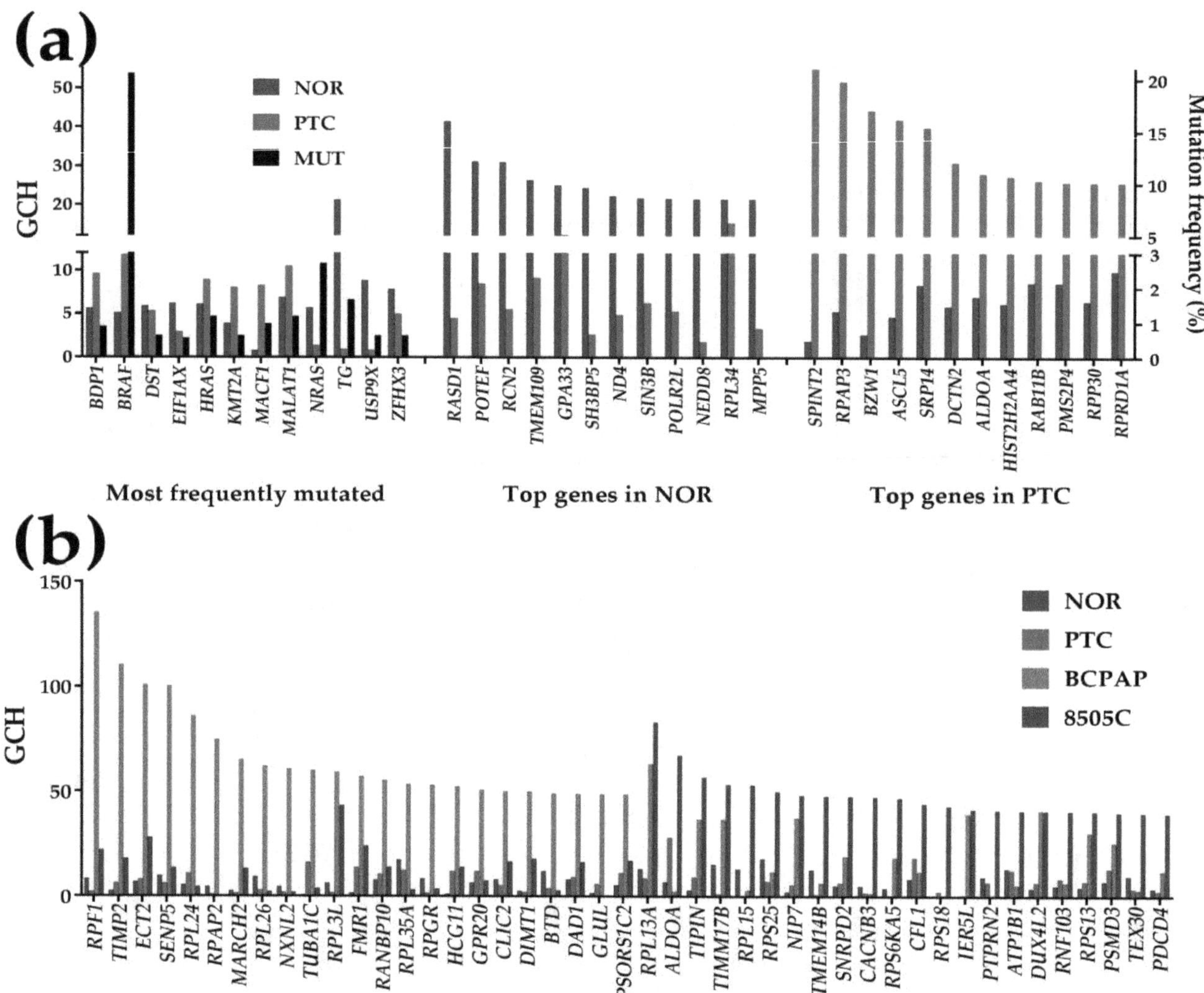

Figure 6. Gene Commanding Height (GCH). (**a**) GCH and mutation frequency of the 12 reported most frequently mutated genes and the top 12 genes in the normal tissue (NOR) and the papillary nodule (PTC). The mutation frequency is plotted on the right axis. (**b**) GCH of the top 23 genes in the papillary (BCPAP) and anaplastic (8505C) thyroid cancer cell lines and their scores in NOR and PTC. Top 3 genes in NOR: RAS, dexamethasone-induced 1 (*RASD1*), POTE ankyrin domain family, member F (*POTEF*), reticulocalbin 2, EF-hand calcium binding domain (*RCN2*). Top 3 genes in PTC: serine peptidase inhibitor, Kunitz type, 2 (*SPINT2*), RNA polymerase II associated protein 3 (*RPAP3*), basic leucine zipper and W2 domains 1 (*BZW1*). Top 3 genes in BCPAP cells: ribosome production factor 1 homolog (S. cerevisiae) (*RPF1*), TIMP metallopeptidase inhibitor 2 (*TIMP2*), epithelial cell transforming 2 (*ECT2*). Top 3 genes in 8505C cells: ribosomal protein L13a (*RPL13A*), aldolase A, fructose-bisphosphate (*ALDOA*), TIMELESS interacting protein (*TIPIN*).

3.8. The Gene Master Regulator at Play

Our study identified *SPINT2*, a not regulated gene in the investigated PTA, as the GMR of this patient's malignancy. What are the mechanisms by which experimental alteration of *SPINT2* expression might selectively kill the cancer cells but not the normal ones? *SPINT2* is highly coordinated with numerous genes from almost all major functional pathways. However, we considered that apoptosis might be the best candidate to evaluate (from a bioinformatics point of view) the effects of *SPINT2* manipulation. Therefore, we analyzed the expression coordination of *SPINT2* with the 112 apoptosis genes quantified in the two regions. Table 1 presents the apoptosis genes that are significantly up/down regulated in PTC or/and significantly synergistically/antagonistically/independently expressed with *SPINT2* in NOR or/and PTC.

Table 1. Apoptosis genes that are significantly up(U)/down(D) regulated in PTC with respect to NOR or/and significantly synergistically (S)/antagonistically (A)/independently (I) expressed with *SPINT2* in NOR or/and PTC.

GENE	DESCRIPTION	NOR	PTC	REG
ACTG1	actin, γ 1	S		
AKT1	v-akt murine thymoma viral oncogene homolog 1			U
AKT3	v-akt murine thymoma viral oncogene homolog 3		S	
ATF4	activating transcription factor 4	A		
ATM	ataxia telangiectasia mutated		S	
BAK1	BCL2-antagonist/killer 1		S	
BAX	BCL2-associated X protein			U
BBC3	BCL2 binding component 3		S	U
BCL2	B-cell CLL/lymphoma 2	I		
BCL2A1	BCL2-related protein A1			U
BCL2L1	BCL2-like 1		S	
BCL2L11	BCL2-like 11		S	
BID	BH3 interacting domain death agonist			U
BIRC5	baculoviral IAP repeat containing 5			U
CAPN1	calpain 1, (mu/I) large subunit		S	
CASP2	caspase 2, apoptosis-related cysteine peptidase		S	
CASP3	caspase 3, apoptosis-related cysteine peptidase			U
CASP6	caspase 6, apoptosis-related cysteine peptidase		S	
CASP9	caspase 9, apoptosis-related cysteine peptidase	S		
CFLAR	CASP8 and FADD-like apoptosis regulator		S	
CTSC	cathepsin C			U
CTSD	cathepsin D		S	
CTSH	cathepsin H			U
CTSK	cathepsin K			D
CTSL	cathepsin L	S		
CTSV	cathepsin V		S	
CYCS	cytochrome c, somatic	S		D
DAB2IP	DAB2 interacting protein		S	U
DFFA	DNA fragmentation factor		S	
DIABLO	diablo, IAP-binding mitochondrial protein		S	U
EIF2AK3	eukaryotic translation initiation factor 2-α kinase 3		S	
EIF2S1	eukaryotic translation initiation factor 2, subunit 1 α		S	
FAS	Fas cell surface death receptor			U
FOS	FBJ murine osteosarcoma viral oncogene homolog			D
GZMB	granzyme B (granzyme 2, cytotoxic T-lymphocyte-associated serine esterase 1)		S	D
IKBKB	inhibitor of kappa light polypeptide gene enhancer in B-cells, kinase β	I	S	
ITPR2	inositol 1,4,5-trisphosphate receptor, type 2			U
JUN	jun proto-oncogene			D
LMNA	lamin A/C			U
LMNB2	lamin B2		S	
MAP2K1	mitogen-activated protein kinase kinase 1			U
MAP2K2	mitogen-activated protein kinase kinase 2		S	
MAP3K9	mitogen-activated protein kinase kinase kinase 9		S	
MAPK1	mitogen-activated protein kinase 1		S	
MAPK3	mitogen-activated protein kinase 3		S	
NFKB1	nuclear factor of kappa light polypeptide gene enhancer in B-cells 1	S		
NFKBIA	nuclear factor of kappa light polypeptide gene enhancer in B-cells inhibitor, α			D
NRAS	neuroblastoma RAS viral (v-ras) oncogene homolog		S	
PARP1	poly (ADP-ribose) polymerase 1			U
PARP4	poly (ADP-ribose) polymerase family, member 4		S	
PDPK1	3-phosphoinositide dependent protein kinase 1		S	
PIK3CA	phosphatidylinositol-4,5-bisphosphate 3-kinase, catalytic subunit α		S	

Table 1. *Cont.*

GENE	DESCRIPTION	NOR	PTC	REG
PIK3R1	phosphoinositide-3-kinase, regulatory subunit 1			D
PIK3R2	phosphoinositide-3-kinase, regulatory subunit 2		S	U
PMAIP1	phorbol-12-myristate-13-acetate-induced protein 1		S	U
RAF1	v-raf-1 murine leukemia viral oncogene homolog 1	S		
RELA	v-rel avian reticuloendotheliosis viral oncogene homolog A		S	
TNFRSF10B	tumor necrosis factor receptor superfamily, member 10b			U
TNFRSF1A	tumor necrosis factor receptor superfamily, member 1A		S	U
TRAF2	TNF receptor-associated factor 2		S	
TUBA1C	tubulin, α 1b	I		
TUBA3D	tubulin, α 3c	I		
TUBA4A	tubulin, α 4a			U
XIAP	X-linked inhibitor of apoptosis		S	

In PTC (21 significantly up-regulated andseven down-regulated apoptosis genes), we found *SPINT2* to be significantly synergistically expressed with 34 apoptosis genes, but with no significant antagonistically or independently expressed partners. This is a substantial increase from the six synergistically, one antagonistically and four independently expressed apoptosis partners of *SPINT2* in NOR. Interestingly, none of the significant correlations in NOR (with: *ACTG1, ATF4, CASP9, CTSL, CYCS, NFKB1*) were maintained in PTC.

What effect the overexpression of an otherwise stably expressed but not regulated gene in PTC (*SPINT2*) may have on cancer cells? Most probably, owing to the substantial expression synergistic coordination with apoptosis genes, the experimental overexpression of *SPINT2* would up-regulate many of these genes, forcing the commanded (PTC) cells to enter programmed death.

There was no way to validate this hypothesis on the patient from whom we had profiled the thyroid tumor. However, we tested the general hypothesis that expression coordination with one gene predicts expression regulation when the expression of that gene is experimentally manipulated. For this purpose, we analyzed the transcriptomes of the TC cell lines BCPAP and 8505C cells before and after stable lentiviral transfection with either *DDX19B, NEMP1, PANK2* or *UBALD1* [8]. Figure 7a,b plots the correlation coefficient with *DDX19B* in the untreated cells against the fold-changes (negative for down-regulation) of the genes in the transfected cells. They clearly show that expression coordination predicts (>86%) the expression regulation with reasonable accuracy. Similar validation (83–91%) was obtained for the same cell lines transfected with either *NEMP1, PANK2* or *UBALD1*. Based on this validation, Figure 7c illustrates the predicted regulations of apoptosis genes if the expression level of *SPINT2* in PTC is significantly increased.

In Figure 7c, we used the uniform contribution of the significantly altered genes to the percentages of (up-/down-) regulated genes. Note that from 21 up-regulated and six down-regulated genes in untreated PTC, overexpression of *SPINT2* may result in 48 up-regulated and six down-regulated genes. The expression of six genes, *BBC3, DAB2IP, DIABLO, PIK3R2, PMAIP1, TNFRSF1A*, which are already up-regulated in PTC may be further increased by treatment, while the down-regulation of *GZMB* in untreated PTC may be recovered by overexpressing *SINT2*.

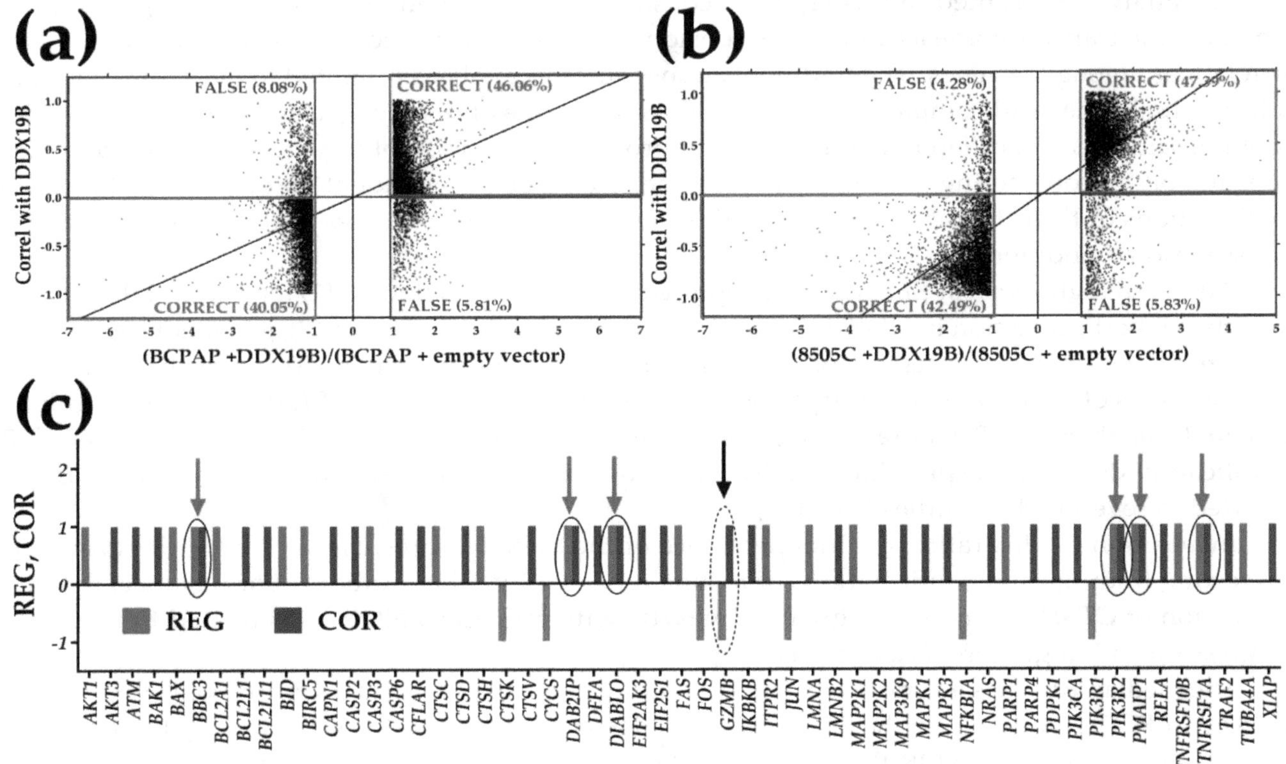

Figure 7. Prediction of the ripple effects of experimental gene regulation. (**a**) Expression coordination with *DDX19B* in untreated BCAP cells accurately predicts 86.11% (40.05 + 46.06) the type of the expression regulation in BCAP cells stably transfected with *DDX19B*; (**b**) Expression coordination with *DDX19B* in untreated 8505C cells accurately predicts 89.88% (42.49 + 47.39) of the type of the expression regulation in 8505C cells stably transfected with *DDX19B*; (**c**) Predicted regulation (1 for up-regulation and −1 for down-regulation) of apoptotic genes in PTC following experimental overexpression of *SPINT2*. REG = significant (1 = up-regulation, −1 = down-regulation). COR = significant expression synergism. Only the regulated genes in the untreated PTC and those expected to be regulated in treated PTC are represented. Red arrows indicate combined effect in treated tumor of regulation and expression synergism in untreated PTC. The black arrow indicates the down-regulation in untreated PTC expected to be compensated by the overexpression of *SPINT2*.

4. Discussion

Although with no molecular biology validation, the bioinformatics analysis of the gene expression profiles in the cancer nodule and surrounding normal tissue of a surgically removed papillary tumor produced some very interesting results, out of which the most important are:

1. Each cell phenotype from the tumor is governed by a different gene hierarchy and a distinct organization of its transcriptome;
2. As selected from the most altered genes in a large population of cancer patients, the biomarkers have low GCH and therefore little therapeutic value;
3. The GMR of the cancer nodule is the most legitimate target of the gene therapy because it is the most influential gene for cancer cells while having very little role in the surrounding normal cells;
4. *SPINT2* was identified as the GMR of the PTC nodule of the profiled tumor and a gene with very low GCH score in NOR;
5. The up-regulation of the synergistically expressed apoptosis genes in untreated PTC following the experimental *SPINT2* overexpression was identified as a potential mechanism of selectively killing the cancer cells.

The analysis presented in this report is consistent with the genomic fabric paradigm [11] that considers the transcriptome as a multi-dimensional object subjected to a dynamic set of expression correlations among the genes. The traditional transcriptomic analysis is limited to the expression level of individual genes and comparisons of the expression levels of distinct genes in the same condition or of the same gene in different conditions. Our procedure considerably enlarges the transcriptomic information by considering for each gene not one, but three independent features and all possible combinations of these features to compare the genes and groups of genes in the same condition or across various conditions.

Although high levels of *EEF1A1* were reported in renal cell carcinoma [27], we found this gene to have the highest expression in NOR and one of the highest levels in PTC (68.47), albeit not significantly down-regulated. A high expression of *NPC2* and its significant elevation in PTC were also detected in meta-analyses of public PTC transcriptomes [28]. Overexpression of *CHI3L1*, the most up-regulated gene in the analyzed PTC, was reported as associated with metastatic PTC [29] and its recurrence [30]. Significantly decreased expression of *TFF3*, the most down-regulated gene in our study, was also reported in several other studies (e.g., [31]).

In addition to illustrating the independence of the three features, Figure 1 provides also some interesting findings and confirmations of results reported by other authors. For instance, the high expression of *CTSH* in PTC (up-regulated by 6.78x with respect to NOR) was related to the tumor progression and migration of cancer cells [32].

The median REV has a statistically significant (p-value = 7.79×10^{-5}) decrease from 39.75 in NOR to 38.69 in PTC. According to the Second Law of Thermodynamics, the significantly larger overall expression variability in NOR than in PTC indicates not only relaxed control by the homeostatic mechanisms (average $REC_{NOR} = 0.084$, average $REC_{PTC} = 0.113$), but also that NOR is closer to the thermodynamic (here physiological) equilibrium. Supporting this assertion is the reduction in the median REV observed by us in all other gene expression studies on animal models of human diseases (e.g., [33–35]) and in tissues of animals subjected to various stresses (e.g., [36–38] or to genetic manipulations (e.g., [39,40]). The high expression variability of *CFLAR* (a key anti-apoptosis regulator [41]) in NOR (REV = 102.93) may explain the adaptability of the apoptosis pathway to a large spectrum of environmental conditions. The *CFLAR* REV dramatic reduction in PTC (REV = 29.41) shows the need for tighter control of resisting apoptosis in cancer. Moreover, its reduction in expression level (in PTC by −1.64x) was associated with delayed apoptosis [41].

The observed down-regulation of *FOS* in PTC (Figure 2) confirms the findings of some groups [42,43] but contradicts its frequent (however not 100%) up-regulation reported by another group in 40 patients with thyroid cancer and 20 with benign thyroid diseases [44]. Let us analyze what measure of regulation is the most informative and use the examples of *FOS* and *KIT* (another gene down-regulated in thyroid cancer [45]). Although both genes account as units for the percentage of the down-regulated genes, they contribute −2.06x and −8.15x as expression ratios and −46.28 and −3.76 as WIRs. Since WIR is a more comprehensive measure, *FOS* regulation appears to be the most important factor in the alteration of this group of genes. Indeed, FOS protein is an important player in cell proliferation, differentiation, transformation and apoptotic cell death.

Among the significantly regulated genes from the KEGG-derived THS pathway (Figure 3), only *PAX8* (−1.94x) was previously related to the thyroid cancer, albeit to the follicular form. Moreover, we found that peroxisome proliferator-activated receptor γ (*PPARG*) whose fusion with *PAX8* is considered an important trigger of the FTC [46], was likewise significantly down-regulated (−4.99x). Interestingly, in Figure 3, the two glutathione peroxidases, *GPX1* (1.60x) and *GPX3* (−1.84x), were oppositely regulated. Since the down-regulation of *GPX1* was reported to augment the pro-inflammatory cytokine-induced redox signaling and endothelial cell activation [47], one may assume that up-regulation of *GPX1* will do the opposite, i.e., diminish the pro-inflammatory cytokine-induced redox signaling. As such, the PTC cells will become more resistant to the inflammatory response.

According to the KEGG map hsa04110, some of the regulated cell-cycle genes (Figure 4) were associated with a wide diversity of cancers. Thus, up-regulation of *CDKN1A* was associated with cervical cancer [48] and down-regulation of *CDKN1C* with gastric cancer [49]. As stated in [3], up-regulation/mutation of *CDKN2A* was detected in numerous cancer forms: neoplasms (squamous cell, ductal, lobular, cystic, mucinous, serous, mesothelial, lipomathous, myomathous, thymic epithelial, complex, mixed), adenomas, adenocarcionmas, gliomas, nevi and melanomas, transitional cell papillomas and carcinomas, mature B-cell lymphomas, soft tissue tumors and sarcomas. *CDKN2B* was associated with malignant pleural mesothelioma, osteosarcoma and meningioma. However, we found no report associating these genes with thyroid cancer. Unfortunately, one of the most cancer-related genes, *TP53* [50], was not quantified in this experiment due to the corrupted probing spot in one of the microarrays, which can be seen as a major limitation of the study.

As illustrated in Figure 5 for interlinks between the five complexes of the oxidative phosphorylation, cancer remodels the gene networks, profoundly perturbing the mitochondrial function [51]. Among others, 10 synergistically expressed gene pairs in NOR are switched into antagonistically expressed pairs in PTC: *NDUFA10-SDHD, CYC1-COX1, COX10-ATP6V0B, COX10-ATP6V0C, COX5B-LHPP, COX6A1-ATV1B2, COX6A1-LHPP, COX6A2-ATP6V0B, COX6A2-ATP6V1A, COX7C-ATP6V1G2.* These switches, the cancellation of all significant antagonisms and the added synergisms increase the expression synchrony of the pathway genes [17] and remove the controlling bottlenecks. In a synergistic pair, the up-regulation of one gene triggers the up-regulation of the other. Although in this experiment we did not detect significantly altered expressions of *NDUFA10* and *SDHD*, their significant synergism in PTC may explain why they are both up-regulated in oral cancer [52].

Given the never-repeatable set of risk factors, each patient is unique and therefore their gene hierarchy is unique. Although the chance of finding the same GMR in two persons is about 1/20,000 and that of the first two genes is 1/400 million, from the first three genes up, the number of possibilities (7.9988×10^{12}) exceeds by far the Earth human population. Therefore, the top three genes are enough to uniquely represent the cancer of each person at a given time. In our studied PTC, the top three genes were: *SPINT2, RPAP3* and *BZW,1* with none of them significantly regulated with respect to NOR.

SPINT2, the identified GMR of the profiled PTC (Figure 6), was previously reported by several groups to be involved in the development and progression of a wide diversity of forms of cancer [53]. Among others, *SPINT2* was associated with metastatic osteosarcoma [54], ovarian cancer [55], glioma/glioblastoma [56,57], prostate cancer [58] and non-small lung cancer [59], leukemia [60] and cervical carcinoma [61]. *RPAP3*, essential for assembling chaperone complexes [62], was linked to hypoxia-adapted cancer cells [63] and *BZW,1* was associated with ovarian [64], lung [65] and salivary gland [66] cancers. However, we found no mention in the literature about the role of these first three genes in any form of thyroid cancer.

In Figure 7 and Table 1, we tested whether expression synergism with apoptosis genes may be one of the mechanisms by which manipulation of *SPINT2* expression is lethal to the PTC cells but not to the NOR cells. First, we determined the significant coordination of *SPINT2* with apoptosis genes in both NOR and PTC and found a substantial increase in the expression synergism in PTC. Then, we tested the predictive value of the expression coordination by profiling two standard human TC cell lines before and after stable transfection with four genes selected, only to have substantially different GCHs in the two cell lines. Although *DDX19B* and *PANK2* (but not *NEMP1* and *UBALD1*) were synergistically expressed with *SPINT2* in PTC, there are no reports relating these genes with *SPINT2* in any form of cancer. As mentioned in [8], *NEMP1* and *PANK2* had higher GCHs and induced larger transcriptomic alterations in the BCPAP than in the 8505C cells. In contrast, *DDX19B* and *UBALD1* had higher GCHs and induced larger transcriptomic alterations in the 8505C than in the BCPAP cells. Figure 7a,b confirms our previous findings that expression correlation with one gene predicts what genes are regulated when the expression of that gene is manipulated. A similar conclusion was drawn in [67], where we had shown that most genes are synergistically/antagonistically expressed with *Gja* (encoding the gap junction protein Cx43) in the brain and hearts of wildtype mice are down-/up-regulated in the brain and hearts of Cx43KO mice. Therefore, as illustrated in Figure 7c, we expect that, due to the synergism, the overexpression of *SPINT2* will force the PTC cells into programmed death by up-regulating numerous apoptosis genes.

5. Conclusions

Owing to the matchless set of conditioning factors, each human is unique and, despite all similarities, the transcriptomes of one person's cell phenotypes can never be identical with those of another person. In a profiled metastatic clear cell renal cell carcinoma [34], we found that even the transcriptomes of two cancer nodules isolated from the same kidney and categorized with the same Fuhrman grade 3 were largely different from each other. Moreover, some of the gene expression conditioning factors (environment, exposure to stress and toxins, medical treatment, diet, ageing etc.) are not constant, forcing the transcriptomes of cancer cells to continuously adapt. By consequence, the gene hierarchy is not only unique for each person and in each of his/her cancer nodules, but it changes over time. As such, this study provides strong reasons in favor of a really personalized and time-sensitive cancer gene therapy based on the manipulation of the gene master regulators.

References

1. Cancer Org Portal. Available online: https://www.cancer.org/cancer/thyroid-cancer (accessed on 26 July 2020).
2. Thyroid Cancer Portal. Available online: https://www.thyroid.org/thyroid-cancer/ (accessed on 26 July 2020).
3. Cancer Gov. Available online: https://portal.gdc.cancer.gov (accessed on 26 July 2020).
4. 1000 Genomes Project Consortium; Auton, A.; Brooks, L.D.; Durbin, R.M.; Garrison, E.P.; Kang, H.M.; Korbel, J.O.; Marchini, J.L.; McCarthy, S.; McVean, G.A.; et al. A global reference for human genetic variation. *Nature* **2015**, *526*, 68–74. [CrossRef] [PubMed]
5. Alexander, E.K.; Kennedy, G.C.; Baloch, Z.W.; Cibas, E.S.; Chudova, D.; Diggans, J.; Friedman, L.; Kloos, R.T.; LiVolsi, V.A.; Mandel, S.J.; et al. Preoperative diagnosis of benign thyroid nodules with indeterminate cytology. *N. Engl. J. Med.* **2012**, *367*, 705–715. [CrossRef] [PubMed]
6. Abdullah, M.I.; Junit, S.M.; Ng, K.L.; Jayapalan, J.J.; Karikalan, B.; Hashim, O.H. Papillary Thyroid Cancer: Genetic Alterations and Molecular Biomrker Investigations. *Int. J. Med. Sci.* **2019**, *16*, 450–460. [CrossRef]
7. Foundation Medicine. Available online: https://www.foundationmedicine.com/genomic-testing (accessed on 12 July 2020).
8. Iacobas, D.A.; Tuli, N.; Iacobas, S.; Rasamny, J.K.; Moscatello, A.; Geliebter, J.; Tiwari, R.K. Gene master regulators of papillary and anaplastic thyroid cancer phenotypes. *Oncotarget* **2018**, *9*, 2410–2424. [CrossRef] [PubMed]
9. Iacobas, S.; Ede, N.; Iacobas, D.A. The Gene Master Regulators (GMR) Approach Provides Legitimate Targets for Personalized, Time-Sensitive Cancer Gene Therapy. *Genes* **2019**, *10*, 560. [CrossRef] [PubMed]
10. Iacobas, D.A. Commentary on "The Gene Master Regulators (GMR) Approach Provides Legitimate Targets for Personalized, Time-Sensitive Cancer Gene Therapy. *J. Cancer Immunol.* **2019**, *1*, 31–33. [CrossRef]
11. Iacobas, D.A. The Genomic Fabric Perspective on the Transcriptome between Universal Quantifiers and Personalized Genomic Medicine. *Biol. Theory* **2016**, *11*, 123–137. [CrossRef]
12. National Center for Biotechnology Information. Available online: https://www.ncbi.nlm.nih.gov/gds/?term=iacobas (accessed on 26 July 2020).
13. Zhang, H.; Xing, Z.; Mani, S.K.; Bancel, B.; Durantel, D.; Zoulim, F.; Tran, E.J.; Merle, P.; Andrisani, O. RNA helicase DEAD box protein 5 regulates Polycomb repressive complex 2/Hox transcript antisense intergenic RNA function in hepatitis B virus infection and hepatocarcinogenesis. *Hepatology* **2016**, *64*, 1033–1048. [CrossRef]
14. Liu, Y.; Tong, C.; Cao, J.; Xiong, M. NEMP1 Promotes Tamoxifen Resistance in Breast Cancer Cells. *Biochem. Genet.* **2019**, *57*, 813–826. [CrossRef]

15. Liu, Y.; Cheng, Z.; Li, Q.; Pang, Y.; Cui, L.; Qian, T.; Quan, L.; Dai, Y.; Jiao, Y.; Zhang, Z.; et al. Prognostic significance of the PANK family expression in acute myeloid leukemia. *Ann. Transl. Med.* **2019**, *7*, 261. [CrossRef]
16. Iacobas, D.A.; Iacobas, S.; Stout, R.; Spray, D.C. Cellular environment remodels the genomic fabrics of functional pathways in astrocytes. *Genes* **2020**, *11*, 520. [CrossRef]
17. Iacobas, D.A.; Iacobas, S.; Lee, P.R.; Cohen, J.E.; Fields, R.D. Coordinated Activity of Transcriptional Networks Responding to the Pattern of Action Potential Firing in Neurons. *Genes* **2019**, *10*, 754. [CrossRef] [PubMed]
18. Iacobas, D.A.; Iacobas, S.; Spray, D.C. Connexin43 and the brain transcriptome of the newborn mice. *Genomics* **2007**, *89*, 113–123. [CrossRef]
19. Mathew, R.; Huang, J.; Iacobas, S.; Iacobas, D.A. Pulmonary Hypertension Remodels the Genomic Fabrics of Major Functional Pathways. *Genes* **2020**, *11*, 126. [CrossRef] [PubMed]
20. Iacobas, D.A.; Iacobas, S.; Tanowitz, H.B.; de Carvalho, A.C.; Spray, D.C. Functional genomic fabrics are remodeled in a mouse model of Chagasic cardiomyopathy and restored following cell therapy. *Microbes Infect.* **2018**, *20*, 185–195. [CrossRef] [PubMed]
21. Kanehisa, M.; Furumichi, M.; Tanabe, M.; Sato, Y.; Morishima, K. KEGG: New perspectives on genomes, pathways, diseases and drugs. *Nucleic Acids Res.* **2017**, *45*, D353–D361. [CrossRef]
22. Kyoto Encyclopedia of Genes and Genomes. Available online: http://www.genome.jp/kegg/ (accessed on 21 June 2020).
23. Liu, Y.C.; Yeh, C.T.; Lin, K.H. Molecular Functions of Thyroid Hormone Signaling in Regulation of Cancer Progression and Anti-Apoptosis. *Int. J. Mol. Sci.* **2019**, *20*, 4986. [CrossRef]
24. Bai, J.W.; Wei, M.; Li, J.W.; Zhang, G.J. Notch Signaling Pathway and Endocrine Resistance in Breast Cancer. *Front. Pharmacol.* **2020**, *11*, 924. [CrossRef]
25. Yuan, Y.; Ju, Y.S.; Kim, Y.; Li, J.; Wang, Y.; Yoon, C.J.; Yang, Y.; Martincorena, I.; Creighton, C.J.; Weinstein, J.N.; et al. Comprehensive molecular characterization of mitochondrial genomes in human cancers. *Nat. Genet.* **2020**, *52*, 342–352. [CrossRef]
26. Kobawala, T.P.; Trivedi, T.I.; Gajjar, K.K.; Patel, D.H.; Patel, G.H.; Ghosh, N.R. Significance of Interleukin-6 in Papillary Thyroid Carcinoma. *J. Thyroid. Res.* **2016**, 6178921. [CrossRef]
27. Bao, Y.; Zhao, T.L.; Zhang, Z.Q.; Liang, X.L.; Wang, Z.X.; Xiong, Y.; Lu, X.; Wang, L.H. High eukaryotic translation elongation factor 1 alpha 1 expression promotes proliferation and predicts poor prognosis in clear cell renal cell carcinoma. *Neoplasma* **2020**, *67*, 78–84. [CrossRef] [PubMed]
28. Wu, C.C.; Lin, J.D.; Chen, J.T.; Chang, C.M.; Weng, H.F.; Hsueh, C.; Chien, H.P.; Yu, J.S. Integrated analysis of fine-needle-aspiration cystic fluid proteome, cancer cell secretome, and public transcriptome datasets for papillary thyroid cancer biomarker discovery. *Oncotarget* **2018**, *9*, 12079–12100. [CrossRef] [PubMed]
29. Luo, D.; Chen, H.; Lu, P.; Li, X.; Long, M.; Peng, X.; Huang, M.; Huang, K.; Lin, S.; Tan, L.; et al. CHI3L1 overexpression is associated with metastasis and is an indicator of poor prognosis in papillary thyroid carcinoma. *Cancer Biomark.* **2017**, *18*, 273–284. [CrossRef] [PubMed]
30. Cheng, S.P.; Lee, J.J.; Chang, Y.C.; Lin, C.H.; Li, Y.S.; Liu, C.L. Overexpression of chitinase-3-like protein 1 is associated with structural recurrence in patients with differentiated thyroid cancer. *J. Pathol.* **2020**, e5503. [CrossRef]
31. Oczko-Wojciechowska, M.; Pfeifer, A.; Jarzab, M.; Swierniak, M.; Rusinek, D.; Tyszkiewicz, T.; Kowalska, M.; Chmielik, E.; Zembala-Nozynska, E.; Czarniecka, A.; et al. Impact of the Tumor Microenvironment on the Gene Expression Profile in Papillary Thyroid Cancer. *Pathobiology* **2020**, *87*, 143–154. [CrossRef] [PubMed]
32. Jevnikar, Z.; Rojnik, M.; Jamnik, P.; Doljak, B.; Fonovic, U.P.; Kos, J. Cathepsin H mediates the processing of talin and regulates migration of prostate cancer cells. *J. Biol. Chem.* **2013**, *288*, 2201–2209. [CrossRef]
33. Iacobas, D.A.; Iacobas, S.; Werner, P.; Scemes, E.; Spray, D.C. Alteration of transcriptomic networks in adoptive-transfer experimental autoimmune encephalomyelitis. *Front. Integr. Neurosci.* **2007**, *1*. [CrossRef]
34. Iacobas, D.A.; Iacobas, S. Towards a Personalized Cancer Gene Therapy: A Case of Clear Cell Renal Cell Carcinoma. *Cancer Oncol. Res.* **2017**, *5*, 45–52. [CrossRef]
35. Frigeri, A.; Iacobas, D.A.; Iacobas, S.; Nicchia, G.P.; Desaphy, J.-F.; Camerino, D.C.; Svelto, M.; Spray, D.C. Effect of microagravity on brain gene expression in mice. *Exp. Brain Res.* **2008**, *191*, 289–300. [CrossRef]
36. Iacobas, D.A.; Fan, C.; Iacobas, S.; Spray, D.C.; Haddad, G.G. Transcriptomic changes in developing kidney exposed to chronic hypoxia. *Biochem. Biophys. Res. Commun.* **2006** *349*, 329–338. [CrossRef]

37. Iacobas, D.A.; Fan, C.; Iacobas, S.; Haddad, G.G. Integrated transcriptomic response to cardiac chronic hypoxia: Translation regulators and response to stress in cell survival. *Funct. Integr. Genom.* **2008**, *8*, 265–275. [CrossRef] [PubMed]

38. Iacobas, D.A.; Iacobas, S.; Haddad, G.G. Heart rhythm genomic fabric in hypoxia. *Biochem. Biophys. Res. Commun.* **2010**, *391*, 1769–1774. [CrossRef] [PubMed]

39. Iacobas, D.A.; Urban, M.; Iacobas, S.; Scemes, E.; Spray, D.C. Array analysis of gene expression in connexin43 null astrocytes. *Physiol. Genom.* **2003**, *15*, 177–190. [CrossRef] [PubMed]

40. Iacobas, D.A.; Iacobas, S.; Urban-Maldonado, M.; Scemes, E.; Spray, D.C. Similar transcriptomic alterations in Cx43 knock-down and knock-out astrocytes. *Cell Commun. Adhes.* **2008**, *15*, 195–206. [CrossRef] [PubMed]

41. Surmiak, M.; Hubalewska-Mazgaj, M.; Wawrzycka-Adamczyk, K.; Musiał, J.; Sanak, M. Delayed neutrophil apoptosis in granulomatosis with polyangiitis: Dysregulation of neutrophil gene signature and circulating apoptosis-related proteins. *Scand. J. Rheumatol.* **2020**, *49*, 57–67. [CrossRef]

42. Zhao, Y.; Liu, X.; Zhong, L.; He, M.; Chen, S.; Wang, T.; Ma, S. The combined use of miRNAs and mRNAs as biomarkers for the diagnosis of papillary thyroid carcinoma. *Int. J. Mol. Med.* **2015**, *36*, 1097–1103. [CrossRef]

43. Deligiorgi, M.V.; Mahaira, H.; Eftychiadis, C.; Kafiri, G.; Georgiou, G.; Theodoropoulos, G.; Konstadoulakis, M.M.; Zografos, E.; Zografos, G.C. RANKL, OPG, TRAIL, KRas, and c-Fos expression in relation to central lymph node metastases in papillary thyroid carcinoma. *J. BU ON Off. J. Balk. Union Oncol.* **2018**, *23*, 1029–1040.

44. Kataki, A.; Sotirianakos, S.; Memos, N.; Karayiannis, M.; Messaris, E.; Leandros, E.; Manouras, A.; Androulakis, G. P53 and C-FOS overexpression in patients with thyroid cancer: An immunohistochemical study. *Neoplasma* **2003**, *50*, 26–30.

45. Franceschi, S.; Lessi, F.; Panebianco, F.; Tantillo, E.; La Ferla, M.; Menicagli, M.; Aretini, P.; Apollo, A.; Naccarato, A.G.; Marchetti, I.; et al. Loss of c-KIT expression in thyroid cancer cells. *PLoS ONE* **2017**, *12*, e0173913. [CrossRef]

46. Chu, Y.H.; Sadow, P.M. Noninvasive Follicular Thyroid Neoplasm with Papillary-Like Nuclear Features (NIFTP): Diagnostic Updates and Molecular Advances. In *Seminars in Diagnostic Pathology*; WB Saunders: Philadelphia, PA, USA, 2020.

47. Lubos, E.; Kelly, N.J.; Oldebeken, S.R.; Leopold, J.A.; Zhang, Y.Y.; Loscalzo, J.; Handy, D.E. Glutathione peroxidase-1 deficiency augments proinflammatory cytokine-induced redox signaling and human endothelial cell activation. *J. Biol. Chem.* **2011**, *286*, 35407–35417. [CrossRef]

48. Cardoso, M.F.S.; Castelletti, C.H.M.; Lima-Filho, J.L.; Martins, D.B.G.; Teixeira, J.A.C. Putative biomarkers for cervical cancer: SNVs, methylation and expression profiles. *Mutat. Res.* **2017**, *773*, 161–173. [CrossRef] [PubMed]

49. Mei, L.; Shen, C.; Miao, R.; Wang, J.Z.; Cao, M.D.; Zhang, Y.S.; Shi, L.H.; Zhao, G.H.; Wang, M.H.; Wu, L.S.; et al. RNA methyltransferase NSUN2 promotes gastric cancer cell proliferation by repressing p57Kip2 by an m5C-dependent manner. *Cell Death Dis.* **2020**, *11*, 270. [CrossRef] [PubMed]

50. Matsuda, S.; Murakami, M.; Ikeda, Y.; Nakagawa, Y.; Tsuji, A.; Kitagishi, Y. Role of tumor suppressor molecules in genomic perturbations and damaged DNA repair involved in the pathogenesis of cancer and neurodegeneration (Review). *Biomed. Rep.* **2020**, *13*, 10. [CrossRef]

51. Księżakowska-Łakoma, K.; Żyła, M.; Wilczyński, J.R. Mitochondrial dysfunction in cancer. *Prz. Menopauzalny* **2014**, *13*, 136–144. [CrossRef]

52. Huang, Y.P.; Chang, N.W. PPARα modulates gene expression profiles of mitochondrial energy metabolism in oral tumorigenesis. *Biomedicine* **2016**, *6*, 3. [CrossRef]

53. Roversi, F.M.; Olalla Saad, S.T.; Machado-Neto, J.A. Serine peptidase inhibitor Kunitz type 2 (SPINT2) in cancer development and progression. *Biomed. Pharmacother.* **2018**, *101*, 278–286. [CrossRef]

54. Guan, X.; Guan, Z.; Song, C. Expression profile analysis identifies key genes as prognostic markers for metastasis of osteosarcoma. *Cancer Cell Int.* **2020**, *20*, 104. [CrossRef]

55. Graumann, J.; Finkernagel, F.; Reinartz, S.; Stief, T.; Brödje, D.; Renz, H.; Jansen, J.M.; Wagner, U.; Worzfeld, T.; Pogge von Strandmann, E.; et al. Multi-platform affinity proteomics identify proteins linked to metastasis and immune suppression in ovarian cancer plasma. *Front. Oncol.* **2019**, *9*, 1150. [CrossRef] [PubMed]
56. Liu, F.; Cox, C.D.; Chowdhury, R.; Dovek, L.; Nguyen, H.; Li, T.; Li, S.; Ozer, B.; Chou, A.; Nguyen, N.; et al. SPINT2 is hypermethylated in both IDH1 mutated and wild-type glioblastomas, and exerts tumor suppression via reduction of c-Met activation. *J. Neurooncol.* **2019**, *142*, 423–434. [CrossRef] [PubMed]
57. Pereira, M.S.; Celeiro, S.P.; Costa, Â.M.; Pinto, F.; Popov, S.; de Almeida, G.C.; Amorim, J.; Pires, M.M.; Pinheiro, C.; Lopes, J.M.; et al. Loss of SPINT2 expression frequently occurs in glioma, leading to increased growth and invasion via MMP2. *Cell. Oncol.* **2020**, *43*, 107–121. [CrossRef] [PubMed]
58. Wu, L.; Shu, X.; Bao, J.; Guo, X.; Kote-Jarai, Z.; Haiman, C.A.; Eeles, R.A.; Zheng, W.; PRACTICAL, CRUK, BPC3, CAPS, PEGASUS Consortia. Analysis of Over 140,000 European Descendants Identifies Genetically Predicted Blood Protein Biomarkers Associated with Prostate Cancer Risk. *Cancer Res.* **2019**, *79*, 4592–4598. [CrossRef] [PubMed]
59. Ma, Z.; Liu, D.; Li, W.; Di, S.; Zhang, Z.; Zhang, J.; Xu, L.; Guo, K.; Zhu, Y.; Han, J.; et al. STYK1 promotes tumor growth and metastasis by reducing SPINT2/HAI-2 expression in non-small cell lung cancer. *Cell Death Dis.* **2019**, *10*, 435. [CrossRef] [PubMed]
60. Roversi, F.M.; Cury, N.M.; Lopes, M.R.; Ferro, K.P.; Machado-Neto, J.A.; Alvarez, M.C.; Dos Santos, G.P.; Giardini Rosa, R.; Longhini, A.L.; Duarte, A.D.S.S.; et al. Up-regulation of SPINT2/HAI-2 by Azacytidine in bone marrow mesenchymal stromal cells affects leukemic stem cell survival and adhesion. *J. Cell. Mol. Med.* **2019**, *23*, 1562–1571. [CrossRef] [PubMed]
61. Wang, N.; Che, Y.; Yin, F.; Yu, F.; Bi, X.; Wang, Y. Study on the methylation status of SPINT2 gene and its expression in cervical carcinoma. *Cancer Biomark.* **2018**, *22*, 435–442. [CrossRef] [PubMed]
62. Rodríguez, C.F.; Llorca, O. RPAP3 C-Terminal Domain: A Conserved Domain for the Assembly of R2TP Co-Chaperone Complexes. *Cells* **2020**, *9*, 1139. [CrossRef] [PubMed]
63. Kawachi, T.; Tanaka, S.; Fukuda, A.; Sumii, Y.; Setiawan, A.; Kotoku, N.; Kobayashi, M.; Arai, M. Target identification of the marine natural products Dictyoceratin-A and -C as selective growth inhibitors in cancer cells adapted to hypoxic environments. *Mar. Drugs* **2019**, *17*, 163. [CrossRef]
64. Liu, F.; Zhao, H.; Gong, L.; Yao, L.; Li, Y.; Zhang, W. MicroRNA-129-3p functions as a tumor suppressor in serous ovarian cancer by targeting BZW1. *Int. J. Clin. Exp. Pathol.* **2018**, *11*, 5901–5908.
65. Chiou, J.; Chang, Y.C.; Jan, Y.H.; Tsai, H.F.; Yang, C.J.; Huang, M.S.; Yu, Y.L.; Hsiao, M. Overexpression of BZW1 is an independent poor prognosis marker and its down-regulation suppresses lung adenocarcinoma metastasis. *Sci. Rep.* **2019**, *9*, 14624. [CrossRef]
66. Li, S.; Chai, Z.; Li, Y.; Liu, D.; Bai, Z.; Li, Y.; Li, Y.; Situ, Z. BZW1, a novel proliferation regulator that promotes growth of salivary muocepodermoid carcinoma. *Cancer Lett.* **2009**, *284*, 86–94. [CrossRef]
67. Iacobas, D.A.; Iacobas, S.; Spray, D.C. Connexin-dependent transcellular transcriptomic networks in mouse brain. *Prog. Biophys. Mol. Biol.* **2007**, *94*, 168–184. [CrossRef]

9

Histogram Analysis of Diffusion Weighted Imaging at 3T is Useful for Prediction of Lymphatic Metastatic Spread, Proliferative Activity and Cellularity in Thyroid Cancer

Stefan Schob [1,*], Hans Jonas Meyer [2], Julia Dieckow [3], Bhogal Pervinder [4], Nikolaos Pazaitis [5], Anne Kathrin Höhn [6], Nikita Garnov [2], Diana Horvath-Rizea [4], Karl-Titus Hoffmann [1] and Alexey Surov [2]

1 Department for Neuroradiology, University Hospital Leipzig, Leipzig 04103, Germany; karl-titus.hoffmann@medizin.uni-leipzig.de
2 Department for Diagnostic and Interventional Radiology, University Hospital Leipzig, Leipzig 04103, Germany; jonas90.meyer@web.de (H.J.M.); nikita@garnov.de (N.G.); alexey.surov@medizin.uni-leipzig.de (A.S.)
3 Department for Ophthalmology, University Hospital Leipzig, Leipzig 04103, Germany; julia@dieckow.de
4 Department for Diagnostic and Interventional Neuroradiology, Katharinenhospital Stuttgart, Stuttgart 70174, Germany; bhogalweb@aol.com (B.P.); dihorvath@freenet.de (D.H.-R.)
5 Institute for Pathology, University Hospital Halle-Wittenberg, Martin-Luther-University Halle-Wittenberg, Halle 06112, Germany; nikolaos.pazaitis@uk-halle.de
6 Institute for Pathology, University Hospital Leipzig, Leipzig 04103, Germany; annekathrin.hoehn@medizin.uni-leipzig.de
* Correspondence: stefan.schob@medizin.uni-leipzig.de

Academic Editor: Daniela Gabriele Grimm

Abstract: Pre-surgical diffusion weighted imaging (DWI) is increasingly important in the context of thyroid cancer for identification of the optimal treatment strategy. It has exemplarily been shown that DWI at 3T can distinguish undifferentiated from well-differentiated thyroid carcinoma, which has decisive implications for the magnitude of surgery. This study used DWI histogram analysis of whole tumor apparent diffusion coefficient (ADC) maps. The primary aim was to discriminate thyroid carcinomas which had already gained the capacity to metastasize lymphatically from those not yet being able to spread via the lymphatic system. The secondary aim was to reflect prognostically important tumor-biological features like cellularity and proliferative activity with ADC histogram analysis. Fifteen patients with follicular-cell derived thyroid cancer were enrolled. Lymph node status, extent of infiltration of surrounding tissue, and Ki-67 and p53 expression were assessed in these patients. DWI was obtained in a 3T system using b values of 0, 400, and 800 s/mm^2. Whole tumor ADC volumes were analyzed using a histogram-based approach. Several ADC parameters showed significant correlations with immunohistopathological parameters. Most importantly, ADC histogram skewness and ADC histogram kurtosis were able to differentiate between nodal negative and nodal positive thyroid carcinoma. Conclusions: histogram analysis of whole ADC tumor volumes has the potential to provide valuable information on tumor biology in thyroid carcinoma. However, further studies are warranted.

Keywords: thyroid carcinoma; diffusion weighted imaging; lymphatic metastatic spread; ADC histogram analysis; histopathologic features; Ki-67; p53

1. Introduction

The incidence of thyroid cancer, being the most abundant endocrine malignancy, is rapidly increasing [1]. The vast majority of thyroid neoplasms is follicular cell-derived and subsumed under the umbrella categories of papillary thyroid cancer, follicular thyroid cancer, poorly differentiated thyroid cancer, and anaplastic thyroid cancer [2]. Although the overall five-year survival rates of thyroid cancer are 94% in women and 85% in men [3], certain entities of the disease are perpetually associated with poor outcomes (for example the tall cell variant of papillary thyroid cancer and undifferentiated thyroid cancer [1]). Some of the differentiated entities—most of all papillary thyroid cancer variants—frequently metastasize locally via the lymphatic system [4], and resultant local recurrence is not an uncommon scenario [5], leading to significant morbidity.

A variety of therapeutic options is available for thyroid cancer [6], but surgery still remains the predominant treatment [7]. Radical surgery is the most important form of therapy for undifferentiated thyroid cancer [8], and surgical treatment of significant nodal disease in well differentiated thyroid cancer is widely accepted to be associated with improved outcomes in terms of survival and recurrence rates [9]. Nonetheless, extensive surgery in this specific context carries a high risk of therapy-related morbidity like phrenic nerve palsy, brachial plexus palsy, cranial nerve injury, chyle leak, and pneumothorax [10].

Considering the broad spectrum of aggressiveness in thyroid cancer and the resulting necessity for customized treatment, employing presurgical imaging is of great importance, as it allows the thyroid surgeon to identify disease subtypes being associated with increased mortality and morbidity such as metastasizing and undifferentiated thyroid cancer.

Diffusion-weighted magnetic resonance imaging (DWI) has the potential to reveal tumor architectural details like cellular density and proliferative activity in different malignant entities [11,12]. Using a standard echo-planar imaging (EPI) technique, DWI has the capability to differentiate between malignant and benign thyroid nodules [13]. Furthermore, DWI can distinguish manifestations of papillary thyroid cancer with extra-glandular growth from those confined to the thyroid [14]. Using a RESOLVE sequence (which is less prone to susceptibility and motion-induced phase artifacts, has less T2* blurring and provides higher resolution than standard EPI DWI, [15]) in a 3T scanner, DWI even has the capability to distinguish between differentiated and undifferentiated subtypes of thyroid carcinoma [16].

However, in the clinical setting, obtained DWI data is commonly analyzed using a two-dimensional region of interest in the slice of the apparent diffusion coefficient (ADC) map representing the maximum diameter of the tumor. This approach does not account for the regularly encountered heterogeneity of whole tumors and certainly does not reflect the complex micro-architectural properties of malignantly transformed tissue.

An enhanced approach using every voxel of the tumor to compute a histogram of intensity levels could help to further increase prediction of histological features of tumors by magnetic resonance imaging (MRI) [17]. This way, the magnitude of tumor heterogeneity probably is revealed in a fashion superior to the commonly used two-dimensional method [17].

To the best of the authors' knowledge, only one study used ADC histogram analysis in thyroid cancer to differentiate benign from malignant nodules and furthermore reveal extra-thyroidal growth of papillary thyroid cancer [18]. So far, no studies demonstrated predictability of lymph node involvement by ADC histogram analysis of the primary tumor. Therefore, the primary aim of this study was to investigate the potential of ADC histogram analysis (including percentiles, entropy, skewness, and kurtosis) on data obtained with RESOLVE DWI to distinguish between nodal-negative and nodal-positive thyroid cancer. The discriminability of metastatic from non-metastatic thyroid cancer is of great clinical importance. Hence, this study investigated a promising translational approach that might have the potential to significantly increase the value of clinical-oncological imaging. The secondary aim was to correlate ADC histogram parameters with expression of important prognostic markers like p53 and Ki-67. Last, it aimed to compare our findings with the results of previous studies, which investigated the potential of DWI to predict histopathological features in thyroid cancer.

2. Results

2.1. *Diffusion Weighted Imaging and Immunohistopathology of Thyroid Carcinoma*

For reasons of clarity and comprehensibility, results of MRI and histopathology were organized in tables. Figure 1 shows MRI findings of a patient with follicular thyroid carcinoma, presenting as heterogeneous enlargement of the right thyroid lobe. The corresponding immunohistological images are shown in Figure 2. The calculated DWI parameters of all investigated thyroid carcinomas are summarized in Table 1 and the corresponding histopathological data is given in Table 2.

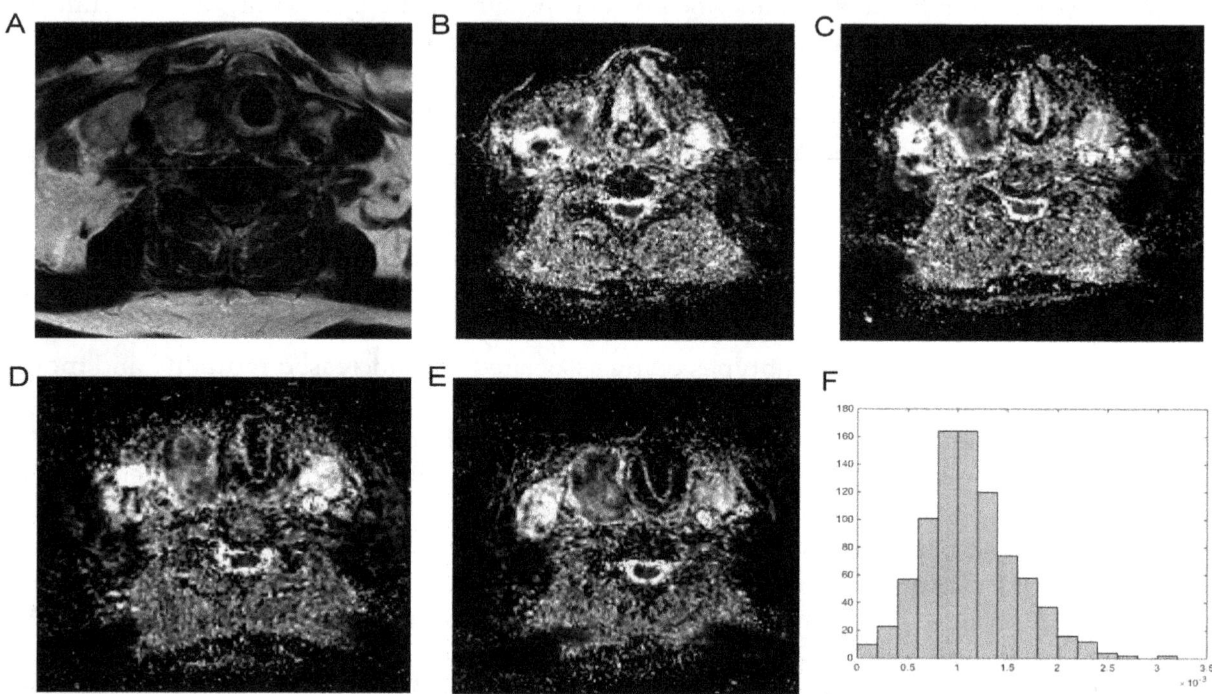

Figure 1. Imaging findings in a patient with follicular thyroid carcinoma. (**A**) Magnetic resonance imaging (T2w axial section) showing a massive inhomogenous enlargement of the right thyroid lobe; (**B–E**) represent the apparent diffusion coefficient (ADC) maps of the tumor; (**F**) is the ADC histogram of the whole lesion. The calculated ADC parameters ($\times 10^{-5}$ $mm^2 \cdot s^{-1}$) are as follows: ADC_{min} = 18.2; ADC_{mean} = 113.3; ADC_{max} = 315.0, mode = 114.4, ADC_{median} = 108.1, P10 = 58.2, P25 = 83.2, P75 = 138.7, and P90 = 176.6. Histogram based parameters are as follows: skewness = 0.59, kurtosis = 3.88, and entropy = 3.21. The *z*-axis in Figure 1F gives the voxel count.

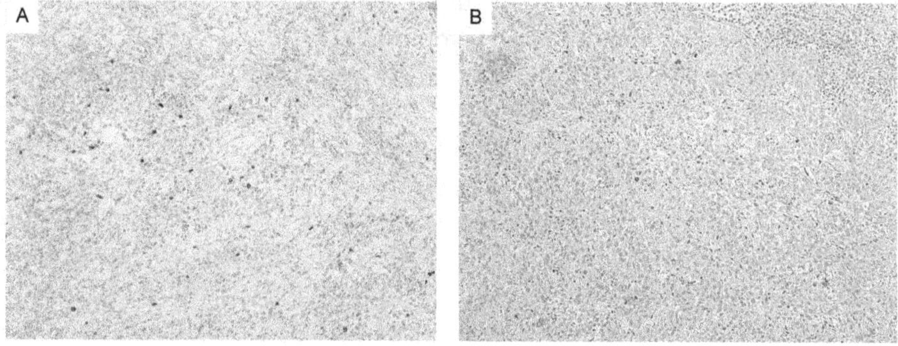

Figure 2. Immunohistochemistry of follicular thyroid carcinoma. (**A**) Shows Ki-67 staining (cell count: 1407, Ki-67 immunoreactiviy: 11%) and (**B**) shows p53 staining (cell count: 1811, p53 immunoreactivity: 36%) of the tumor displayed in Figure 1.

Table 1. Diffusion weighted imaging and related histogram parameters of thyroid carcinoma based on $n = 15$ patients.

DWI Related Parameters	Median	Range	Minimum–Maximum
ADC_{mean}, $\times10^{-5}$ $mm^2 \cdot s^{-1}$	124.30	90	73–163
ADC_{min}, $\times10^{-5}$ $mm^2 \cdot s^{-1}$	14.90	53	0.2–53
ADC_{max}, $\times10^{-5}$ $mm^2 \cdot s^{-1}$	250.70	179	147–325
P10 ADC, $\times10^{-5}$ $mm^2 \cdot s^{-1}$	72.10	85	30–114
P25 ADC, $\times10^{-5}$ $mm^2 \cdot s^{-1}$	91.90	84	52–136
P75 ADC, $\times10^{-5}$ $mm^2 \cdot s^{-1}$	140.40	99	93–192
P90 ADC, $\times10^{-5}$ $mm^2 \cdot s^{-1}$	172.82	116	97–213
Median ADC, $\times10^{-5}$ $mm^2 \cdot s^{-1}$	118.00	94	71–165
Mode ADC, $\times10^{-5}$ $mm^2 \cdot s^{-1}$	101.40	88	53–141
Kurtosis	3.64	1.90	2.89–4.79
Skewness	0.30	1.79	−0.97–0.81
Entropy	3.27	1.98	2.75–4.72

Table 2. Estimated immunohistopathological parameters of thyroid carcinoma ($n = 15$).

Parameters	Median	Range	Minimum–Maximum
Cell count, n	1407	1808	439–2247
Ki 67, %	32.0	90	9–99
p53, %	4.0	94	0–94
Total nuclear area, μm^2	71,735	148,620	14,649–163,269
Average nuclear area, μm^2	53.0	61	33–94

2.2. Correlation Analysis

Table 3 displays results of the correlation analysis between immunohistopathological parameters and ADC fractions as well as histogram related parameters. Correlation analysis identified the following, significant correlations: ADC_{mean} with p53 ($r = 0.548$, $p = 0.034$), ADC_{max} with Ki67 ($r = -0.646$, $p = 0.009$) and p53 ($r = 0.645$, $p = 0.009$), ADCp75 with p53 ($r = 0.537$, $p = 0.025$), ADCp90 with Ki67 ($r = -0.568$, $p = 0.027$) and p53 ($r = 0.588$, $p = 0.021$), ADC_{median} with p53 ($r = 0.556$, $p = 0.032$), ADC_{modus} with p53 ($r = 0.534$, $p = 0.040$), and kurtosis with cell count ($r = -0.571$, $p = 0.026$). Figure 3 summarizes the significant correlations graphically and displays them as dot plots.

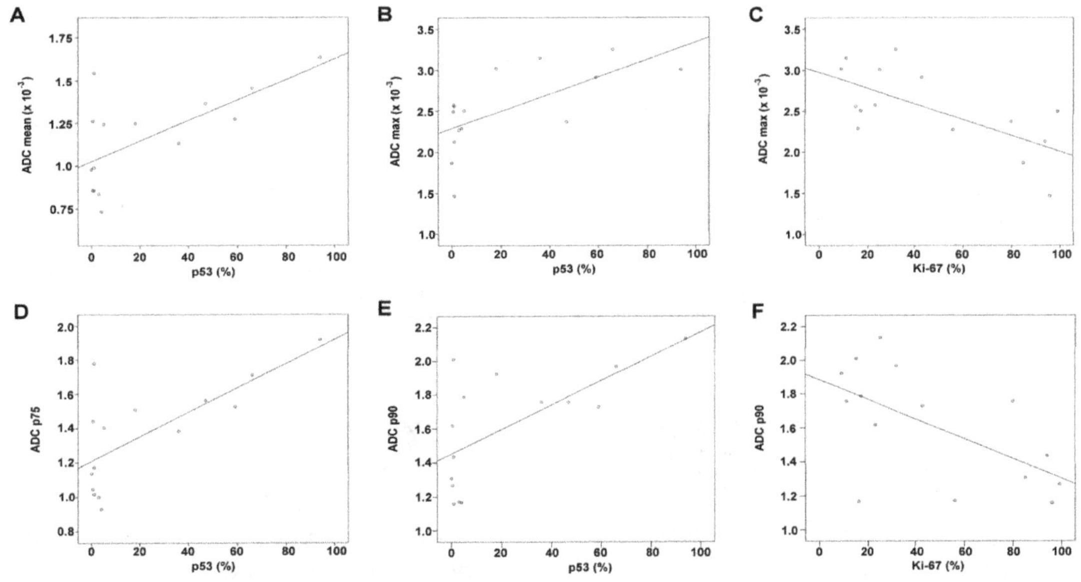

Figure 3. *Cont.*

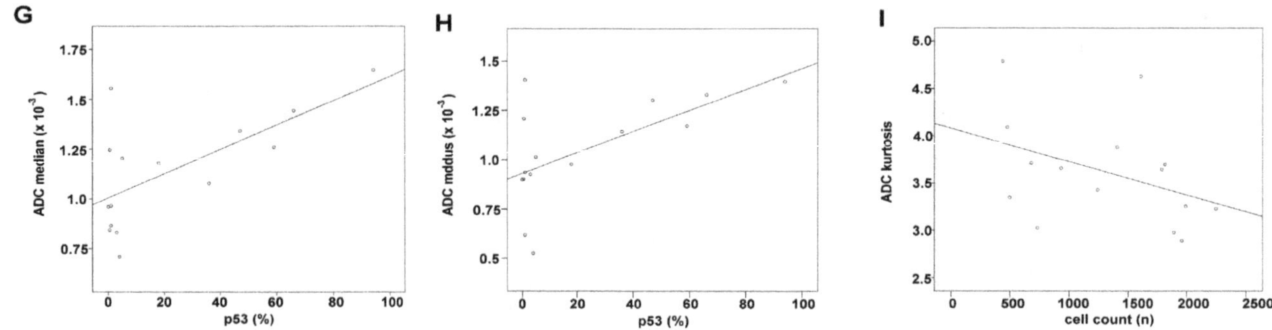

Figure 3. Graphic summary of the significant correlations between imaging and immunohistological findings. R^2-values for the plots shown in Figure 3 are as follows; (**A**) ADC_{mean} & p53: $r^2 = 0.438$; (**B**) ADC_{max} & p53: $r^2 = 0.425$; (**C**) ADC_{max} & Ki-67: $r^2 = 0.464$; (**D**) ADCp75 & p53: $r^2 = 0.499$; (**E**) ADCp90 & p53: $r^2 = 0.431$; (**F**) ADCp90 & Ki-67: $r^2 = 0.360$; (**G**) ADC_{median} & p53: $r^2 = 0.440$; (**H**) ADC_{modus} & p53: $r^2 = 0.377$; (**I**) $ADC_{kurtosis}$ & cell count: $r^2 = 0.160$.

Table 3. Results of Spearman's rank order correlation analysis between DWI and immunohistological parameters ($n = 15$).

ADC Parameters and Histogram Values	Cell Count	p53	Ki-67	Total Nuclear Area	Average Nuclear Area
ADC_{mean}, $\times 10^{-3}$ $mm^2 \cdot s^{-1}$	$r = 0.429$ $p = 0.111$	$r = 0.548$ $p = 0.034$	$r = -0.325$ $p = 0.237$	$r = 0.389$ $p = 0.152$	$r = 0.034$ $p = 0.904$
ADC_{min}, $\times 10^{-3}$ $mm^2 \cdot s^{-1}$	$r = 0.256$ $p = 0.358$	$r = 0.244$ $p = 0.381$	$r = -0.241$ $p = 0.386$	$r = 0.163$ $p = 0.562$	$r = -0.208$ $p = 0.456$
ADC_{max}, $\times 10^{-3}$ mm^2 s^{-1}	$r = 0.372$ $p = 0.173$	$r = 0.645$ $p = 0.009$	$r = -0.646$ $p = 0.009$	$r = 0.461$ $p = 0.084$	$r = 0.155$ $p = 0.580$
ADC p10, $\times 10^{-3}$ $mm^2 \cdot s^{-1}$	$r = 0.361$ $p = 0.187$	$r = 0.409$ $p = 0.130$	$r = 0.289$ $p = 0.296$	$r = 0.275$ $p = 0.321$	$r = -0.079$ $p = 0.781$
ADC p25, $\times 10^{-3}$ $mm^2 \cdot s^{-1}$	$r = 0.375$ $p = 0.168$	$r = 0.509$ $p = 0.053$	$r = 0.361$ $p = 0.187$	$r = 0.311$ $p = 0.260$	$r = -0.064$ $p = 0.820$
ADC p75, $\times 10^{-3}$ $mm^2 \cdot s^{-1}$	$r = 0.450$ $p = 0.092$	$r = 0.537$ $p = 0.025$	$r = -0.343$ $p = 0.211$	$r = 0.411$ $p = 0.128$	$r = 0.055$ $p = 0.845$
ADC p90, $\times 10^{-3}$ $mm^2 \cdot s^{-1}$	$r = 0.289$ $p = 0.296$	$r = 0.588$ $p = 0.021$	$r = -0.568$ $p = 0.027$	$r = 0.300$ $p = 0.277$	$r = 0.075$ $p = 0.790$
Median ADC, $\times 10^{-3}$ $mm^2 \cdot s^{-1}$	$r = 0.414$ $p = 0.125$	$r = 0.556$ $p = 0.032$	$r = -0.314$ $p = 0.254$	$r = 0.361$ $p = 0.187$	$r = -0.020$ $p = 0.945$
Mode ADC, $\times 10^{-3}$ $mm^2 \cdot s^{-1}$	$r = 0.496$ $p = 0.060$	$r = 0.534$ $p = 0.040$	$r = -0.357$ $p = 0.191$	$r = 0.432$ $p = 0.108$	$r = -0.149$ $p = 0.682$
Kurtosis	$r = -0.571$ $p = 0.026$	$r = -0.262$ $p = 0.346$	$r = -0.314$ $p = 0.254$	$r = -0.411$ $p = 0.128$	$r = -0.182$ $p = 0.516$
Skewness	$r = -0.229$ $p = 0.413$	$r = -0.004$ $p = 0.990$	$r = -0.389$ $p = 0.152$	$r = 0.011$ $p = 0.970$	$r = 0.186$ $p = 0.507$
Entropy	$r = 0.243$ $p = 0.383$	$r = -0.240$ $p = 0.389$	$r = 0.289$ $p = 0.296$	$r = 0.225$ $p = 0.420$	$r = 0.316$ $p = 0.251$

2.3. Group Comparisons

Histogram analysis derived ADC values are compared between the nodal negative and the nodal positive group in Figure 4. Levene's Test revealed homoscedasticity for the nodal-negative and the nodal-positive group only regarding $ADC_{skewness}$ ($p = 0.015$). For all remaining ADC derived histogram parameters, Levene's Test showed heterogeneity of variance when comparing the nodal-negative and the nodal-positive group. Hence, group comparisons were performed using unpaired *t*-test for $ADC_{skewness}$ and Mann-Whitney-U Test for all remaining parameters. The corresponding *p*-values are given in Table 4. Statistically significant differences were only identified for skewness ($p = 0.031$) and kurtosis ($p = 0.028$). No other significant differences or trends were delineable when comparing thyroid carcinoma patients with restricted vs. advanced infiltration pattern (results not presented).

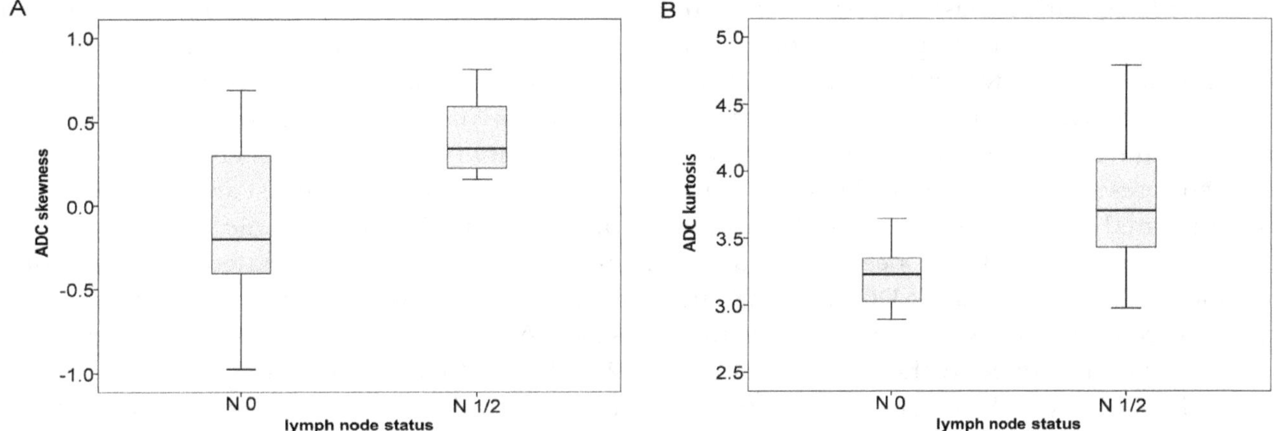

Figure 4. Graphically summarizes the differences in histogram parameters between nodal negative and nodal positive patients with thyroid carcinoma. (**A**) Shows significantly increased ADC histogram skewness in noda-positive compared to nodal-negative patients; (**B**) demonstrates significantly increased values of ADC histogram kurtosis in nodal-positive compared to nodal negative thyroid carcinomas.

Table 4. Group comparison of ADC and histogram parameters of thyroid carcinomas with (N1/2, $n = 10$ patients) and without lymphatic metastatic dissemination (N0, $n = 5$ patients).

ADC Parameters and Histogram Values	N0 Mean ± SD		N1/2 Mean ± SD		Group Comparison: *p*-Values
ADC_{mean}, $\times 10^{-5}$ $mm^2 \cdot s^{-1}$	125.25	34.1	111.41	25.00	0.513
ADC_{min}, $\times 10^{-5}$ $mm^2 \cdot s^{-1}$	28.26	17.30	14.02	16.90	0.075
ADC_{max}, $\times 10^{-5}$ $mm^2 \cdot s^{-1}$	238.44	69.40	259.43	38.50	0.768
P10 ADC, $\times 10^{-5}$ $mm^2 \cdot s^{-1}$	82.15	26.17	69.14	23.50	0.371
P25 ADC, $\times 10^{-5}$ $mm^2 \cdot s^{-1}$	102.25	30.00	89.19	23.30	0.440
P75 ADC, $\times 10^{-5}$ $mm^2 \cdot s^{-1}$	147.26	39.14	131.75	26.43	0.440
P90 ADC, $\times 10^{-5}$ $mm^2 \cdot s^{-1}$	170.69	44.15	156.55	28.50	0.440
Median ADC, $\times 10^{-5}$ $mm^2 \cdot s^{-1}$	124.14	34.86	109.19	25.50	0.513
Mode ADC, $\times 10^{-5}$ $mm^2 \cdot s^{-1}$	112.32	25.56	101.39	27.50	0.594
Kurtosis	3.23	0.29	3.81	0.57	*0.028*
Skewness	−0.12	0.64	0.41	0.21	0.031
Entropy	3.56	0.66	3.5	0.71	0.768

3. Discussion

This study aimed to investigate the potential of 3T RESOLVE DWI using an ADC histogram analysis approach to distinguish between limited and advanced thyroid cancer with reference to the status of lymphatic metastatic dissemination. To the author's best knowledge, this work is the first to show differences in ADC histogram parameters between nodal-positive and nodal-negative thyroid cancer.

In detail, skewness and kurtosis of the ADC histograms were significantly increased in nodal-positive compared to nodal-negative thyroid cancer. This finding corresponds to previous studies in other malignant tumors, exemplarily clear cell renal cell carcinoma, and rectal cancer, which revealed that increased skewness of ADC histograms is associated with a more advanced disease stage [19,20]. Furthermore, an increase in ADC histogram skewness was observed in patients suffering from recurrent high grade glioma who showed disease progress under anti-proliferative chemotherapy, indicating ongoing proliferation of glioma cells within the tumor [21]. The association between changes in ADC values and altered cellularity in tumors is a well-known phenomenon [22]. Considering this, the findings of the aforementioned studies and our results we hypothesize that the process of lymphatic metastatic spread of thyroid cancer is linked to profound changes in the tissue microarchitecture, related to proliferation of distinct tumor cell clusters and subsequent migration via the lymphatic system, which finds its reflection in corresponding changes of the ADC histogram.

Additionally, this study found significant correlations between ADC histogram analysis derived values of thyroid cancer and corresponding immune-reactivity for p53. p53 has great importance as tumor suppressor and controls cell fate via induction of apoptosis, cell cycle arrest and senescence [23]. Under normal conditions, p53 remains undetectable for its rapid proteasomic degradation [23]. In thyroid cancer, p53 has been used as prognostic marker being associated with favorable outcome [24,25]. ADC mean, ADC max, ADC median, ADC modus, ADC p75 and ADC p90 correlated significantly with p53 expression. In general, increased ADC values of tumors have been shown to be associated with good therapeutic responses [26]. It was thereupon concluded that increased ADC values of thyroid cancer—in consent with previously published work—indicate a favorable prognosis. Furthermore, a clear inverse correlation of ADC max and ADC p90 with Ki-67 expression was identified. Ki-67 is a nuclear protein strictly associated with cell division and widely used in the clinical routine to assess proliferative activity [27].

Increased proliferation of cells, as indicated by increased expression of Ki-67, consecutively decreases the corresponding extracellular space in a given volume of tissue and thereupon reduces water diffusibility, which is reflected by decreased ADC values [22]. Thus—in accordance to other malignancies [11,28,29]—decreased ADC values are associated with an increased proliferation rate within thyroid cancer tissue.

This study furthermore identified a significant inverse correlation between cell count and kurtosis. Only few studies investigated the potential of ADC kurtosis to reflect histological properties, for example Chandarana and colleagues were able to differentiate clear cell from papillary subtype of renal cell cancer by means of ADC kurtosis [30]. It is therefore concluded that ADC histogram kurtosis provides additional insight in tumor-architectural details, but further studies are necessary to validate this finding in order to further elaborate the significance of this parameter. Conventionally, ADC_{mean} and ADC_{min} were used to investigate histopathological features like cellularity of tumors in vivo [22]. However, classical ADC parameters like ADC_{mean} and ADC_{min} are strongly scanner-dependent and cannot be used to compare patients investigated in different MRI devices without normalization. In contrary, histogram parameters estimate characteristics of the ADC distribution, which is not scanner-dependent like the absolute ADC values. Therefore, ADC derived histogram parameters (skewness, entropy, kurtosis) might be superior when investigating histopathological features in vivo using more than one MRI scanner in a singular study.

This study suffers from few limitations. The major limitation is the small number of patients included in this study. Furthermore, this study did not include all clinically relevant subtypes of thyroid cancer, exemplarily medullary thyroid carcinomas were not investigated. Therefore, future works including greater cohorts with different histopathological subtypes have to confirm these findings and further elucidate the relationship between histopathological findings and ADC alterations. Also, ADC histogram analysis was performed by a single, experienced reader. The suitability of histogram analysis for the clinical routine necessitates assessment of inter-reader and intra-reader variability including readers with different levels of experience. A future work needs to investigate these phenomena in a larger cohort.

ADC histogram analysis can provide more detailed information on diffusion characteristics of tumors than commonly obtained ADC parameters. For example, a previously published study demonstrated that common ADC parameters (mean, max, and min) did not reflect histopathological features like cellularity and proliferative activity in thyroid carcinoma [16]. In contrast, this study demonstrated that certain ADC histogram parameters reflect distinct histopathological features very well. Although it has proven to be a very sensitive tool for detection of microstructural changes, the specificity of ADC histogram parameters for the underlying histological changes is unclear. Characteristic changes of ADC histogram parameters in different tumor entities might be related to very different histological changes. Therefore, the significance of ADC histogram analysis should be investigated in a tumor-specific manner.

4. Materials and Methods

This retrospective study was approved (No. 2014-99) by the local research ethics committee of the Martin-Luther-University Halle-Wittenberg.

4.1. Patients

The radiological database for thyroid carcinoma was reviewed. In total, 20 patients were identified, but only 15 patients with histopathologically confirmed thyroid carcinoma had received proper DWI (using the RESOLVE sequence) and were therefore enrolled in our study.

The patient group was comprised of one male and 14 female patients. The mean age was 67 years (with a standard deviation of 12.9 years). The distribution of histopathological subtypes was as follows; follicular thyroid carcinoma: $n = 4$, papillary thyroid carcinoma: $n = 5$, anaplastic thyroid carcinoma: $n = 6$. Five patients were diagnosed with nodal negative thyroid cancer, and 10 patients had pathologically confirmed lymph node metastases. One patient was diagnosed with distant metastatic disease (pulmonary and pleural manifestation). Infiltration pattern ranged from restriction to the thyroid gland to advanced infiltration including infiltration of the trachea, esophagus, and internal jugular vein. An overview of demographic, clinical and pathological information is given in Table 5.

Table 5. Demographic and pathological data of the investigated thyroid carcinoma patients.

Case	Age	Gender	Histological Subtype	Infiltration Pattern	M Stage	N Stage
1	91	female	anaplastic	trachea	0	1
2	60	female	papillary	trachea	0	1
3	73	male	papillary	trachea, esophagus	0	1
4	68	female	papillary	trachea, esophagus internal jugular vein	0	0
5	73	female	papillary	trachea	0	1
6	67	female	anaplastic	Trachea internal jugular vein	1	2
7	73	female	anaplastic	trachea, esophagus	0	0
8	41	female	follicular	trachea	0	1
9	72	female	anaplastic	none	0	1
10	59	female	anaplastic	trachea	0	1
11	83	female	papillary	trachea	0	0
12	77	female	follicular	trachea	0	1
13	52	female	anaplastic	trachea	0	0
14	51	female	follicular	trachea	0	0
15	66	female	anaplastic	trachea	0	1

4.2. MRI

MRI of the neck was performed for all patients using a 3T device (Magnetom Skyra, Siemens, Erlangen, Germany). The imaging protocol included the following sequences:

1. axial T2 weighted (T2w) turbo spin echo (TSE) sequence (TR/TE: 4000/69, flip angle: 150°, slice thickness: 4 mm, acquisition matrix: 200 × 222, field of view: 100 mm);
2. axial T1 weighted (T1w) turbo spin echo (TSE) sequences (TR/TE: 765/9.5, flip angle: 150°, slice thickness: 5 mm, acquisition matrix: 200 × 222, field of view: 100 mm) before and after intravenous application of contrast medium (gadopentate dimeglumine, Magnevist®, Bayer Schering Pharma, Leverkusen, Germany);

3. axial DWI (readout-segmented, multi-shot EPI sequence; TR/TE: 5400/69, flip angle 180°, slice thickness: 4 mm, acquisition matrix: 200 × 222, field of view: 100 mm) with b values of 0, 400 and 800 s/mm^2. ADC maps were generated automatically by the implemented software package and analyzed as described previously [28].

All images were available in digital form and were analyzed by an experienced radiologist without knowledge of the histopathological diagnosis on a PACS workstation (Centricity PACS, GE Medical Systems, Milwaukee, WI, USA). Figure 1 shows a representative axial T2 weighted image of follicular thyroid carcinoma and corresponding axial ADC images of the whole tumor, which were used for histogram analysis (also displayed in Figure 1).

4.3. Histogram Analysis of ADC Values

DWI data was transferred in DICOM format and processed offline with a custom-made Matlab-based application (The Mathworks, Natick, MA, USA) on a standard windows operated system. The ADC maps were displayed within a graphical user interface (GUI) that enables the reader to scroll through the slices and draw a volume of interest (VOI) at the tumor's boundary. The VOI was created by manually drawing regions of interest (ROIs) along the margin of the tumor using all slices displaying the tumor (whole lesion measure). All measures were performed by one author (AS). The ROIs were modified in the GUI and saved (in Matlab-specific format) for later processing. After setting the ROIs, the following parameters were calculated and given in a spreadsheet format: ROI volume (cm^3), mean (ADC_{mean}), maximum (ADC_{max}), minimum (ADC_{min}), median (ADC_{median}), modus (ADC_{modus}), and the following percentils: 10th (ADCp10), 25th (ADCp25), 75th (ADCp75), and 90th (ADCp90). Additionally, histogram-based characteristics of the VOI—kurtosis, skewness, and entropy—were computed. All calculations were performed using in-build Matlab functions.

4.4. Histopathology and Immunohistochemistry

All thyroid carcinomas were surgically resected and histopathologically analysed. In every case, the proliferation index was estimated on Ki-67 antigen stained specimens using MIB-1 monoclonal antibody (DakoCytomation, Glostrup, Denmark) as reported previously [31]. Furthermore, p53 index was estimated using monoclonal antibody p57, clone DO-7 (DakoCytomation). Two high power fields (0.16 mm^2 per field, ×400) were analysed. The area with the highest number of positive nuclei was selected. Figure 2 exemplarily shows Ki-67 and p53 immunostaining of a follicular thyroid carcinoma. Additionally, cellular density was calculated for each tumor as average cell count per five high power fields (×400). Furthermore, average nuclear area and total nuclear area were estimated using ImageJ package 1.48v (National Institute of Health, Bethesda, MD, USA) as described previously [11]. All histopathological sections were analysed using a research microscope Jenalumar equipped with a Diagnostic instruments camera 4.2 (Zeiss, Jena, Germany).

4.5. Statistical Analysis

Statistical analysis was performed using IBM SPSS 23™ (SPSS Inc., Chicago, IL, USA). Collected data was first evaluated by means of descriptive statistics. Correlative analysis was then performed using Spearman's correlation coefficient in order to analyze associations between histogram analysis derived values of ADC and (immuno-) histopathological parameters. Subsequently, Levene's Test for homogeneity of variance was performed to assess the equality of variances of ADC derived histogram parameters between different groups of thyroid carcinoma patients in order to identify the suitable test for group comparisons. In case of homoscedasticity, unpaired t test was performed to compare values among different (e.g., the metastatic and the non-metastatic) groups. In case of heteroscedasticity, Mann-Whitney-*U* test was performed to compare values among the different groups. Group comparisons were performed for nodal negative vs. nodal positive patients and patients with restricted (thyroid gland and trachea) vs. advanced (trachea, esophagus, jugular vein) infiltration pattern. Since only one patient with distant metastatic disease was included, a sufficient group comparison between M0 and M1 patients could not be performed. p-Values ≤ 0.05 were considered as statistically significant.

5. Conclusions

This exploratory study revealed significant differences in ADC histogram skewness and kurtosis comparing nodal negative and nodal positive thyroid cancer. Significant correlations between different ADC parameters were identified with p53, Ki-67, and cell count, substantiating the potential of ADC as an important prognostic imaging biomarker. This information certainly has the potential to aid thyroid surgeons in identifying the optimal treatment strategy for patients with thyroid cancer. Further studies investigating a greater cohort of patients are necessary to confirm these findings.

Acknowledgments: We acknowledge funding by the German Research Foundation (DFG) and University Leipzig within the program of open access publishing.

Author Contributions: Stefan Schob and Alexey Surov conceived and designed the experiments and wrote the paper; Nikolaos Pazaitis and Anne Kathrin Höhn performed the immunohistopathological experiments; Diana Horvath-Rizea and Bhogal Pervinder analyzed the data; Nikita Garnov contributed the histogram analysis tool; Hans Jonas Meyer digitalized the immunohistological slides and performed image analysis; Karl-Titus Hoffmann performed MRI; Julia Dieckow wrote the paper.

Abbreviations

MDPI	Multidisciplinary Digital Publishing Institute
DOAJ	Directory of Open Access Journals
TLA	Three Letter Acronym
LD	linear Dichroism

References

1. Katoh, H.; Yamashita, K.; Enomoto, T.; Watanabe, M. Classification and general considerations of thyroid cancer. *Ann. Clin. Pathol.* **2015**, *3*, 1–9.
2. Dralle, H.; Machens, A.; Basa, J.; Fatourechi, V.; Franceschi, S.; Hay, I.D.; Nikiforov, Y.E.; Pacini, F.; Pasieka, J.L.; Sherman, S.I. Follicular cell-derived thyroid cancer. *Nat. Rev. Dis. Prim.* **2015**, *1*, 15077. [CrossRef] [PubMed]
3. Paschke, R.; Lincke, T.; Müller, S.P.; Kreissl, M.C.; Dralle, H.; Fassnacht, M. The treatment of well-differentiated thyroid carcinoma. *Dtsch. Arztebl. Int.* **2015**, *112*, 452–458. [PubMed]
4. Nixon, I.J.; Shaha, A.R. Management of regional nodes in thyroid cancer. *Oral Oncol.* **2013**, *49*, 671–675. [CrossRef] [PubMed]
5. Shaha, A.R. Recurrent differentiated thyroid cancer. *Endocr. Pract.* **2012**, *18*, 600–603. [CrossRef] [PubMed]
6. Ferrari, S.M.; Fallahi, P.; Politti, U.; Materazzi, G.; Baldini, E.; Ulisse, S.; Miccoli, P.; Antonelli, A. Molecular targeted therapies of aggressive thyroid cancer. *Front Endocrinol.* **2015**, *6*, 176. [CrossRef] [PubMed]
7. Cabanillas, M.E.; Dadu, R.; Hu, M.I.; Lu, C.; Gunn, G.B.; Grubbs, E.G.; Lai, S.Y.; Williams, M.D. Thyroid gland malignancies. *Hematol. Oncol. Clin. N. Am.* **2015**, *29*, 1123–1143. [CrossRef] [PubMed]
8. Wendler, J.; Kroiss, M.; Gast, K.; Kreissl, M.C.; Allelein, S.; Lichtenauer, U.; Blaser, R.; Spitzweg, C.; Fassnacht, M.; Schott, M.; et al. Clinical presentation, treatment and outcome of anaplastic thyroid carcinoma: Results of a multicenter study in Germany. *Eur. J. Endocrinol.* **2016**, *175*, 521–529. [CrossRef] [PubMed]
9. Asimakopoulos, P.; Nixon, I.J.; Shaha, A.R. Differentiated and medullary thyroid cancer: Surgical management of cervical lymph nodes. *Clin. Oncol.* **2017**, *29*, 283–289. [CrossRef] [PubMed]
10. Mizrachi, A.; Shaha, A.R. Lymph node dissection for differentiated thyroid cancer. *Mol. Imaging Radionucl. Ther.* **2016**, *26*, 10–15. [CrossRef] [PubMed]
11. Schob, S.; Meyer, J.; Gawlitza, M.; Frydrychowicz, C.; Müller, W.; Preuss, M.; Bure, L.; Quäschling, U.; Hoffmann, K.-T.; Surov, A. Diffusion-weighted MRI reflects proliferative activity in primary CNS lymphoma. *PLoS ONE* **2016**, *11*, e0161386. [CrossRef] [PubMed]

12. Surov, A.; Stumpp, P.; Meyer, H.J.; Gawlitza, M.; Höhn, A.-K.; Boehm, A.; Sabri, O.; Kahn, T.; Purz, S. Simultaneous ^{18}F-FDG-PET/MRI: Associations between diffusion, glucose metabolism and histopathological parameters in patients with head and neck squamous cell carcinoma. *Oral Oncol.* **2016**, *58*, 14–20. [CrossRef] [PubMed]
13. Khizer, A.T.; Raza, S.; Slehria, A.-U.-R. Diffusion-weighted MR imaging and ADC mapping in differentiating benign from malignant thyroid nodules. *J. Coll. Physicians Surg. Pak.* **2015**, *25*, 785–788. [PubMed]
14. Lu, Y.; Moreira, A.L.; Hatzoglou, V.; Stambuk, H.E.; Gonen, M.; Mazaheri, Y.; Deasy, J.O.; Shaha, A.R.; Tuttle, R.M.; Shukla-Dave, A. Using diffusion-weighted MRI to predict aggressive histological features in papillary thyroid carcinoma: A novel tool for pre-operative risk stratification in thyroid cancer. *Thyroid* **2015**, *25*, 672–680. [CrossRef] [PubMed]
15. Porter, D.A.; Heidemann, R.M. High resolution diffusion-weighted imaging using readout-segmented echo-planar imaging, parallel imaging and a two-dimensional navigator-based reacquisition. *Magn. Reson. Med.* **2009**, *62*, 468–475. [CrossRef] [PubMed]
16. Schob, S.; Voigt, P.; Bure, L.; Meyer, H.J.; Wickenhauser, C.; Behrmann, C.; Höhn, A.; Kachel, P.; Dralle, H.; Hoffmann, K.-T.; Surov, A. Diffusion-weighted imaging using a readout-segmented, multishot EPI sequence at 3T distinguishes between morphologically differentiated and undifferentiated subtypes of thyroid carcinoma—A preliminary study. *Transl. Oncol.* **2016**, *9*, 403–410. [CrossRef] [PubMed]
17. Just, N. Improving tumour heterogeneity MRI assessment with histograms. *Br. J. Cancer* **2014**, *111*, 2205–2213. [CrossRef] [PubMed]
18. Hao, Y.; Pan, C.; Chen, W.; Li, T.; Zhu, W.; Qi, J. Differentiation between malignant and benign thyroid nodules and stratification of papillary thyroid cancer with aggressive histological features: Whole-lesion diffusion-weighted imaging histogram analysis. *J. Magn. Reson. Imaging* **2016**, *44*, 1546–1555. [CrossRef] [PubMed]
19. Kierans, A.S.; Rusinek, H.; Lee, A.; Shaikh, M.B.; Triolo, M.; Huang, W.C.; Chandarana, H. Textural differences in apparent diffusion coefficient between low- and high-stage clear cell renal cell carcinoma. *Am. J. Roentgenol.* **2014**, *203*, W637–W644. [CrossRef] [PubMed]
20. Liu, L.; Liu, Y.; Xu, L.; Li, Z.; Lv, H.; Dong, N.; Li, W.; Yang, Z.; Wang, Z.; Jin, E. Application of texture analysis based on apparent diffusion coefficient maps in discriminating different stages of rectal cancer. *J. Magn. Reson. Imaging* **2016**. [CrossRef] [PubMed]
21. Nowosielski, M.; Recheis, W.; Goebel, G.; Güler, O.; Tinkhauser, G.; Kostron, H.; Schocke, M.; Gotwald, T.; Stockhammer, G.; Hutterer, M. ADC histograms predict response to anti-angiogenic therapy in patients with recurrent high-grade glioma. *Neuroradiology* **2011**, *53*, 291–302. [CrossRef] [PubMed]
22. Chen, L.; Liu, M.; Bao, J.; Xia, Y.; Zhang, J.; Zhang, L.; Huang, X.; Wang, J. The correlation between apparent diffusion coefficient and tumor cellularity in patients: A meta-analysis. *PLoS ONE* **2013**, *8*, e79008. [CrossRef] [PubMed]
23. Wang, Z.; Sun, Y. Targeting p53 for novel anticancer therapy. *Transl. Oncol.* **2010**, *3*, 1–12. [CrossRef] [PubMed]
24. Godballe, C.; Asschenfeldt, P.; Jørgensen, K.E.; Bastholt, L.; Clausen, P.P.; Hansen, T.P.; Hansen, O.; Bentzen, S.M. Prognostic factors in papillary and follicular thyroid carcinomas: P53 expression is a significant indicator of prognosis. *Laryngoscope* **1998**, *108*, 243–249. [CrossRef] [PubMed]
25. Bachmann, K.; Pawliska, D.; Kaifi, J.; Schurr, P.; Zörb, J.; Mann, O.; Kahl, H.J.; Izbicki, J.R.; Strate, T. P53 is an independent prognostic factor for survival in thyroid cancer. *Anticancer Res.* **2006**, *27*, 3993–3997.
26. Padhani, A.R.; Liu, G.; Mu-Koh, D.; Chenevert, T.L.; Thoeny, H.C.; Takahara, T.; Dzik-Jurasz, A.; Ross, B.D.; Van Cauteren, M.; Collins, D.; et al. Diffusion-weighted magnetic resonance imaging as a cancer biomarker: Consensus and recommendations. *Neoplasia* **2009**, *11*, 102–125. [CrossRef] [PubMed]
27. Schlüter, C.; Duchrow, M.; Wohlenberg, C. The cell proliferation-associated antigen of antibody Ki-67: A very large, ubiquitous nuclear protein with numerous repeated elements, representing a new kind of cell cycle-maintaining proteins. *J. Cell Biol.* **1993**, *123*, 1–10. [CrossRef]
28. Surov, A.; Caysa, H.; Wienke, A.; Spielmann, R.P.; Fiedler, E. Correlation between different ADC fractions, cell count, Ki-67, total nucleic areas and average nucleic areas in meningothelial meningiomas. *Anticancer Res.* **2015**, *35*, 6841–6846. [PubMed]
29. Chen, L.; Zhang, J.; Chen, Y.; Wang, W.; Zhou, X.; Yan, X.; Wang, J. Relationship between apparent diffusion coefficient and tumour cellularity in lung cancer. *PLoS ONE* **2014**, *9*, e99865. [CrossRef] [PubMed]

30. Chandarana, H.; Rosenkrantz, A.B.; Mussi, T.C.; Kim, S.; Ahmad, A.A.; Raj, S.D.; McMenamy, J.; Melamed, J.; Babb, J.S.; Kiefer, B.; et al. Histogram analysis of whole-lesion enhancement in differentiating clear cell from papillary subtype of renal cell cancer. *Radiology* **2012**, *265*, 790–798. [CrossRef] [PubMed]
31. Surov, A.; Gottschling, S.; Mawrin, C.; Prell, J.; Spielmann, R.P.; Wienke, A.; Fiedler, E. Diffusion-weighted imaging in meningioma: Prediction of tumor grade and association with histopathological parameters. *Transl. Oncol.* **2015**, *8*, 517–523. [CrossRef] [PubMed]

10

Micronuclei Formation upon Radioiodine Therapy for Well-Differentiated Thyroid Cancer: The Influence of DNA Repair Genes Variants

Luís S. Santos [1,2], Octávia M. Gil [3], Susana N. Silva [1,*], Bruno C. Gomes [1], Teresa C. Ferreira [4], Edward Limbert [5] and José Rueff [1]

1 Centre for Toxicogenomics and Human Health (ToxOmics), Genetics, Oncology and Human Toxicology, NOVA Medical School; Faculdade de Ciências Médicas, Universidade Nova de Lisboa, 1169-056 Lisboa, Portugal; lsilvasantos@gmail.com (L.S.S.); bruno.gomes@nms.unl.pt (B.C.G.); jose.rueff@nms.unl.pt (J.R.)

2 Institute of Health Sciences (ICS), Center for Interdisciplinary Research in Health (CIIS), Universidade Católica Portuguesa, 3504-505 Viseu, Portugal

3 Centro de Ciências e Tecnologias Nucleares, Instituto Superior Técnico, Universidade de Lisboa, 2695-066 Bobadela, Loures, Portugal; ogil@ctn.tecnico.ulisboa.pt

4 Serviço de Medicina Nuclear, Instituto Português de Oncologia de Lisboa (IPOLFG), 1099-023 Lisboa, Portugal; teresa.ferreira_medical@yahoo.com

5 Serviço de Endocrinologia, Instituto Português de Oncologia de Lisboa (IPOLFG), 1099-023 Lisboa, Portugal; elimbert@ipolisboa.min-saude.pt

* Correspondence: snsilva@nms.unl.pt

Abstract: Radioiodine therapy with ^{131}I remains the mainstay of standard treatment for well-differentiated thyroid cancer (DTC). Prognosis is good but concern exists that ^{131}I-emitted ionizing radiation may induce double-strand breaks in extra-thyroidal tissues, increasing the risk of secondary malignancies. We, therefore, sought to evaluate the induction and 2-year persistence of micronuclei (MN) in lymphocytes from 26 ^{131}I-treated DTC patients and the potential impact of nine homologous recombination (HR), non-homologous end-joining (NHEJ), and mismatch repair (MMR) polymorphisms on MN levels. MN frequency was determined by the cytokinesis-blocked micronucleus assay while genotyping was performed through pre-designed TaqMan® Assays or conventional PCR-restriction fragment length polymorphism (RFLP). MN levels increased significantly one month after therapy and remained persistently higher than baseline for 2 years. A marked reduction in lymphocyte proliferation capacity was also apparent 2 years after therapy. *MLH1* rs1799977 was associated with MN frequency (absolute or net variation) one month after therapy, in two independent groups. Significant associations were also observed for *MSH3* rs26279, *MSH4* rs5745325, *NBN* rs1805794, and tumor histotype. Overall, our results suggest that ^{131}I therapy may pose a long-term challenge to cells other than thyrocytes and that the individual genetic profile may influence ^{131}I sensitivity, hence its risk-benefit ratio. Further studies are warranted to confirm the potential utility of these single nucleotide polymorphisms (SNPs) as radiogenomic biomarkers in the personalization of radioiodine therapy.

Keywords: thyroid cancer; Iodine-131; chromosome-defective micronuclei; DNA repair; micronucleus assay; single nucleotide polymorphism; pharmacogenomic variants; pharmacogenetics; precision medicine

---

1. Introduction

Thyroid cancer (TC) is the most common endocrine malignancy, accounting for approximately 2.1% of cancers diagnosed all over the world. TC incidence is about two to four times higher in women than in men and is one of the most common malignancies in adolescent and young adults (ages 15–39 years), with the median age at diagnosis being lower than that for most other types of cancer [1–3]. TC incidence has been steadily increasing, over the last three decades [1], most likely because of "surveillance bias" and overdiagnosis resulting from increased detection of small stationary lesions of limited clinical relevance. A true rise in the number of TC cases (e.g., due to increasing exposure to ionizing radiation (IR) from medical sources) is, however, also possible [2–4].

Papillary (PTC) and follicular (FTC) thyroid carcinoma represent 85–90% and 5–10% of TC cases, respectively. These tumor histotypes retain their morphologic features, being often referred to as differentiated thyroid carcinoma (DTC) [3,4]. The best-established modifiable risk factor for DTC is IR exposure during childhood and adolescence (radioiodines including ^{131}I, X-radiation, γ-radiation) [2–5] and the standard treatment consists of surgical resection (total or near-total thyroidectomy) accompanied by post-thyroidectomy radioiodine (RAI) therapy and TSH suppression [3,4]. The majority of DTC cases is indolent in nature, iodine-avid, and responds favorably to standard therapy. Overall prognosis is thus generally good, translating into high long-term survival and low disease-specific mortality [4].

The widespread use of RAI therapy in the management of DTC relies on the ability of ^{131}I to be preferentially taken up and concentrated in normal or neoplastic thyroid follicular cells, taking advantage of these cells' specialized mechanism for iodide uptake and accumulation [3,6,7]. Thyrocyte-accumulated ^{131}I undergoes [β and γ] decay and releases high-energy electrons that inflict devastating DNA damage locally. Thyroid cell death through radiation cytotoxicity ensues, allowing for the ablation of remnant normal thyroid tissue and the eradication of any residual tumor foci [3,6]. Unfortunately, since other tissues may also concentrate ^{131}I, its DNA damaging effects may not be limited to the thyroid gland, increasing the risk of RAI-associated secondary malignancies such as soft tissue tumors, colorectal cancer, salivary tumors, and leukemia [3,7]. Since the rising incidence of TC is mostly driven by increased detection of stationary subclinical lesions, concern exists that DTC overdiagnosis may result in potentially harmful overtreatment [2]. Indeed, if we consider the indolent behavior of the disease, its long-term survival rate, and its mean age of diagnosis, such therapy-related morbidity may not be justified, as most patients will have many years to experience its negative effects [2]. The revised American Thyroid Association (ATA) clinical practice guidelines for the management of DTC [8] reflect such concern for the first time, recommending a more cautious diagnosis and treatment approach in order to reduce RAI use (hence, radiation exposure) particularly in younger ages. This includes, for example, more stringent criteria for diagnosis upon nodule detection, molecular-based risk stratification for improved treatment decisions, personalized disease management and long-term surveillance strategies and, most importantly, use of lower RAI doses (30–50 mCi) in patients with low-risk DTC [2,8,9].

The most relevant types of DNA damage inflicted upon IR exposure are double-strand breaks (DSBs). Such lesions are predominantly processed by DNA repair enzymes of the homologous recombination (HR) and non-homologous end-joining (NHEJ) repair pathways, despite mismatch repair (MMR) pathway enzymes have also been implicated [10,11]. The activity of such DNA repair enzymes determines the capacity of cells to repair DSBs which, in turn, influences their sensitivity to IR. Lower DNA repair capacity, therefore, increases the extent of IR-induced DNA damage, increasing both the likelihood of cell death through IR-induced cytotoxicity and the likelihood of malignant transformation upon IR exposure [12,13].

Single nucleotide polymorphisms (SNPs) in DNA repair enzymes across these three pathways have been identified and some have been demonstrated to affect the DNA repair capacity [14,15]. Such DNA repair SNPs may therefore modulate sensitivity to IR and many have indeed been associated with TC or, more specifically, DTC susceptibility (for which IR exposure is the best-established risk factor) [16–21]. It is likely that such functional DNA repair SNPs, through interference with the extent of IR-induced DSBs on thyrocytes, could influence the cytotoxic potential of RAI therapy, hence its efficacy on DTC treatment. Likewise, through a similar effect on other cells that take up and concentrate ^{131}I, such SNPs could also modify the risk of secondary malignancies, hence the safety of RAI therapy.

Identifying these variants is, therefore, an important challenge with clinical relevance. However, to our knowledge, the issue has not been addressed in prior studies.

We have previously demonstrated that therapy with 70 mCi ^{131}I in DTC patients is consistently associated with increased DNA damage levels in peripheral lymphocytes [22,23]. With this study, we aimed to confirm, through the use of the cytokinesis-blocked micronucleus (CBMN) assay, our prior findings in a new group of DTC patients submitted to RAI therapy with 100 mCi. Further, we sought to extend our analysis at 24 months after ^{131}I administration so that the long-term persistence of ^{131}I-induced DNA damage could be better characterized. Finally, the potential influence of HR, NHEJ, and MMR polymorphisms on the micronuclei (MN) frequency in RAI-treated DTC patients was also investigated.

Understanding the role of repair SNPs on the extent and persistence of ^{131}I-induced DNA damage will contribute to the identification of genetic biomarkers that influence the individual response to ^{131}I-based RAI therapy and thus modulate the risk-benefit ratio of RAI therapy in DTC patients. Such efforts may provide the basis for improved, personalized, therapeutic decisions in the context of DTC therapy, with impact on disease prognosis and patient safety.

2. Materials and Methods

2.1. Study Population

Twenty-six DTC patients proposed for radioiodine therapy at the Department of Nuclear Medicine of the Portuguese Oncology Institute of Lisbon (Portugal) were selected according to criteria published elsewhere [22]. All participants were treated according to current practice, consisting of total thyroidectomy followed by oral administration of ^{131}I, 70 mCi (15 patients) or 100 mCi (11 patients), to ablate thyroid remnant cells. Patients were followed for two years unless they had to be submitted to further treatment. In such cases, patients were no longer elective for cytogenetic analysis and had to be excluded from further analysis. A mixed cross-sectional and longitudinal study design was used, respectively, for comparisons among genotypes or dose groups at each time point and across different time points. In the latter case, pre-treatment values allowed each patient to serve as his own control.

To characterize the study population and account for potential confounding factors, all participants were interviewed and completed a detailed questionnaire covering standard demographic characteristics, personal and family medical history, lifestyle habits, and prior IR exposure. For the purpose of smoking status, former smokers who had quit smoking at least 2 years prior to diagnosis were considered as non-smokers. Clinical and pathological examination was also performed.

Peripheral blood samples were collected from each patient into both 10 mL heparinized tubes (for cytogenetic analysis) and citrated tubes (for genotype analysis). For cytogenetic analysis, blood samples were drawn (1) prior to ^{131}I administration as well as 1, 6, and 24 months after therapy in patients submitted to a 70 mCi dose and (2) prior to ^{131}I administration as well as 1 and 3 months afterward in patients submitted to a 100 mCi dose. For genotype analysis, blood samples were stored at −80 °C until further use.

All subjects gave their informed consent for inclusion before they participated in the study. The study was conducted in accordance with the Declaration of Helsinki, and the protocol was approved by the Ethics Committee of Instituto Português de Oncologia Francisco Gentil (GIC/357) and by the Ethics Committee of Faculdade Ciências Médicas (CE-5/2008).

2.2. Genotype Analysis

Genomic DNA was isolated from blood samples using the commercially available QIAamp® DNA mini kit (QIAamp® DNA mini kit; Qiagen GmbH, Hilden, Germany), according to the manufacturer's recommendations. The fluorimetric Quant-iT™ Picogreen® dsDNA Assay Kit (Invitrogen, Waltham, MA, USA) was used to quantify and ensure uniformity in DNA concentration (2.5 ng/μL). DNA samples were kept at −20 °C until further use.

SNPs were selected from those already analyzed by our team in a cohort of 106 DTC patients, according to selection criteria published elsewhere [18–21]. Due to sample size limitations, only SNPs presenting a minor allele frequency (MAF) > 0.15 in the original pool of patients were considered. *MLH3* rs175080 was excluded *a posteriori* for insufficient genotype frequency ($n \leq 1$) in at least one of the ^{131}I dose groups (Table S1). Overall, a total of 9 DNA repair SNPs across 3 DNA repair pathways (HR, NHEJ, and MMR) were considered for further analysis (Table 1).

Table 1. Selected SNPs and detailed information on the corresponding base and amino acid changes, minor allele frequency, and Applied Biosystems (AB) assay used for genotyping.

Gene	Location	DB SNP Cluster ID (RS NO.)	Base Change	Amino Acid Change	MAF (%) [a]	AB Assay ID
MLH1	3p22.2	rs1799977	A → G	Ile219Val	23.3	C___1219076_20
MSH3	5q14.1	rs26279	A → G	Thr1045Ala	27.1	C____800002_1_
MSH4	1p31.1	rs5745325	G → A	Ala97Thr	26.0	C___3286081_10
PMS1	2q32.2	rs5742933	G → C	– [b]	23.4	C__29329633_10
MSH6	2p16.3	rs1042821	C → T	Gly39Glu	18.2	C___8760558_10
RAD51	15q15.1	rs1801321	G → T	– [b]	33.2	C___7482700_10
NBN	8q21.3	rs1805794	G → C	Glu185Gln	34.7	C__26470398_30
XRCC3	14q32.33	rs861539	C → T	Thr241Met	29.0	– [d]
XRCC5	2q35	rs2440	C → T	– [c]	36.3	C___3231046_10

[a] MAF, minor allele frequency, according to the Genome Aggregation Database (gnomAD), v2.1.1, available at https://gnomad.broadinstitute.org/. [b] SNP located on 5′ UTR. [c] SNP located on 3′ UTR. [d] not applicable (genotyping performed by PCR-RFLP). SNPs, single nucleotide polymorphisms.

Genotyping was performed mostly by real-time polymerase chain reaction (RT-PCR): amplification and allelic discrimination were carried out on a 96-well ABI 7300 Real-Time PCR system thermal cycler (Applied Biosystems; Thermo Fisher Scientific, Inc., Waltham, MA, USA), following the manufacturer's instructions, with the use of the commercially available TaqMan® SNP Genotyping Assays (Applied Biosystems) identified in Table 1. For *XRCC3* rs861539 (HR pathway), genotyping was performed by conventional PCR-restriction fragment length polymorphism (RFLP) techniques. Primer sequences, PCR, and digestion conditions as well as expected electrophoretic patterns have been described [19]. To confirm genotyping and ensure accurate results, inconclusive samples were reanalyzed and genotyping was repeated in 10–15% of randomly chosen samples, with 100% concordance.

2.3. Cytogenetic Analysis

The cytokinesis-block micronucleus assay (CBMN) was used to analyze DNA damage and conducted according to standard methods. The methodology was performed and published as described previously [22–24]. The frequency of binucleated cells carrying micronuclei (BNMN), defined as the number of cells with MN per 1000 binucleated lymphocytes, is expressed as a count per thousand (‰). The Cytokinesis-Block Proliferation Index (CBPI) was determined according to the formula CBPI = [MI + 2MII + 3(MIII + MIV)]/N, where MI-MIV correspond to the number of human lymphocytes with one to four nuclei, respectively, and N is the total number of cells analyzed.

2.4. Statistical Analysis

All analyses were done with SPSS 22.0 (IBM SPSS Statistics for Windows, version 22.0, IBM Corp, Armonk, NY, USA) except for deviation of genotype distributions from Hardy–Weinberg equilibrium (HWE) and linkage disequilibrium (LD) analysis between SNPs on the same chromosome, which were performed with SNPstats [25].

Categorical variables, presented as frequencies and percentages, were compared between dose groups and with the original cohort of DTC patients by the Pearson's Chi-square (χ^2) test or the two-sided Fisher's exact test whenever 2 × 2 contingency tables were possible. For continuous variables (BNMN frequency, CBPI, and their net variation from baseline), presented as mean ± standard deviation, the normality and homogeneity of variances were evaluated by the Shapiro-Wilk and Levene tests, respectively. Longitudinal comparisons were performed by the paired sample t test (whenever a normal distribution could not be excluded) or the Wilcoxon signed-rank test (remaining cases) while the parametric Student t test (normal distributions) or the nonparametric Mann-Whitney U test (non-normal distributions) for independent samples were used for cross-sectional comparisons between the two ^{131}I dose groups and between different gender, age class, smoking status, histological type of tumor, and genotype categories.

Variable transformation was considered, when practically useful: DTC patients were dichotomized according to age, with the cut-off point being defined as the median age of all patients included (54 years). Due to limited sample size (hence, low frequency of homozygous variant genotypes), a dominant model of inheritance was assumed for all SNPs. Moreover, the net variation in BNMN frequency (i.e., therapy-induced BNMN) was calculated by subtracting the background (pre-treatment) BNMN frequency from the corresponding post-treatment values.

This is an exploratory 'proof of concept' study, not a conclusive final one. As such, the Bonferroni adjustment was deemed as not necessary as it is too conservative. Furthermore, the complement of the false-negative rate β to compute the power of a test (1-β) was not taken into account at this stage since larger studies are needed to change this preliminary study into a confirmatory one. Statistical significance was set at $p < 0.05$.

3. Results

3.1. Characteristics of the Study Population

A general description of the study population is presented in Table 2. The age of DTC patients submitted to ^{131}I therapy ranged from 32 to 73 years, with a mean of 52.54 ± 11.62 years. As expected, female patients (88.5%, n = 23) greatly outnumbered male patients (11.5%, n = 3) and papillary carcinoma cases (PTC, 69.2%, n = 18) were also more frequent than follicular ones (FTC, 30.8%, n = 8), in agreement with gender and histotype distributions commonly reported for DTC [1,2,4]. Overall, 15.4% (n = 4) of patients were smokers. No significant differences in patient age, gender, histological type of tumor, and smoking status were observed between groups submitted to different ^{131}I doses (Table 2) nor between any of these groups (separated or together) and our original DTC population [18].

Table 2. General characteristics for differentiated thyroid carcinoma (DTC) patients treated with 70 mCi (n = 15) and 100 mCi (n = 11) ^{131}I.

Characteristics	Study Population n (%)	70 mCi n (%)	100 mCi n (%)	p Value [c]
Gender				
Male	3 (11.5)	1 (6.7)	2 (18.2)	0.556
Female	23 (88.5)	14 (93.3)	9 (81.8)	
Age [a]	52.54 ± 11.62 [b]	52.07 ± 10.26 [b]	53.18 ± 13.76 [b]	0.815
≤54	14 (53.8)	8 (53.3)	6 (54.5)	1.000
>54	12 (46.2)	7 (46.7)	5 (45.5)	
Smoking habits				
Non-smokers	22 (84.6)	13 (86.7)	9 (81.8)	1.000
Smokers	4 (15.4)	2 (13.3)	2 (18.2)	
Histology				
Papillary	18 (69.2)	10 (66.7)	8 (72.7)	1.000
Follicular	8 (30.8)	5 (33.3)	3 (27.3)	

[a] For age categorization purposes, the median age of all patients included in the study (54 years) was defined as the cut-off point. [b] mean ± S.D. [c] p value for 70 mCi *versus* 100 mCi groups determined by two-sided Fisher's exact test (gender, smoking habits, and age categories) or Student t test (age mean ± S.D.).

3.2. Cytogenetic Data

The frequency of BNMN (mean ± S.D.) in the 26 DTC patients submitted to ^{131}I therapy and included in this study is illustrated in Figure 1 and summarized in Table S2. Pre-treatment and post-treatment values are presented, stratified by dose group.

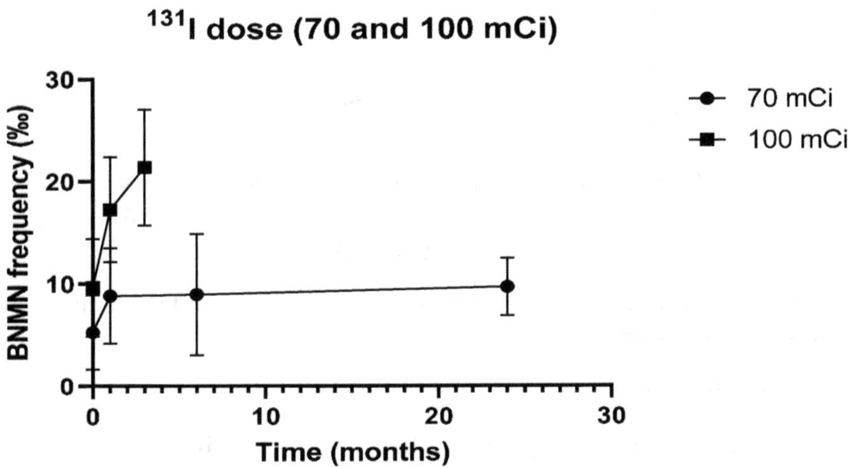

Figure 1. Binucleated cells carrying micronuclei (BNMN) frequency (‰, mean ± S.D.) in DTC patients before and after (1, 3/6, and 24 months) therapy with different doses of ^{131}I (70 and 100 mCi).

The results from the 70 mCi dose group until 6 months after ^{131}I administration have been published before [22]. As it was not possible to collect genotyping data on 4 of the original 19 patients, these patients were excluded and the data were re-analyzed. Longitudinal results in this dose group are, nevertheless, similar to those originally reported [22]: as evident from Figure 1, BNMN frequency in these patients increases significantly 1 month after ^{131}I therapy (from 5.27 ± 3.63‰ to 8.80 ± 4.65‰, $p = 0.039$) and stabilizes at 6 months after ^{131}I therapy (8.93 ± 5.92‰, $p = 0.944$ vs. 1 month after therapy), remaining persistently higher than before treatment ($p = 0.041$).

To investigate the long-term persistence of such therapy-induced damage, the study of these patients at 2 years after therapy was extended (Table S2 and Figure 1). Cytogenetic data at such time point was available for 11 patients only. The frequency of BNMN remained stable (9.64 ± 2.80‰, similar to values at 1 and 6 months, $p = 0.460$ and $p = 0.328$, respectively) and persistently higher than baseline ($p = 0.005$).

To confirm these findings and check for a possible dose effect, the study was replicated in an independent group of patients administered with 100 mCi. As expected, BNMN frequency was significantly higher in the 100 mCi group than in the 70 mCi group, irrespective of the time point (Table S2 and Figure 1), suggesting a dose-effect association (hence, a cause-effect relation) between iodine dose and BNMN levels. Apart from this quantitative difference, the effect of either dose on BNMN frequency was qualitatively similar, BNMN in the 100 mCi group increasing significantly 1 month after therapy (from 9.64 ± 4.78‰ to 17.27 ± 5.14‰, $p = 0.011$) and remaining persistently higher than baseline at 3 months (21.40 ± 5.66‰, $p < 0.001$ and $p = 0.054$ compared to pre-treatment and 1 month post-treatment values, respectively) (Table S2).

Moreover, of notice, the BNMN increment (net balance) after ^{131}I therapy was more pronounced in the 100 mCi group than in the 70 mCi group, despite the difference was not significant ($p > 0.05$).

Finally, the CBPI (mean ± S.D.) was also determined for the 15 DTC patients submitted to therapy with 70 mCi ^{131}I. As depicted in Figure 2, this index, which indicates the proliferation capacity of lymphocytes and may be used to calculate cytotoxicity [26], did not change appreciably at 1 and 6 months after ^{131}I administration but was markedly reduced at 24 months after therapy (from 1.78 ± 0.13 to 1.53 ± 0.09, $p = 0.001$).

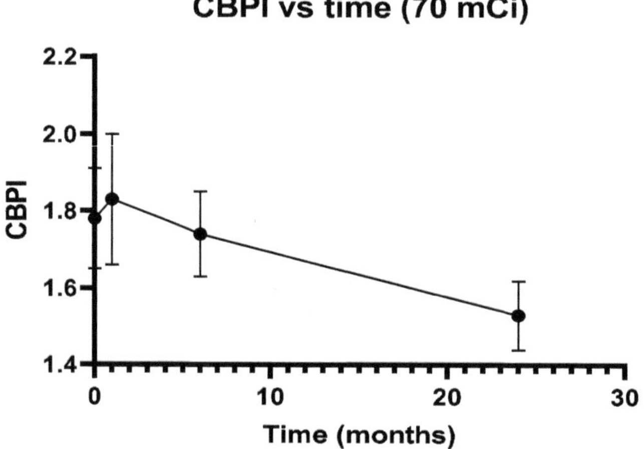

Figure 2. Cytokinesis-Block Proliferation Index (CBPI) (mean ± S.D.) in DTC patients before and after (1, 6, and 24 months) therapy with ^{131}I (70 mCi).

3.3. Characteristics of the Study Population and Cytogenetic Data

The potential influence of the demographic, lifestyle, and clinical characteristics of the study population on cytogenetic data was also evaluated. As depicted in Figure 3, in patients treated with 70 mCi, histology interfered with both pre-treatment BNMN levels and its net balance 1 month after ^{131}I therapy (Figure 3): basal BNMN frequency was significantly higher in FTC than in PTC patients (8.20 ± 3.11‰ vs. 3.80 ± 3.01‰, $p = 0.020$) but, 1 month after therapy, increased only in PTC patients, resulting in a significantly different net balance between the two histotypes (+6.20 ± 5.05‰ in PTC vs. −1.80 ± 3.96‰ in FTC, $p = 0.009$). Such effect was not observed in 100 mCi-treated patients nor when both dose groups were considered together. Likewise, no significant effect of gender, age, or smoking habits on BNMN levels or its net balance was detected, irrespective of the time point or dose group. Furthermore, except maybe for gender, no significant effect on CBPI was observed for any of these variables in the 70 mCi dose group. Baseline CBPI values were borderline higher in female compared to male patients ($p = 0.045$) but such finding should not be overvalued as only one male patient was included in this dose group.

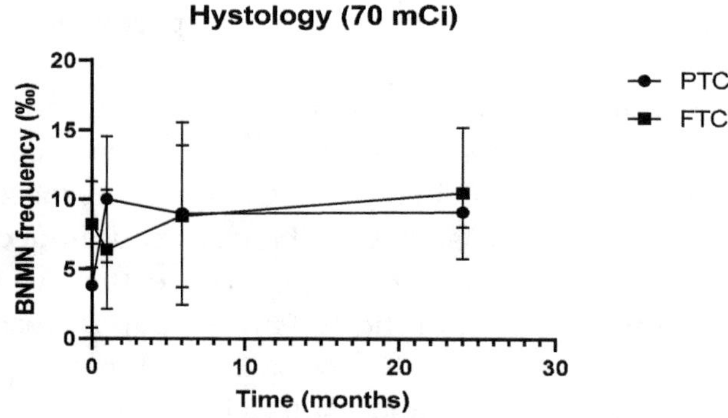

Figure 3. BNMN frequency (‰, mean ± S.D.) in DTC patients before and after (1, 6, and 24 months) therapy with 70 mCi ^{131}I, according to tumor histotype (papillary thyroid carcinoma (PTC) and follicular thyroid carcinoma (FTC)).

3.4. Distribution of DNA Repair SNPs in the Study Population

Table 3 reports the allele frequency and genotype distribution of 9 DNA repair SNPs among our sample of ^{131}I-treated patients. Genotype distributions were consistent with HWE in either dose group or their combination ($p > 0.05$) and, except for *MSH3* rs26279, did not differ significantly from those described in our previously studied DTC population ([c]). For *MSH3* rs26279, non-uniform distribution was observed, with the common allele being overrepresented in the study sample compared to the original population ($p = 0.048$, in the dominant model, Table S1). Moreover, importantly, no significant differences in genotype distributions were detected between dose groups, for any of the SNPs, irrespective of the model of inheritance assumed (Table 3). No relevant linkage association was observed between any of the SNPs.

Table 3. Allele and genotype frequencies in DTC patients submitted to ^{131}I therapy.

Genotype	70 mCi (n = 15)		100 mCi (n = 11)		TOTAL (n = 26)	
	MAF	Genotype Frequency n (%)	MAF	Genotype Frequency n (%)	MAF	Genotype Frequency n (%)
MLH1 rs1799977						
Ile/Ile	G: 0.30	7 (46.7)	G: 0.45	3 (27.3)	G: 0.37	10 (38.5)
Ile/Val		7 (46.7)		6 (54.5)		13 (50.0)
Val/Val		1 (6.7)		2 (18.2)		3 (11.5)
Ile/Val+Val/Val		8 (53.3)		8 (72.7)		16 (61.5)
MSH3 rs26279						
Thr/Thr	G: 0.23	10 (66.7)	G: 0.14	8 (72.7)	G: 0.19	18 (69.2)
Thr/Ala		3 (20.0)		3 (27.3)		6 (23.1)
Ala/Ala		2 (13.3)		0 (0.0)		2 (7.7)
Thr/Ala+Ala/Ala		5 (33.3)		3 (27.3)		8 (30.8)
MSH4 rs5745325						
Ala/Ala	A: 0.13	11 (73.3)	A: 0.32	4 (36.4)	A: 0.21	15 (57.7)
Ala/Thr		4 (26.7)		7 (63.6)		11 (42.3)
Thr/Thr		0 (0.0)		0 (0.0)		0 (0.0)
Ala/Thr+Thr/Thr		4 (26.7)		7 (63.6)		11 (42.3)
PMS1 rs5742933						
G/G	C: 0.18	10 (71.4)	C: 0.14	9 (81.8)	C: 0.16	19 (76.0)
G/C		3 (21.4)		1 (9.1)		4 (16.0)
C/C		1 (7.1)		1 (9.1)		2 (8.0)
G/C+C/C		4 (28.6)		2 (18.2)		6 (24.0)
MSH6 rs1042821						
Gly/Gly	T: 0.17	10 (66.7)	T: 0.09	9 (81.8)	T: 0.13	19 (73.1)
Gly/Glu		5 (33.3)		2 (18.2)		7 (26.9)
Glu/Glu		0 (0.0)		0 (0.0)		0 (0.0)
Gly/Glu+Glu/Glu		5 (33.3)		2 (18.2)		7 (26.9)
RAD51 rs1801321						
T/T	G: 0.50	4 (26.7)	G: 0.45	4 (36.4)	G: 0.48	8 (30.8)
T/G		7 (46.7)		4 (36.4)		11 (42.3)
G/G		4 (26.7)		3 (27.3)		7 (26.9)
T/G+G/G		11 (73.3)		7 (63.6)		18 (69.2)
NBN rs1805794						
Glu/Glu	C: 0.30	7 (46.7)	C: 0.14	8 (72.7)	C: 0.23	15 (57.7)
Glu/Gln		7 (46.7)		3 (27.3)		10 (38.5)
Gln/Gln		1 (6.7)		0 (0.0)		1 (3.8)
Glu/Gln+Gln/Gln		8 (53.3)		3 (27.3)		11 (42.3)
XRCC3 rs861539						
Thr/Thr	C: 0.47	5 (33.3)	T: 0.36	5 (45.5)	T: 0.46	10 (38.5)
Thr/Met		4 (26.7)		4 (36.4)		8 (30.8)
Met/Met		6 (40.0)		2 (18.2)		8 (30.8)
Thr/Met+Met/Met		10 (66.7)		6 (54.5)		16 (61.5)
XRCC5 rs2440						
T/T	C: 0.47	5 (33.3)	C: 0.50	2 (22.2)	C: 0.48	7 (29.2)
T/C		6 (40.0)		5 (55.6)		11 (45.8)
C/C		4 (26.7)		2 (22.2)		6 (25.0)
T/C+C/C		10 (66.7)		7 (77.8)		17 (70.8)

MAF, minor allele frequency. All comparisons of genotype distributions were performed by the two-sided Fisher's exact test (whenever 2 × 2 contingency tables are possible) or the χ^2 test (remaining cases). No significant differences among the 70 and 100 mCi dose groups were observed.

3.5. DNA Repair SNPs and Cytogenetic Data

The influence of DNA repair SNPs on BNMN frequencies and the corresponding variation from pre-treatment values is shown in Figure 4, Table 4, Table 5 and Tables S3–S5.

Prior to ^{131}I administration, BNMN frequency was higher in patients carrying the *MLH1* rs1799977 variant allele than in those homozygous for the common allele, with the difference being significant in the 100 mCi dose group ($p = 0.012$) and in the pool of both groups ($p = 0.019$).

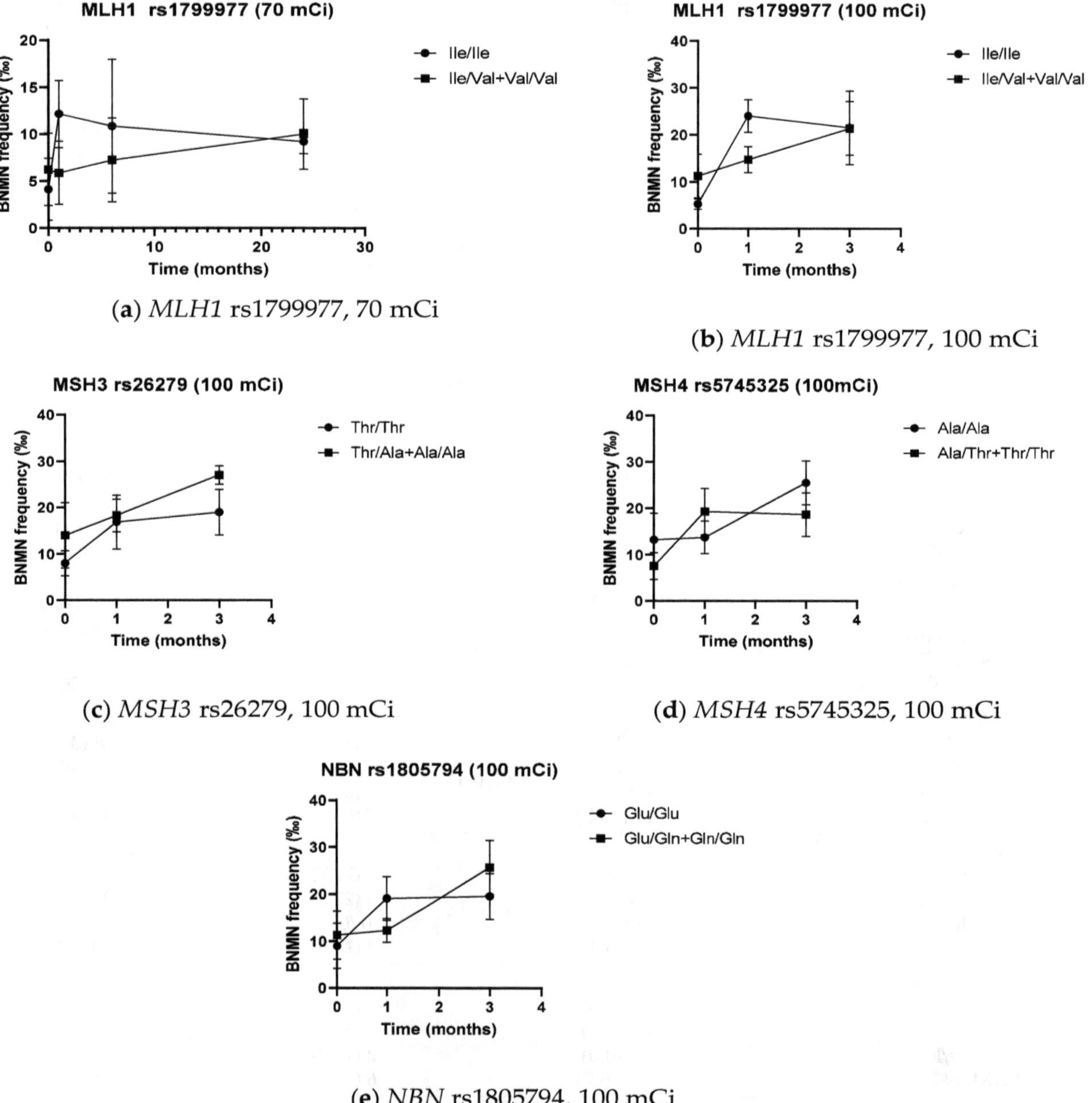

(**a**) *MLH1* rs1799977, 70 mCi

(**b**) *MLH1* rs1799977, 100 mCi

(**c**) *MSH3* rs26279, 100 mCi

(**d**) *MSH4* rs5745325, 100 mCi

(**e**) *NBN* rs1805794, 100 mCi

Figure 4. BNMN frequency (‰, mean ± S.D.) in DTC patients before and after (1, 3/6, and 24 months) therapy with ^{131}I, according to genotype and ^{131}I dose group: (**a**) *MLH1* rs1799977, 70 mCi; (**b**) *MLH1* rs1799977, 100 mCi; (**c**) *MSH3* rs26279, 100 mCi; (**d**) *MSH4* rs5745325, 100 mCi; (**e**) *NBN* rs1805794, 100 mCi.

Table 4. Frequency of micronucleated cells (‰BNMN, mean ± SD) in each ^{131}I dose group at t_0, t_1, t_3/t_6, and t_{24}, according to genotype (only SNPs presenting significant findings are shown).

Genotype	70 mCi Group (*n* = 15), ‰BNMN (Mean ± SD)				100 mCi Group (*n* = 11), ‰BNMN (Mean ± SD)			70 + 100 mCi Groups (*n* = 26), ‰BNMN (Mean ± SD)	
	t_0	t_1	t_6	t_{24}	t_0	t_1	t_3	t_0	t_1
MLH1 rs1799977									
Ile/Ile	4.14 ± 3.29	**12.14 ± 3.58**	10.86 ± 7.11	9.20 ± 1.30	**5.33 ± 1.16**	**24.00 ± 3.46**	21.50 ± 7.78	**4.50 ± 2.80**	**15.70 ± 6.63**
Ile/Val + Val/Val	6.25 ± 3.85	**5.88 ± 3.36** *	7.25 ± 4.46	10.00 ± 3.74	**11.25 ± 4.62** *	**14.75 ± 2.77** *	21.38 ± 5.71	**8.75 ± 4.85** *	**10.31 ± 5.46** *
MSH3 rs26279									
Thr/Thr	5.50 ± 3.63	8.90 ± 3.81	9.90 ± 7.09	10.13 ± 1.64	8.00 ± 2.73	16.88 ± 5.79	**19.00 ± 4.93**	6.61 ± 3.42	12.44 ± 6.18
Thr/Ala + Ala/Ala	4.80 ± 4.03	8.60 ± 6.54	7.00 ± 1.58	8.33 ± 5.13	14.00 ± 7.00	18.33 ± 3.51	**27.00 ± 2.00** *	8.25 ± 6.78	12.25 ± 7.31
MSH4 rs5745325									
Ala/Ala	5.18 ± 3.79	8.91 ± 5.07	9.09 ± 6.64	9.63 ± 3.34	13.25 ± 5.68	13.75 ± 3.50	25.50 ± 4.73	7.33 ± 5.55	**10.20 ± 5.09**
Ala/Thr + Thr/Thr	5.50 ± 3.70	8.50 ± 3.87	8.50 ± 4.04	9.67 ± 0.58	7.57 ± 2.88	19.29 ± 4.99	18.67 ± 4.68	6.82 ± 3.19	**15.36 ± 7.00** *
NBN rs1805794									
Glu/Glu	5.43 ± 4.61	10.00 ± 4.51	8.14 ± 4.56	9.86 ± 2.12	9.00 ± 4.84	**19.13 ± 4.64**	19.57 ± 4.89	7.33 ± 4.92	**14.87 ± 6.46**
Glu/Gln + Gln/Gln	5.13 ± 2.85	7.75 ± 4.80	9.63 ± 7.15	9.25 ± 4.11	11.33 ± 5.13	**12.33 ± 2.52** *	25.67 ± 5.77	6.82 ± 4.40	**9.00 ± 4.69** *

* $p < 0.05$; *p*-value for variant allele carriers *versus* common allele homozygotes determined by the Student *t* test (whenever a normal distribution could not be excluded through the Shapiro-Wilk test) or the Mann-Whitney U test (remaining cases). Significant findings highlighted in bold.

Table 5. Variation in the frequency of micronucleated cells from baseline (‰BNMN, mean ± SD) in each ^{131}I dose group at t_1, t_3/t_6, and t_{24}, according to genotype (only SNPs presenting significant findings are shown).

Genotype	70 mCi Group (n = 15), ‰BNMN (mean ± SD)			100 mCi Group (n = 11), ‰BNMN (mean ± SD)		70 + 100 mCi Groups (n = 26), ‰BNMN (mean ± SD)
	Δt_1	Δt_6	Δt_{24}	Δt_1	Δt_3	Δt_1
MLH1 rs1799977						
Ile/Ile	**8.00 ± 4.97**	6.71 ± 6.85	5.00 ± 3.39	**18.67 ± 3.06**	16.50 ± 6.36	**11.20 ± 6.71**
Ile/Val + Val/Val	**−0.38 ± 3.70** *	1.00 ± 4.90	3.50 ± 4.37	**3.50 ± 4.57** *	10.13 ± 5.28	**1.56 ± 4.49** *
MSH4 rs5745325						
Ala/Ala	3.73 ± 6.83	3.91 ± 7.05	4.13 ± 3.91	**0.50 ± 3.11**	12.25 ± 5.32	**2.87 ± 6.13**
Ala/Thr + Thr/Thr	3.00 ± 3.56	3.00 ± 4.90	4.33 ± 4.51	**11.71 ± 7.27** *	10.83 ± 6.49	**8.55 ± 7.41** *

* $p < 0.05$; p-value for variant allele carriers *versus* common allele homozygotes determined by the Student t test (whenever a normal distribution could not be excluded through the Shapiro-Wilk test) or the Mann-Whitney U test (remaining cases). Significant findings highlighted in bold.

One month after ^{131}I administration, *MLH1* rs1799977 variant allele carriers always presented significantly lower BNMN levels than patients homozygous for the common allele, either when considering absolute values ($p = 0.004$, $p = 0.012$ and $p = 0.034$ in the 70 mCi, 100 mCi, and in the pool of both groups, respectively) or the net variation from baseline ($p = 0.002$, $p = 0.001$ and $p < 0.001$ in the 70 mCi, 100 mCi and in the pool of both groups, respectively). BNMN frequency one month after therapy was also significantly lower in carriers of the variant allele for *NBN* rs1805794 ($p = 0.043$ in the 100 mCi group and $p = 0.017$ in the pool of both groups), with the difference in net BNMN values almost being significant ($p = 0.099$ in the 100 mCi dose group and $p = 0.058$ in the pool of both groups). Further, carriers of at least one *MSH4* rs5745325 variant allele exhibited higher levels of ^{131}I-induced BNMN than patients homozygous for the common allele ($p = 0.018$ in the 100 mCi group, $p = 0.043$ in the combination of both groups), with the difference in absolute BNMN frequencies being significant in the pooled analysis of both groups ($p = 0.039$) and almost significant in the 100 mCi group ($p = 0.084$).

Three months after therapy, significantly higher BNMN frequencies were found in patients from the 100 mCi group carrying the *MSH3* rs26279 variant allele ($p = 0.030$).

No other significant difference in either absolute or therapy-induced BNMN frequencies was found between the different genotypes of the DNA repair SNPs, at any time point. Likewise, no influence of genotype in CBPI, either absolute or relative to baseline values, was detected for any of the DNA repair SNPs considered in this study, at any time point (Table S6).

4. Discussion

We have previously demonstrated a significant increase in BNMN frequency in peripheral lymphocytes from 19 DTC patients treated with 70 mCi ^{131}I [22]. In the present exploratory study, in order to confirm these findings, to evaluate the long-term persistence of such ^{131}I-induced DNA damage and to determine whether it may be influenced by DNA repair SNPs, we extended our analysis at 2 years after ^{131}I administration in this group of patients, included a new group of patients submitted to RAI therapy with 100 mCi and profiled 9 DNA repair SNPs in patients from both groups.

In line with our previously reported results, we observed, in the 100 mCi dose group, a significant and persistent increase in BNMN frequency after ^{131}I therapy, with mean levels being always higher than in the 70 mCi group, irrespective of the time point considered. Replication across two independent sets of patients and observation of a dose effect strongly suggests a causal relation between RAI therapy and systemic chromosomal damage in lymphocytes, as assessed by the MNCB assay. Such correlation has been repeatedly demonstrated (both in thyroid patients following RAI therapy [27–32] and in other settings where exposure to low levels of low-LET (linear energy transfer) ionizing radiation occurs [28,33]) and is expected since ^{131}I may be taken up by extra-thyroidal cells [7] and emit β- and γ-radiation capable of inducing dose-dependent chromosomal damage detectable by cytogenetic analysis (e.g., micronuclei) [27,28,32]. The ability of ^{131}I to induce cytogenetic damage in peripheral lymphocytes in a dose-dependent manner is, in fact, clear and well-established, allowing BNMN frequency to be used as a valid, highly sensitive, and specific biomarker of effect for biological dosimetry of RAI therapy and, hence, to predict its associated genotoxic risk in dividing mammalian cells [27,28,32,34,35].

A less clear picture exists, however, concerning the long-term persistence (kinetics of the recovery) of such IR-induced cytogenetic damage. Our results from the 70 mCi dose group suggest that ^{131}I-induced damage in peripheral lymphocytes persists for at least 2 years. Despite negative results have also been published [36,37], our results are in line with most prior follow-up studies on RAI therapy or other low-dose IR exposures (e.g., for diagnostic purposes) [28,29,38–41]. Considering the half-life of ^{131}I (ranging from 1 to 8 days in thyroidectomized and non-thyroidectomized TC patients, respectively) [28] and of circulating lymphocytes (about 3 years) [28,38], such repeated demonstration of persistent cytogenetic damage is somehow surprising and challenge the widely held views about the mechanisms of IR-induced DNA damage. Possible explanations for the long-term genomic instability of lymphocytes from ^{131}I-exposed subjects include the introduction, upon irradiation, of DNA damage and cytogenetic alterations (1) in a subset of long-lived naïve T lymphocytes, quiescent cells that survive for prolonged periods of time in a resting stage, retaining the initially inflicted DNA damage and expressing it as micronuclei when stimulated to proliferate in the CBMN assay [38,42,43], (2) in hematopoietic stem and progenitor cells that, through clonal expansion, may give rise to mature T lymphocytes with stable and unstable aberrations, perpetuating genomic instability in time (transgenerational effect) [38,42,43], and (3) in non-irradiated lymphocytes (a delayed non-targeted effect), as a result of the long-term production and plasma secretion of soluble clastogenic factors by irradiated cells (oxidative stress by-products such as ROS (reactive oxygen species) and inflammatory cytokines such as TNF-α) that may further extend IR-induced cytogenetic damage in time ("bystander effect") [44]. The two latter explanations are generally favored, as a large number of studies exist demonstrating either the high frequency of gene mutations and chromosomal aberrations in the progeny of irradiated cells or the production and plasma release of factors with clastogenic activity by irradiated cells (including one on ^{131}I-treated patients) [37]. Overall, current evidence [44–47] supports the notion that a potent long-term inflammatory-type response develops upon IR exposure, irradiated cells producing danger signals (oxidative stress by-products and inflammatory cytokines) capable of exerting an array of persistent bystander effects in non-irradiated cells (altered levels of damage-inducible and stress-related proteins), leading to delayed genomic instability (chromosomal aberrations, sister chromatid exchanges, micronuclei formation/induction or mutations), hence, predisposing to malignancy (altered proliferation or transformation). Such long-term inflammatory-type response could also be responsible for the marked reduction in CBPI that we observed at 24 months after ^{131}I therapy.

In this study, complying with current recommendations, we also investigated the role of potential confounding factors on BNMN frequency. As reviewed elsewhere [48–50] and demonstrated through meta-analysis in the International Human MicroNucleus (HUMN) Project [51], age and gender are well-established factors, with increasing age and female gender being consistently associated with higher BNMN levels in peripheral blood lymphocytes. The influence of age has been demonstrated, in particular, in ^{131}I-treated patients [28,31]. Data on the potential role of smoking status on BNMN levels are somewhat more inconsistent, and many studies failing to find an association except, maybe, in heavy smokers and in those with relevant occupational exposures [48–51]. In this study, no significant effect of gender, age, or smoking habits on BNMN levels or its net balance was detected, irrespective of the time point or dose group. The study was probably underpowered to detect such effects. It is also possible that the effect of these variables may have been masked by the impact of internal IR exposure after ^{131}I administration.

We did observe, however, in the 70 mCi group only, differences on BNMN levels between the two TC histotypes, as FTC patients presented significantly higher basal BNMN frequency than PTC patients but significantly lower therapy-induced BNMN levels at one month after ^{131}I administration. This is suggestive of higher background genomic instability in FTC but higher sensitivity to the DNA damaging effects of IR in PTC. Considering the small sample size and the non-reproducibility of the findings between the two dose groups, extreme caution must be taken in the interpretation of these results. Nevertheless, the available evidence supports both findings: PTC usually presents as a microsatellite stable tumor, with no appreciable levels of either loss of heterozygosity (LOH) or aneuploidy (stable chromosome profile) [52–54]. On the contrary, a considerable degree of chromosomal instability appears to be a hallmark feature of FTC, which presents a consistently higher frequency of chromosomal abnormalities, LOH, allelic loss, and a higher mutational burden compared to PTC [52,53,55–57]. Microsatellite instability (MSI), despite uncommon in TC, also appears to be more frequent in FTC than in PTC [53–55]. The available evidence thus largely supports our observation of higher background genomic instability in FTC. Moreover, considering that activating *RAS* mutations are commonly observed in FTC but not in PTC [53,58,59], the association between increased *RAS* expression and decreased frequency of IR-induced MN reported by Miller et al. [60] is coherent with our own observation of lower ^{131}I-induced BNMN frequency in FTC, supporting the idea that this histotype is less sensitive to the DNA damaging effects of IR than PTC. Such hypothesis (i.e., higher sensitivity to

IR in PTC) is further reinforced by a recent observation, through meta-analysis, of increased efficacy of RAI therapy in PTC patients, compared to FTC [61] but more studies are needed for a solid conclusion to be drawn.

Moreover, in the present study, we further evaluated the potential impact of selected HR, NHEJ, and MMR pathway SNPs on BNMN levels, before and after the administration of ^{131}I. To our knowledge, this is the first study doing so. Significant genotype effects on MN frequency and/or its net balance were observed for HR (*NBN*) and MMR (*MLH1, MSH3, MSH4*) repair pathway SNPs across different time points. This was expected because (1) IR exposure results in increased DNA damage, most notably, single- and double-strand breaks, oxidative lesions (e.g., 8-oxoG), DNA-protein crosslinks (DPCs) and clustered DNA lesions [62–67]; (2) the HR pathway, acting in the S/G2 stages of the cell cycle, is the major DNA repair pathway involved in the error-free correction of DSBs [11,33,35,68]; (3) MMR proteins, besides their canonical actions on the post-replication repair of mispaired nucleotides and insertion–deletion loops, have also been demonstrated to play an important role on the damage response to IR-induced DSBs, either through cooperation with HR or through signaling for cell-cycle arrest and apoptosis [64,69–71]; (4) DSBs, if left unrepaired, e.g., due to the presence of SNPs that reduce the DNA repair capacity, may give rise to chromosome breakage and MN formation upon replication [28,33,35,72]. The potential influence of functional DSB repair SNPs on ^{131}I-induced BNMN frequency is, therefore, fully justified. A literature review on the functional impact of these SNPs and their putative association with response to radio and/or chemotherapy was performed and is presented below (Table 6).

Table 6. Literature review on the functional impact of the studied SNPs and their putative association with radio and/or chemosensitivity (only SNPs presenting significant findings in the present study are shown).

Gene	DB SNP Cluster ID (RS NO.)	Functional Impact	Clinical Association Studies (Radio and/or Chemosensitivity)
MLH1	rs1799977	Missense SNP located in a highly conserved N-terminal ATPase domain, vital for MLH1 function [73]; G allele associated with reduced expression [74–77].	GG genotype associated with increased radiosensitivity in cancer patients, translating into increased efficacy [78] or toxicity [79] of radiotherapy (alone or combined with chemotherapy).
MSH3	rs26279	Missense SNP located in the ATPase domain, critical for protein activity [80]; altered expression has been suggested [81] but not confirmed [82].	GG genotype associated with decreased incidence of radiation dermatitis in breast cancer patients receiving radiotherapy [83], decreased overall survival in head and neck squamous cell carcinoma patients submitted to radiochemotherapy [81] and decreased response to platinum-based chemotherapy in advanced non-small cell lung cancer patients [84].
MSH4	rs5745325	Missense SNP located in the N-terminal domain, involved in the interaction with eIF3f [85].	None to be reported.
NBN	rs1805794	Missense SNP located in the BRCT domain, a region involved in the interaction with BRCA1 [86–89]; conflicting results from functional studies [88,90–92].	No association detected in most studies focusing on response to radiotherapy [79,93–96] or chemotherapy [97–99]; conflicting results also reported as the C allele has been associated with either improved [86,100] or worse [68,101] prognosis upon platinum-based chemotherapy; increased frequency of binucleated lymphocytes with nucleoplasmic bridges in Glu/Gln children with high IR exposure, opposite to Gln/Gln children [102].

MLH1, together with PMS2, forms the MutLα heterodimer, a complex critical for the maintenance of genomic integrity [103,104]. The common rs1799977 (c.665A>G, Ile219Val) missense SNP is located in a region that codes for a highly conserved N-terminal ATPase domain, vital for MLH1 function. However, since both alleles code for nonpolar pH-neutral amino acids, the substitution is considered conservative and not expected to result in drastic changes in protein properties and function [73].

Several functional studies support this hypothesis [73,74,105–107] but the existence of a more subtle effect should not be excluded [73,106,108,109] as an association between the G variant allele and reduced MLH1 expression has been demonstrated repeatedly in cancer patients [74–77]. Moreover, two recent meta-analyses have associated this variant with increased risk of colorectal cancer [110,111]. Considering the important role that MLH1 plays in the maintenance of genome integrity and cancer avoidance, both observations are compatible with our own observation of increased baseline BNMN levels in TC patients carrying the G allele. A different picture emerges, however, upon IR exposure: as previously stated, MMR proteins such as MLH1 play a dual role in the DNA damage response to IR, triggering cell-cycle arrest and allowing for either DSB repair or apoptosis [11,64]. MMR proficiency is thus expected to result in higher repair efficiency of IR-induced damage (hence, lower cytogenetic levels) and, simultaneously, higher cytotoxicity upon IR exposure (hence, increased sensitivity to radiotherapy). Indeed, alongside with increased cancer susceptibility, the *MLH1* rs1799977 variant GG genotype has been associated with increased radiosensitivity in cancer patients, translating into increased efficacy [78] or toxicity [79] of radiotherapy (alone or combined with chemotherapy). This is suggestive of increased MMR proficiency in such patients and supports our own observation of significantly lower BNMN levels, one month after ^{131}I therapy, in TC patients carrying the G allele. How the same allele may be associated with decreased function under basal conditions and increased function after IR exposure remains to be explained: MLH1 has been demonstrated to be upregulated upon IR exposure [112,113], it is possible that such upregulation might be more pronounced in G allele carriers, but this is highly speculative. Nevertheless, the high level of significance in our observations (especially when considering the change in MN frequency from baseline) and their cross-validation in independent groups strengthen our conclusions and warrant further studies to clarify this issue.

Two other MMR polymorphisms presented significant findings in our study, *MSH3* rs26279 and *MSH4* rs5745325. Like MLH1, MSH3 also appears to be involved in the repair and damage response to IR-associated lesions such as DSBs and inter-strand crosslinks [84,114]. *MSH3* rs26279 (c.3133A>G; Thr1045Ala) is a common SNP that results in an amino acid change in the ATPase domain of MLH3. This domain is critical for MSH3 activity, suggesting a functional impact for this variant [80]. Such hypothesis remains to be verified as, to the best of our knowledge, functional studies are lacking. An association with altered MSH3 expression levels has been suggested [81] but not confirmed [82]. The *MSH3* rs26279 G allele or GG genotype has been consistently associated with cancer risk in all 3 meta-analysis that we are aware of, particularly for colon and breast cancer [115–117], suggesting decreased DNA repair capacity in G allele carriers. Further, *MSH3* rs26279 GG homozygosity has also been associated with decreased incidence of radiation dermatitis in breast cancer patients receiving radiotherapy [83], decreased overall survival in head and neck squamous cell carcinoma patients submitted to radiochemotherapy [81], and decreased response to platinum-based chemotherapy in advanced non-small cell lung cancer patients [84], suggesting decreased sensitivity to DNA damaging agents such as IR or platinum in GG homozygous individuals. Such phenotype is commonly associated with MMR deficiency [64,69,70,118,119]. If we consider, once again, the dual role that MMR proteins such as MSH3 play in damage repair and apoptosis, these results are compatible with decreased G allele function, resulting in decreased DNA repair and apoptosis, increased damage tolerance, resistance to radio/chemotherapy, and reduced efficacy and cytotoxicity of such therapeutic agents. Our own observation of increased MN levels in TC patients carrying the G allele, 6 months after receiving 100 mCi ^{131}I, fits comfortably into this picture.

Likewise, in our study, MN frequency was also significantly increased (absolute and change from baseline values) in TC patients carrying the A allele of *MSH4* rs5745325, one month after ^{131}I administration. *MSH4* rs5745325 (c.289G>A; Ala97Thr) has only seldom been evaluated: on single SNP analysis, two prior studies by our team failed to detect an association with either thyroid [21] or breast cancer risk [120]. The same was observed in the only two other association studies that we found focusing on this SNP [121,122]. Interestingly, in three out of these four studies, significant associations were detected when interactions with other SNPs—*MSH6* rs1042821 [21], *MLH3* rs175080 [120], and *CHRNA5* rs16969968 [121]—were considered. Besides the important role that MSH4 plays in recombinational repair during meiosis [123], it is also suggested to participate, through interaction with a vast array of binding partners, in DSB-triggered damage response and repair [85,123,124]. It is possible that *MSH4* rs5745325 interferes with the binding properties of MSH4, with impact on its putative contribution to the DNA damage response and repair. The interaction of MSH4 with eIF3f (a subunit of the eIF3 complex implicated in apoptosis regulation and tumor development), for example, occurs at the region comprising the first 150 amino acids of the N-terminal domain of MSH4 (where rs5745325 is located) and has been demonstrated to foster hMSH4 stabilization and to modulate sensitivity to IR-induced DNA damage [85]. This is in line with our own findings.

Finally, we also observed a significant association between *NBN* rs1805794 and BNMN frequency, one month after the administration of 100 mCi ^{131}I. Nibrin plays a pivotal role in the initial steps of the cellular response to DNA damage, directly initiating DSB repair through the RAD51-dependent HR pathway and further contributing to cell cycle checkpoint activation through an ATM-dependent pathway [68,125–127]. Inactivating germline mutations in the *NBN* gene (which encodes for the Nibrin protein) markedly impair DSB repair and cause the Nijmegen breakage syndrome, characterized by chromosomal instability, increased cancer susceptibility, and increased sensitivity to DSB-causing agents such as IR or cisplatin. These features highlight the importance of Nibrin for genome stability (hence, cancer prevention) [86,93,125,127]. NBN overexpression also appears to be associated with poor prognosis in several types of cancer [68], which is consistent with a putative increase in DNA repair efficiency, hence, resistance to cytotoxic therapy. Among the numerous *NBN* polymorphisms, rs1805794 (c.553G>C; Glu185Gln) is the most frequently investigated. This missense variant results in an amino acid change in the BRCT (BRCA1 C Terminus) domain (amino acids 108-196), a domain involved in the interaction of Nibrin with BRCA1. The resulting complex (the BRCA1-associated genome surveillance complex, BASC) is responsible for the recognition and repair of aberrant DNA [86–89]. *NBN* rs1805794 has been suggested to interfere with the interaction properties of Nibrin and thus with DNA repair capacity, sensitivity to DNA damaging agents (such as IR) and cancer susceptibility. Accordingly, *NBN* rs1805794 has been repeatedly associated with cancer risk, as demonstrated by numerous meta-analysis [68,88,89,125,128–132] but conflicting reports exist [126,127,133,134]. Interestingly, the association may vary according to ethnicity [88,130] and tumor site [125], as one of these meta-analysis has demonstrated, for example, increased risk of leukemia, nasopharyngeal, and urinary system cancers but decreased risk of lung, gastric, and digestive system cancers [125]. Furthermore, final conclusive evidence on the significance of *NBN* rs1805794 is still lacking, as the functional studies performed thus far have yielded negative or conflicting results: while lymphocytes from healthy individuals homozygous for the G allele have been reported to present higher DNA damage levels (as assessed by the Comet assay) than lymphocytes from C allele carriers [90], opposite results have been reported in ex vivo X-ray irradiated cells from healthy subjects [88]. Further ex vivo irradiation studies have failed to observe a significant influence of *NBN* rs1805794 on DNA repair capacity and radiosensitivity [91,92]. Furthermore, since a putative functional impact of this SNP on DNA repair capacity could possibly influence patient sensitivity to radio and/or chemotherapy, association studies correlating *NBN* rs1805794 genotype with therapy response, toxicity, or prognosis have also been performed. Again, most studies failed to find an association in radiotherapy [79,93–96] or chemotherapy [97–99] treated patients, while other studies presented opposite findings, associating the *NBN* rs1805794 C allele with either improved [86,100] or worse [68,101] prognosis upon platinum-based chemotherapy. Interestingly, increased frequency of binucleated lymphocytes with nucleoplasmic bridges was observed in peripheral lymphocytes from children with high environmental exposure to IR that were heterozygous for *NBN* rs1805794, while the reverse patter was observed in children homozygous for the Gln allele [102]. This may be suggestive of molecular heterosis, a hypothesis that, considering the high interethnic variability of the *NBN* rs1805794 distribution, could help in explaining such divergent results. Overall, despite extensively investigated, the functional significance of *NBN* rs1805794, as well as its putative role in sensitivity to DNA damaging agents (such as IR) and cancer susceptibility remains elusive, warranting further studies to clarify this issue.

5. Conclusions

In conclusion, our results confirm that BNMN levels in peripheral lymphocytes from DTC patients increase significantly immediately 1 month after ^{131}I therapy and further suggest that these remain stable and persistently higher than baseline for at least 2 years. Furthermore, a marked reduction in CBPI is observed at 24 months after ^{131}I administration. Moreover, HR and MMR SNPs (*MLH1* rs1799977, *MSH3* rs26279, *MSH4* rs5745325, and *NBN* rs1805794) were, for the first time, associated with IR-induced MN, a cytogenetic marker of DNA damage, in TC patients submitted to ^{131}I therapy. Among such findings, a highly significant and independently replicated association was observed for *MLH1* rs1799977, strongly suggesting a role for this particular SNP on the personalization of RAI therapy in TC cancer patients. Baseline and post-therapy MN levels also diverged according to tumor histotype. These results should be regarded as merely suggestive and proof of concept, as the sample was small and the number of tests was high, increasing the likelihood of false-positive results. Nevertheless, our findings suggest that TC therapy with ^{131}I may pose a long-term challenge to cells other than thyrocytes and that the patient genetic profile may influence the individual sensitivity to this therapy. Such hypotheses are of relevance to the efficacy and safety of ^{131}I therapy, a widespread practice in TC patients. As such, extending the benefit already achieved with the latest guidelines on TC treatment in terms of risk/benefit ratio through improved clinical assessment of the potential long-term risks of ^{131}I therapy is desirable. Likewise, despite the micronucleus test is considered the gold standard methodology in genetic toxicology testing and often used as a "stand-alone" test in numerous and relevant papers in this area, other tests should also be employed to validate these results. Furthermore, potential radiogenomic markers such as those suggested here should be evaluated in larger samples, preferentially through multi-center independent studies adequately powered to provide more robust evidence and, eventually, to allow for gene-gene and gene-environment interactions to be assessed. Identifying the most clinically relevant variables, genetic or non-genetic, and accurately estimating their impact on ^{131}I therapy response rate and adverse event risk for each individual TC patient is the ultimate goal, under a personalized medicine approach.

Supplementary Materials

Table S1: Allele and genotype frequencies in thyroid cancer patients submitted to ^{131}I therapy (n = 26) and in the original (reference) DTC population (n = 106), Table S2: BNMN frequency (‰, mean ± S.D.) in DTC patients before and after (1, 3/6, and 24 months) therapy with different doses of ^{131}I (70 and 100 mCi), Table S3: Frequency of micronucleated cells (‰BNMN, mean ± SD) in the 70 mCi dose group at t_0, t_1, t_6 and t_{24}, and corresponding variation, according to genotype, Table S4: Frequency of micronucleated cells (‰BNMN, mean ± SD) in the 100 mCi dose group at t_0, t_1 and t_3, and corresponding variation, according to genotype, Table S5: Frequency of micronucleated cells (‰BNMN, mean ± SD) in the combined dose groups at t_0 and t_1, and corresponding variation, according to genotype, Table S6: Cytokinesis-Block Proliferation Index (CBPI, mean ± SD) in the 70 mCi dose group at t_0, t_1, t_6 and t_{24}, and corresponding variation, according to genotype.

Author Contributions: Conceptualization was mainly developed by J.R., T.C.F., and E.L.; methodology was performed by, O.M.G., L.S.S., and B.C.G.; validation proceedings by L.S.S., B.C.G., and S.N.S.; formal analysis was done by L.S.S. and S.N.S.; investigation was mainly performed by L.S.S. and B.C.G.; resources acquired in restrict collaboration by O.M.G. and T.C.F.; data curation, O.M.G., T.C.F., and E.L.; writing—original draft preparation, L.S.S; writing—review and editing, B.C.G., O.M.G., S.N.S., and J.R.; visualization has been prepared by L.S.S. and S.N.S.; supervision of this project was done by J.R.; project administration, J.R. and E.L.; funding acquisition, J.R. All authors have read and agreed to the published version of the manuscript.

Acknowledgments: The authors warmly acknowledge the generous collaboration of patients and controls in this study as well as of our colleague Ana Paula Azevedo for technical support.

References

1. Ferlay, J.; Ervik, M.; Lam, F.; Colombet, M.; Mery, L.; Piñeros, M.; Znaor, A.; Soerjomataram, I.; Bray, F. Global Cancer Observatory: Cancer Today. Available online: https://gco.iarc.fr/today (accessed on 28 May 2019).
2. Kitahara, C.M.; Sosa, J.A. The changing incidence of thyroid cancer. *Nat. Rev. Endocrinol.* **2016**, *12*, 646–653. [CrossRef] [PubMed]
3. Lebastchi, A.H.; Callender, G.G. Thyroid cancer. *Curr. Probl. Cancer* **2014**, *38*, 48–74. [CrossRef] [PubMed]
4. Khosravi, M.H.; Kouhi, A.; Saeedi, M.; Bagherihagh, A.; Amirzade-Iranaq, M.H. Thyroid Cancers: Considerations, Classifications, and Managements. In *Diagnosis and Management of Head and Neck Cancer*; Akarslan, Z., Ed.; IntechOpen: London, UK, 2017; pp. 57–82. [CrossRef]
5. Wild, C.; Weiderpass, E.; Stewart, B. (Eds.) *World Cancer Report: Cancer Research for Cancer Prevention*; International Agency for Research on Cancer: Lyon, France, 2020.
6. Mayson, S.E.; Yoo, D.C.; Gopalakrishnan, G. The evolving use of radioiodine therapy in differentiated thyroid cancer. *Oncology* **2015**, *88*, 247–256. [CrossRef]
7. Carballo, M.; Quiros, R.M. To treat or not to treat: The role of adjuvant radioiodine therapy in thyroid cancer patients. *J. Oncol.* **2012**, *2012*, 707156. [CrossRef] [PubMed]
8. Haugen, B.R.; Alexander, E.K.; Bible, K.C.; Doherty, G.M.; Mandel, S.J.; Nikiforov, Y.E.; Pacini, F.; Randolph, G.W.; Sawka, A.M.; Schlumberger, M.; et al. 2015 American Thyroid Association Management Guidelines for Adult Patients with Thyroid Nodules and Differentiated Thyroid Cancer: The American Thyroid Association Guidelines Task Force on Thyroid Nodules and Differentiated Thyroid Cancer. *Thyroid Off. J. Am. Thyroid Assoc.* **2016**, *26*, 1–133. [CrossRef] [PubMed]
9. Haugen, B.R. 2015 American Thyroid Association Management Guidelines for Adult Patients with Thyroid Nodules and Differentiated Thyroid Cancer: What is new and what has changed? *Cancer* **2017**, *123*, 372–381. [CrossRef]
10. Chatterjee, N.; Walker, G.C. Mechanisms of DNA damage, repair, and mutagenesis. *Environ. Mol. Mutagenesis* **2017**, *58*, 235–263. [CrossRef]
11. Collins, S.P.; Dritschilo, A. The mismatch repair and base excision repair pathways: An opportunity for individualized (personalized) sensitization of cancer therapy. *Cancer Biol. Ther.* **2009**, *8*, 1164–1166. [CrossRef]
12. Doai, M.; Watanabe, N.; Takahashi, T.; Taniguchi, M.; Tonami, H.; Iwabuchi, K.; Kayano, D.; Fukuoka, M.; Kinuya, S. Sensitive immunodetection of radiotoxicity after iodine-131 therapy for thyroid cancer using gamma-H2AX foci of DNA damage in lymphocytes. *Ann. Nucl. Med.* **2013**, *27*, 233–238. [CrossRef]
13. Eberlein, U.; Scherthan, H.; Bluemel, C.; Peper, M.; Lapa, C.; Buck, A.K.; Port, M.; Lassmann, M. DNA Damage in Peripheral Blood Lymphocytes of Thyroid Cancer Patients After Radioiodine Therapy. *J. Nucl. Med. Off. Publ. Soc. Nucl. Med.* **2016**, *57*, 173–179. [CrossRef]
14. Simonelli, V.; Mazzei, F.; D'Errico, M.; Dogliotti, E. Gene susceptibility to oxidative damage: From single nucleotide polymorphisms to function. *Mutat. Res.* **2012**, *731*, 1–13. [CrossRef] [PubMed]
15. Sameer, A.S.; Nissar, S. XPD-The Lynchpin of NER: Molecule, Gene, Polymorphisms, and Role in Colorectal Carcinogenesis. *Front. Mol. Biosci.* **2018**, *5*, 23. [CrossRef]
16. Adjadj, E.; Schlumberger, M.; de Vathaire, F. Germ-line DNA polymorphisms and susceptibility to differentiated thyroid cancer. *Lancet Oncol.* **2009**, *10*, 181–190. [CrossRef]
17. Gatzidou, E.; Michailidi, C.; Tseleni-Balafouta, S.; Theocharis, S. An epitome of DNA repair related genes and mechanisms in thyroid carcinoma. *Cancer Lett.* **2010**, *290*, 139–147. [CrossRef] [PubMed]
18. Santos, L.S.; Gomes, B.C.; Bastos, H.N.; Gil, O.M.; Azevedo, A.P.; Ferreira, T.C.; Limbert, E.; Silva, S.N.; Rueff, J. Thyroid Cancer: The Quest for Genetic Susceptibility Involving DNA Repair Genes. *Genes* **2019**, *10*, 586. [CrossRef]
19. Bastos, H.N.; Antao, M.R.; Silva, S.N.; Azevedo, A.P.; Manita, I.; Teixeira, V.; Pina, J.E.; Gil, O.M.; Ferreira, T.C.; Limbert, E.; et al. Association of polymorphisms in genes of the homologous recombination DNA repair pathway and thyroid cancer risk. *Thyroid Off. J. Am. Thyroid Assoc.* **2009**, *19*, 1067–1075. [CrossRef]
20. Gomes, B.C.; Silva, S.N.; Azevedo, A.P.; Manita, I.; Gil, O.M.; Ferreira, T.C.; Limbert, E.; Rueff, J.; Gaspar, J.F. The role of common variants of non-homologous end-joining repair genes XRCC4, LIG4 and Ku80 in thyroid cancer risk. *Oncol. Rep.* **2010**, *24*, 1079–1085.
21. Santos, L.S.; Silva, S.N.; Gil, O.M.; Ferreira, T.C.; Limbert, E.; Rueff, J. Mismatch repair single nucleotide polymorphisms and thyroid cancer susceptibility. *Oncol. Lett.* **2018**, *15*, 6715–6726. [CrossRef]

22. Gil, O.M.; Oliveira, N.G.; Rodrigues, A.S.; Laires, A.; Ferreira, T.C.; Limbert, E.; Leonard, A.; Gerber, G.; Rueff, J. Cytogenetic alterations and oxidative stress in thyroid cancer patients after iodine-131 therapy. *Mutagenesis* **2000**, *15*, 69–75. [CrossRef]
23. Monteiro Gil, O.; Oliveira, N.G.; Rodrigues, A.S.; Laires, A.; Ferreira, T.C.; Limbert, E.; Rueff, J. Possible transient adaptive response to mitomycin C in peripheral lymphocytes from thyroid cancer patients after iodine-131 therapy. *Int. J. Cancer* **2002**, *102*, 556–561. [CrossRef]
24. Gil, O.M.; Oliveira, N.G.; Rodrigues, A.S.; Laires, A.; Ferreira, T.C.; Limbert, E.; Rueff, J. No evidence of increased chromosomal aberrations and micronuclei in lymphocytes from nonfamilial thyroid cancer patients prior to radiotherapy. *Cancer Genet. Cytogenet.* **2000**, *123*, 55–60. [CrossRef] [PubMed]
25. Sole, X.; Guino, E.; Valls, J.; Iniesta, R.; Moreno, V. SNPStats: A web tool for the analysis of association studies. *Bioinformatics* **2006**, *22*, 1928–1929. [CrossRef] [PubMed]
26. OECD. *Test No. 487: In Vitro Mammalian Cell Micronucleus Test*; OECD: Paris, France, 2016. [CrossRef]
27. Hernández, A.; Xamena, N.; Gutiérrez, S.; Velázquez, A.; Creus, A.; Surrallés, J.; Galofré, P.; Marcos, R. Basal and induced micronucleus frequencies in human lymphocytes with different GST and NAT2 genetic backgrounds. *Mutat. Res.* **2006**, *606*, 12–20. [CrossRef]
28. Gutiérrez, S.; Carbonell, E.; Galofré, P.; Creus, A.; Marcos, R. Cytogenetic damage after 131-iodine treatment for hyperthyroidism and thyroid cancer. A study using the micronucleus test. *Eur. J. Nucl. Med.* **1999**, *26*, 1589–1596. [CrossRef] [PubMed]
29. Livingston, G.K.; Foster, A.E.; Elson, H.R. Effect of in vivo exposure to iodine-131 on the frequency and persistence of micronuclei in human lymphocytes. *J. Toxicol. Environ. Health* **1993**, *40*, 367–375. [CrossRef] [PubMed]
30. Ramírez, M.J.; Puerto, S.; Galofré, P.; Parry, E.M.; Parry, J.M.; Creus, A.; Marcos, R.; Surrallés, J. Multicolour FISH detection of radioactive iodine-induced 17cen-p53 chromosomal breakage in buccal cells from therapeutically exposed patients. *Carcinogenesis* **2000**, *21*, 1581–1586.
31. Ramírez, M.J.; Surrallés, J.; Galofré, P.; Creus, A.; Marcos, R. Radioactive iodine induces clastogenic and age-dependent aneugenic effects in lymphocytes of thyroid cancer patients as revealed by interphase FISH. *Mutagenesis* **1997**, *12*, 449–455. [CrossRef]
32. Monzen, S.; Mariya, Y.; Wojcik, A.; Kawamura, C.; Nakamura, A.; Chiba, M.; Hosoda, M.; Takai, Y. Predictive factors of cytotoxic damage in radioactive iodine treatment of differentiated thyroid cancer patients. *Mol. Clin. Oncol.* **2015**, *3*, 692–698. [CrossRef]
33. Shakeri, M.; Zakeri, F.; Changizi, V.; Rajabpour, M.R.; Farshidpour, M.R. Cytogenetic effects of radiation and genetic polymorphisms of the XRCC1 and XRCC3 repair genes in industrial radiographers. *Radiat. Environ. Biophys.* **2019**, *58*, 247–255. [CrossRef]
34. Müller, W.U.; Nüsse, M.; Miller, B.M.; Slavotinek, A.; Viaggi, S.; Streffer, C. Micronuclei: A biological indicator of radiation damage. *Mutat. Res.* **1996**, *366*, 163–169. [CrossRef]
35. Sinitsky, M.Y.; Minina, V.I.; Asanov, M.A.; Yuzhalin, A.E.; Ponasenko, A.V.; Druzhinin, V.G. Association of DNA repair gene polymorphisms with genotoxic stress in underground coal miners. *Mutagenesis* **2017**, *32*, 501–509. [CrossRef] [PubMed]
36. Watanabe, N.; Yokoyama, K.; Kinuya, S.; Shuke, N.; Shimizu, M.; Futatsuya, R.; Michigishi, T.; Tonami, N.; Seto, H.; Goodwin, D.A. Radiotoxicity after iodine-131 therapy for thyroid cancer using the micronucleus assay. *J. Nucl. Med. Off. Publ. Soc. Nucl. Med.* **1998**, *39*, 436–440.
37. Ballardin, M.; Gemignani, F.; Bodei, L.; Mariani, G.; Ferdeghini, M.; Rossi, A.M.; Migliore, L.; Barale, R. Formation of micronuclei and of clastogenic factor(s) in patients receiving therapeutic doses of iodine-131. *Mutat. Res.* **2002**, *514*, 77–85. [CrossRef]
38. Livingston, G.K.; Khvostunov, I.K. Cytogenetic effects of radioiodine therapy: A 20-year follow-up study. *Radiat. Environ. Biophys.* **2016**, *55*, 203–213. [CrossRef]
39. Puerto, S.; Marcos, R.; Ramírez, M.J.; Galofré, P.; Creus, A.; Surrallés, J. Equal induction and persistence of chromosome aberrations involving chromosomes 1, 4 and 10 in thyroid cancer patients treated with radioactive iodine. *Mutat. Res.* **2000**, *469*, 147–158. [CrossRef]
40. Fenech, M.; Denham, J.; Francis, W.; Morley, A. Micronuclei in cytokinesis-blocked lymphocytes of cancer patients following fractionated partial-body radiotherapy. *Int. J. Radiat. Biol.* **1990**, *57*, 373–383. [CrossRef]

41. M'Kacher, R.; Légal, J.D.; Schlumberger, M.; Aubert, B.; Beron-Gaillard, N.; Gaussen, A.; Parmentier, C. Sequential biological dosimetry after a single treatment with iodine-131 for differentiated thyroid carcinoma. *J. Nucl. Med. Off. Publ. Soc. Nucl. Med.* **1997**, *38*, 377–380.
42. Livingston, G.K.; Escalona, M.; Foster, A.; Balajee, A.S. Persistent in vivo cytogenetic effects of radioiodine therapy: A 21-year follow-up study using multicolor FISH. *J. Radiat. Res.* **2018**, *59*, 10–17. [CrossRef]
43. Livingston, G.K.; Ryan, T.L.; Smith, T.L.; Escalona, M.B.; Foster, A.E.; Balajee, A.S. Detection of Simple, Complex, and Clonal Chromosome Translocations Induced by Internal Radioiodine Exposure: A Cytogenetic Follow-Up Case Study after 25 Years. *Cytogenet. Genome Res.* **2019**, *159*, 169–181. [CrossRef]
44. Lindholm, C.; Acheva, A.; Salomaa, S. Clastogenic plasma factors: A short overview. *Radiat. Environ. Biophys.* **2010**, *49*, 133–138. [CrossRef]
45. Morgan, W.F. Is there a common mechanism underlying genomic instability, bystander effects and other nontargeted effects of exposure to ionizing radiation? *Oncogene* **2003**, *22*, 7094–7099. [CrossRef] [PubMed]
46. Mavragani, I.V.; Laskaratou, D.A.; Frey, B. Key mechanisms involved in ionizing radiation-induced systemic effects. A current review. *Toxicol. Res.* **2016**, *5*, 12–33. [CrossRef] [PubMed]
47. Lorimore, S.A.; McIlrath, J.M.; Coates, P.J.; Wright, E.G. Chromosomal instability in unirradiated hemopoietic cells resulting from a delayed in vivo bystander effect of gamma radiation. *Cancer Res.* **2005**, *65*, 5668–5673. [CrossRef] [PubMed]
48. Fenech, M.; Bonassi, S. The effect of age, gender, diet and lifestyle on DNA damage measured using micronucleus frequency in human peripheral blood lymphocytes. *Mutagenesis* **2011**, *26*, 43–49. [CrossRef]
49. Fenech, M.; Holland, N.; Zeiger, E.; Chang, W.P.; Burgaz, S.; Thomas, P.; Bolognesi, C.; Knasmueller, S.; Kirsch-Volders, M.; Bonassi, S. The HUMN and HUMNxL international collaboration projects on human micronucleus assays in lymphocytes and buccal cells–past, present and future. *Mutagenesis* **2011**, *26*, 239–245. [CrossRef]
50. Battershill, J.M.; Burnett, K.; Bull, S. Factors affecting the incidence of genotoxicity biomarkers in peripheral blood lymphocytes: Impact on design of biomonitoring studies. *Mutagenesis* **2008**, *23*, 423–437. [CrossRef]
51. Bonassi, S.; Fenech, M.; Lando, C.; Lin, Y.P.; Ceppi, M.; Chang, W.P.; Holland, N.; Kirsch-Volders, M.; Zeiger, E.; Ban, S.; et al. HUman MicroNucleus project: International database comparison for results with the cytokinesis-block micronucleus assay in human lymphocytes: I. Effect of laboratory protocol, scoring criteria, and host factors on the frequency of micronuclei. *Environ. Mol. Mutagenesis* **2001**, *37*, 31–45. [CrossRef]
52. Caria, P.; Vanni, R. Cytogenetic and molecular events in adenoma and well-differentiated thyroid follicular-cell neoplasia. *Cancer Genet. Cytogenet.* **2010**, *203*, 21–29. [CrossRef]
53. Genutis, L.K.; Tomsic, J.; Bundschuh, R.A.; Brock, P.L.; Williams, M.D.; Roychowdhury, S.; Reeser, J.W.; Frankel, W.L.; Alsomali, M.; Routbort, M.J.; et al. Microsatellite Instability Occurs in a Subset of Follicular Thyroid Cancers. *Thyroid Off. J. Am. Thyroid Assoc.* **2019**, *29*, 523–529. [CrossRef]
54. Lazzereschi, D.; Palmirotta, R.; Ranieri, A.; Ottini, L.; Veri, M.C.; Cama, A.; Cetta, F.; Nardi, F.; Colletta, G.; Mariani-Costantini, R. Microsatellite instability in thyroid tumours and tumour-like lesions. *Br. J. Cancer* **1999**, *79*, 340–345. [CrossRef]
55. Migdalska-Sek, M.; Czarnecka, K.H.; Kusinski, M.; Pastuszak-Lewandoska, D.; Nawrot, E.; Kuzdak, K.; Brzezianska-Lasota, E. Clinicopathological Significance of Overall Frequency of Allelic Loss (OFAL) in Lesions Derived from Thyroid Follicular Cell. *Mol. Diagn. Ther.* **2019**, *23*, 369–382. [CrossRef] [PubMed]
56. Ward, L.S.; Brenta, G.; Medvedovic, M.; Fagin, J.A. Studies of allelic loss in thyroid tumors reveal major differences in chromosomal instability between papillary and follicular carcinomas. *J. Clin. Endocrinol. Metab.* **1998**, *83*, 525–530. [CrossRef] [PubMed]
57. Gillespie, J.W.; Nasir, A.; Kaiser, H.E. Loss of heterozygosity in papillary and follicular thyroid carcinoma: A mini review. *VIVO (AthensGreece)* **2000**, *14*, 139–140.
58. Xing, M. Molecular pathogenesis and mechanisms of thyroid cancer. *Nat. Rev. Cancer* **2013**, *13*, 184–199. [CrossRef] [PubMed]
59. Sobrinho-Simoes, M.; Eloy, C.; Magalhaes, J.; Lobo, C.; Amaro, T. Follicular thyroid carcinoma. *Mod. Pathol.* **2011**, *24*, S10–S18. [CrossRef]
60. Miller, A.C.; Gafner, J.; Clark, E.P.; Samid, D. Differences in radiation-induced micronuclei yields of human cells: Influence of ras gene expression and protein localization. *Int. J. Radiat. Biol.* **1993**, *64*, 547–554. [CrossRef]

61. Zhang, X.; Liu, D.S.; Luan, Z.S.; Zhang, F.; Liu, X.H.; Zhou, W.; Zhong, S.F.; Lai, H. Efficacy of radioiodine therapy for treating 20 patients with pulmonary metastases from differentiated thyroid cancer and a meta-analysis of the current literature. *Clin. Transl. Oncol.* **2018**, *20*, 928–935. [CrossRef]
62. Eccles, L.J.; O'Neill, P.; Lomax, M.E. Delayed repair of radiation induced clustered DNA damage: Friend or foe? *Mutat. Res.* **2011**, *711*, 134–141. [CrossRef] [PubMed]
63. Sage, E.; Shikazono, N. Radiation-induced clustered DNA lesions: Repair and mutagenesis. *Free Radic. Biol. Med.* **2017**, *107*, 125–135. [CrossRef]
64. Martin, L.M.; Marples, B.; Coffey, M.; Lawler, M.; Lynch, T.H.; Hollywood, D.; Marignol, L. DNA mismatch repair and the DNA damage response to ionizing radiation: Making sense of apparently conflicting data. *Cancer Treat. Rev.* **2010**, *36*, 518–527. [CrossRef]
65. Nickoloff, J.A.; Sharma, N.; Taylor, L. Clustered DNA Double-Strand Breaks: Biological Effects and Relevance to Cancer Radiotherapy. *Genes* **2020**, *11*, 99. [CrossRef] [PubMed]
66. Zhang, H.; Xiong, Y.; Chen, J. DNA-protein cross-link repair: What do we know now? *Cell Biosci.* **2020**, *10*, 3. [CrossRef] [PubMed]
67. Nakano, T.; Xu, X.; Salem, A.M.H.; Shoulkamy, M.I.; Ide, H. Radiation-induced DNA-protein cross-links: Mechanisms and biological significance. *Free Radic. Biol. Med.* **2017**, *107*, 136–145. [CrossRef] [PubMed]
68. Wang, L.; Cheng, J.; Gao, J.; Wang, J.; Liu, X.; Xiong, L. Association between the NBS1 Glu185Gln polymorphism and lung cancer risk: A systemic review and meta-analysis. *Mol. Biol. Rep.* **2013**, *40*, 2711–2715. [CrossRef]
69. Kinsella, T.J. Coordination of DNA mismatch repair and base excision repair processing of chemotherapy and radiation damage for targeting resistant cancers. *Clin. Cancer Res. Off. J. Am. Assoc. Cancer Res.* **2009**, *15*, 1853–1859. [CrossRef]
70. Edelbrock, M.A.; Kaliyaperumal, S.; Williams, K.J. Structural, molecular and cellular functions of MSH2 and MSH6 during DNA mismatch repair, damage signaling and other noncanonical activities. *Mutat. Res.* **2013**, *743*, 53–66. [CrossRef]
71. Iyama, T.; Wilson, D.M., 3rd. DNA repair mechanisms in dividing and non-dividing cells. *DNA Repair* **2013**, *12*, 620–636. [CrossRef]
72. Iarmarcovai, G.; Bonassi, S.; Botta, A.; Baan, R.A.; Orsière, T. Genetic polymorphisms and micronucleus formation: A review of the literature. *Mutat. Res.* **2008**, *658*, 215–233. [CrossRef]
73. Plotz, G.; Raedle, J.; Spina, A.; Welsch, C.; Stallmach, A.; Zeuzem, S.; Schmidt, C. Evaluation of the MLH1 I219V alteration in DNA mismatch repair activity and ulcerative colitis. *Inflamm. Bowel Dis.* **2008**, *14*, 605–611. [CrossRef]
74. Milanizadeh, S.; Khanyaghma, M.; Haghighi, M.M.; Mohebbi, S.; Damavand, B.; Almasi, S.; Azimzadeh, P.; Zali, M. Molecular analysis of imperative polymorphisms of MLH1 gene in sporadic colorectal cancer. *Cancer Biomark. Sect. A Dis. Markers* **2013**, *13*, 427–432. [CrossRef]
75. Kim, J.C.; Roh, S.A.; Koo, K.H.; Ka, I.H.; Kim, H.C.; Yu, C.S.; Lee, K.H.; Kim, J.S.; Lee, H.I.; Bodmer, W.F. Genotyping possible polymorphic variants of human mismatch repair genes in healthy Korean individuals and sporadic colorectal cancer patients. *Fam. Cancer* **2004**, *3*, 129–137. [CrossRef] [PubMed]
76. Rossi, D.; Rasi, S.; Di Rocco, A.; Fabbri, A.; Forconi, F.; Gloghini, A.; Bruscaggin, A.; Franceschetti, S.; Fangazio, M.; De Paoli, L.; et al. The host genetic background of DNA repair mechanisms is an independent predictor of survival in diffuse large B-cell lymphoma. *Blood* **2011**, *117*, 2405–2413. [CrossRef] [PubMed]
77. Xiao, X.Q.; Gong, W.D.; Wang, S.Z.; Zhang, Z.D.; Rui, X.P.; Wu, G.Z.; Ren, F. Polymorphisms of mismatch repair gene hMLH1 and hMSH2 and risk of gastric cancer in a Chinese population. *Oncol. Lett.* **2012**, *3*, 591–598. [CrossRef] [PubMed]
78. Dreussi, E.; Cecchin, E.; Polesel, J.; Canzonieri, V.; Agostini, M.; Boso, C.; Belluco, C.; Buonadonna, A.; Lonardi, S.; Bergamo, F.; et al. Pharmacogenetics Biomarkers and Their Specific Role in Neoadjuvant Chemoradiotherapy Treatments: An Exploratory Study on Rectal Cancer Patients. *Int. J. Mol. Sci.* **2016**, *17*, 1482. [CrossRef]
79. Damaraju, S.; Murray, D.; Dufour, J.; Carandang, D.; Myrehaug, S.; Fallone, G.; Field, C.; Greiner, R.; Hanson, J.; Cass, C.E.; et al. Association of DNA repair and steroid metabolism gene polymorphisms with clinical late toxicity in patients treated with conformal radiotherapy for prostate cancer. *Clin. Cancer Res. Off. J. Am. Assoc. Cancer Res.* **2006**, *12*, 2545–2554. [CrossRef]

80. Morales, F.; Vásquez, M.; Santamaría, C.; Cuenca, P.; Corrales, E.; Monckton, D.G. A polymorphism in the MSH3 mismatch repair gene is associated with the levels of somatic instability of the expanded CTG repeat in the blood DNA of myotonic dystrophy type 1 patients. *DNA Repair* **2016**, *40*, 57–66. [CrossRef]
81. Nogueira, G.A.; Lourenço, G.J.; Oliveira, C.B.; Marson, F.A.; Lopes-Aguiar, L.; Costa, E.F.; Lima, T.R.; Liutti, V.T.; Leal, F.; Santos, V.C.; et al. Association between genetic polymorphisms in DNA mismatch repair-related genes with risk and prognosis of head and neck squamous cell carcinoma. *Int. J. Cancer* **2015**, *137*, 810–818. [CrossRef]
82. Vogelsang, M.; Wang, Y.; Veber, N.; Mwapagha, L.M.; Parker, M.I. The cumulative effects of polymorphisms in the DNA mismatch repair genes and tobacco smoking in oesophageal cancer risk. *PLoS ONE* **2012**, *7*, e36962. [CrossRef]
83. Mangoni, M.; Bisanzi, S.; Carozzi, F.; Sani, C.; Biti, G.; Livi, L.; Barletta, E.; Costantini, A.S.; Gorini, G. Association between genetic polymorphisms in the XRCC1, XRCC3, XPD, GSTM1, GSTT1, MSH2, MLH1, MSH3, and MGMT genes and radiosensitivity in breast cancer patients. *Int. J. Radiat. Oncol. Biol. Phys.* **2011**, *81*, 52–58. [CrossRef]
84. Xu, X.L.; Yao, Y.L.; Xu, W.Z.; Feng, J.G.; Mao, W.M. Correlation of MSH3 polymorphisms with response and survival in advanced non-small cell lung cancer patients treated with first-line platinum-based chemotherapy. *Genet. Mol. Res. Gmr* **2015**, *14*, 3525–3533. [CrossRef]
85. Chu, Y.L.; Wu, X.; Xu, Y.; Her, C. MutS homologue hMSH4: Interaction with eIF3f and a role in NHEJ-mediated DSB repair. *Mol. Cancer* **2013**, *12*, 51. [CrossRef] [PubMed]
86. Xu, J.L.; Hu, L.M.; Huang, M.D.; Zhao, W.; Yin, Y.M.; Hu, Z.B.; Ma, H.X.; Shen, H.B.; Shu, Y.Q. Genetic variants of NBS1 predict clinical outcome of platinum-based chemotherapy in advanced non-small cell lung cancer in Chinese. *Asian Pac. J. Cancer Prev. Apjcp* **2012**, *13*, 851–856. [CrossRef] [PubMed]
87. Smith, T.R.; Liu-Mares, W.; Van Emburgh, B.O.; Levine, E.A.; Allen, G.O.; Hill, J.W.; Reis, I.M.; Kresty, L.A.; Pegram, M.D.; Miller, M.S.; et al. Genetic polymorphisms of multiple DNA repair pathways impact age at diagnosis and TP53 mutations in breast cancer. *Carcinogenesis* **2011**, *32*, 1354–1360. [CrossRef] [PubMed]
88. Fang, W.; Qiu, F.; Zhang, L.; Deng, J.; Zhang, H.; Yang, L.; Zhou, Y.; Lu, J. The functional polymorphism of NBS1 p.Glu185Gln is associated with an increased risk of lung cancer in Chinese populations: Case-control and a meta-analysis. *Mutat. Res.* **2014**, *770*, 61–68. [CrossRef] [PubMed]
89. Lu, M.; Lu, J.; Yang, X.; Yang, M.; Tan, H.; Yun, B.; Shi, L. Association between the NBS1 E185Q polymorphism and cancer risk: A meta-analysis. *BMC Cancer* **2009**, *9*, 124. [CrossRef]
90. Goricar, K.; Erculj, N.; Zadel, M.; Dolzan, V. Genetic polymorphisms in homologous recombination repair genes in healthy Slovenian population and their influence on DNA damage. *Radiol. Oncol.* **2012**, *46*, 46–53. [CrossRef]
91. Gdowicz-Klosok, A.; Widel, M.; Rzeszowska-Wolny, J. The influence of XPD, APE1, XRCC1, and NBS1 polymorphic variants on DNA repair in cells exposed to X-rays. *Mutat. Res.* **2013**, *755*, 42–48. [CrossRef]
92. Mumbrekar, K.D.; Goutham, H.V.; Vadhiraja, B.M.; Bola Sadashiva, S.R. Polymorphisms in double strand break repair related genes influence radiosensitivity phenotype in lymphocytes from healthy individuals. *Dna Repair* **2016**, *40*, 27–34. [CrossRef]
93. Yin, M.; Liao, Z.; Huang, Y.J.; Liu, Z.; Yuan, X.; Gomez, D.; Wang, L.E.; Wei, Q. Polymorphisms of homologous recombination genes and clinical outcomes of non-small cell lung cancer patients treated with definitive radiotherapy. *PLoS ONE* **2011**, *6*, e20055. [CrossRef]
94. Venkatesh, G.H.; Manjunath, V.B.; Mumbrekar, K.D.; Negi, H.; Fernandes, D.J.; Sharan, K.; Banerjee, S.; Bola Sadashiva, S.R. Polymorphisms in radio-responsive genes and its association with acute toxicity among head and neck cancer patients. *PLoS ONE* **2014**, *9*, e89079. [CrossRef]
95. Chang-Claude, J.; Ambrosone, C.B.; Lilla, C.; Kropp, S.; Helmbold, I.; von Fournier, D.; Haase, W.; Sautter-Bihl, M.L.; Wenz, F.; Schmezer, P.; et al. Genetic polymorphisms in DNA repair and damage response genes and late normal tissue complications of radiotherapy for breast cancer. *Br. J. Cancer* **2009**, *100*, 1680–1686. [CrossRef] [PubMed]
96. Kerns, S.L.; Stock, R.G.; Stone, N.N.; Blacksburg, S.R.; Rath, L.; Vega, A.; Fachal, L.; Gómez-Caamaño, A.; De Ruysscher, D.; Lammering, G.; et al. Genome-wide association study identifies a region on chromosome 11q14.3 associated with late rectal bleeding following radiation therapy for prostate cancer. *Radiother. Oncol. J. Eur. Soc. Ther. Radiol. Oncol.* **2013**, *107*, 372–376. [CrossRef] [PubMed]

97. Ding, C.; Zhang, H.; Chen, K.; Zhao, C.; Gao, J. Genetic variability of DNA repair mechanisms influences treatment outcome of gastric cancer. *Oncol. Lett.* **2015**, *10*, 1997–2002. [CrossRef] [PubMed]
98. Erčulj, N.; Kovač, V.; Hmeljak, J.; Franko, A.; Dodič-Fikfak, M.; Dolžan, V. DNA repair polymorphisms and treatment outcomes of patients with malignant mesothelioma treated with gemcitabine-platinum combination chemotherapy. *J. Thorac. Oncol. Off. Publ. Int. Assoc. Study Lung Cancer* **2012**, *7*, 1609–1617. [CrossRef] [PubMed]
99. Ott, K.; Rachakonda, P.S.; Panzram, B.; Keller, G.; Lordick, F.; Becker, K.; Langer, R.; Buechler, M.; Hemminki, K.; Kumar, R. DNA repair gene and MTHFR gene polymorphisms as prognostic markers in locally advanced adenocarcinoma of the esophagus or stomach treated with cisplatin and 5-fluorouracil-based neoadjuvant chemotherapy. *Ann. Surg. Oncol.* **2011**, *18*, 2688–2698. [CrossRef]
100. Zhou, J.; Liu, Z.Y.; Li, C.B.; Gao, S.; Ding, L.H.; Wu, X.L.; Wang, Z.Y. Genetic polymorphisms of DNA repair pathways influence the response to chemotherapy and overall survival of gastric cancer. *Tumour Biol. J. Int. Soc. Oncodev. Biol. Med.* **2015**, *36*, 3017–3023. [CrossRef]
101. Jiang, Y.H.; Xu, X.L.; Ruan, H.H.; Xu, W.Z.; Li, D.; Feng, J.G.; Han, Q.B.; Mao, W.M. The impact of functional LIG4 polymorphism on platinum-based chemotherapy response and survival in non-small cell lung cancer. *Med. Oncol.* **2014**, *31*, 959. [CrossRef]
102. Sinitsky, M.Y.; Larionov, A.V.; Asanov, M.A.; Druzhinin, V.G. Associations of DNA-repair gene polymorphisms with a genetic susceptibility to ionizing radiation in residents of areas with high radon (222Rn) concentration. *Int. J. Radiat. Biol.* **2015**, *91*, 486–494. [CrossRef]
103. Senghore, T.; Wang, W.C.; Chien, H.T. Polymorphisms of Mismatch Repair Pathway Genes Predict Clinical Outcomes in Oral Squamous Cell Carcinoma Patients Receiving Adjuvant Concurrent Chemoradiotherapy. *Cancers* **2019**, *11*, 598. [CrossRef]
104. Dominguez-Valentin, M.; Drost, M.; Therkildsen, C.; Rambech, E.; Ehrencrona, H.; Angleys, M.; Lau Hansen, T.; de Wind, N.; Nilbert, M.; Juel Rasmussen, L. Functional implications of the p.Cys680Arg mutation in the MLH1 mismatch repair protein. *Mol. Genet. Genom. Med.* **2014**, *2*, 352–355. [CrossRef]
105. Dominguez-Valentin, M.; Wernhoff, P.; Cajal, A.R.; Kalfayan, P.G.; Piñero, T.A.; Gonzalez, M.L.; Ferro, A.; Sammartino, I.; Causada Calo, N.S.; Vaccaro, C.A. MLH1 Ile219Val Polymorphism in Argentinean Families with Suspected Lynch Syndrome. *Front. Oncol.* **2016**, *6*, 189. [CrossRef] [PubMed]
106. Blasi, M.F.; Ventura, I.; Aquilina, G.; Degan, P.; Bertario, L.; Bassi, C.; Radice, P.; Bignami, M. A human cell-based assay to evaluate the effects of alterations in the MLH1 mismatch repair gene. *Cancer Res.* **2006**, *66*, 9036–9044. [CrossRef] [PubMed]
107. Campbell, P.T.; Curtin, K.; Ulrich, C.M.; Samowitz, W.S.; Bigler, J.; Velicer, C.M.; Caan, B.; Potter, J.D.; Slattery, M.L. Mismatch repair polymorphisms and risk of colon cancer, tumour microsatellite instability and interactions with lifestyle factors. *Gut* **2009**, *58*, 661–667. [CrossRef] [PubMed]
108. Valentin, M.D.; Da Silva, F.C.; Santos, E.M.; Da Silva, S.D.; De Oliveira Ferreira, F.; Aguiar Junior, S.; Gomy, I.; Vaccaro, C.; Redal, M.A.; Della Valle, A.; et al. Evaluation of MLH1 I219V polymorphism in unrelated South American individuals suspected of having Lynch syndrome. *Anticancer Res.* **2012**, *32*, 4347–4351.
109. Nejda, N.; Iglesias, D.; Moreno Azcoita, M.; Medina Arana, V.; González-Aguilera, J.J.; Fernández-Peralta, A.M. A MLH1 polymorphism that increases cancer risk is associated with better outcome in sporadic colorectal cancer. *Cancer Genet. Cytogenet.* **2009**, *193*, 71–77. [CrossRef]
110. Li, S.; Zheng, Y.; Tian, T.; Wang, M.; Liu, X.; Liu, K.; Zhai, Y.; Dai, C.; Deng, Y.; Li, S.; et al. Pooling-analysis on hMLH1 polymorphisms and cancer risk: Evidence based on 31,484 cancer cases and 45,494 cancer-free controls. *Oncotarget* **2017**, *8*, 93063–93078. [CrossRef]
111. Zare, M.; Jafari-Nedooshan, J. Relevance of hMLH1 -93G>A, 655A>G and 1151T>A polymorphisms with colorectal cancer susceptibility: A meta-analysis based on 38 case-control studies. *Rev. Assoc. Med. Bras. (1992)* **2018**, *64*, 942–951. [CrossRef]
112. Zhang, Y.; Rohde, L.H.; Emami, K.; Hammond, D.; Casey, R.; Mehta, S.K.; Jeevarajan, A.S.; Pierson, D.L.; Wu, H. Suppressed expression of non-DSB repair genes inhibits gamma-radiation-induced cytogenetic repair and cell cycle arrest. *DNA Repair* **2008**, *7*, 1835–1845. [CrossRef]
113. Bakhtiari, E.; Monfared, A.S.; Niaki, H.A.; Borzoueisileh, S.; Niksirat, F.; Fattahi, S.; Monfared, M.K.; Gorji, K.E. The expression of MLH1 and MSH2 genes among inhabitants of high background radiation area of Ramsar, Iran. *J. Environ. Radioact.* **2019**, *208–209*, 106012. [CrossRef]

114. Yang, J.; Huang, Y.; Feng, Y.; Li, H.; Feng, T.; Chen, J.; Yin, L.; Wang, W.; Wang, S.; Liu, Y.; et al. Associations of Genetic Variations in Mismatch Repair Genes MSH3 and PMS1 with Acute Adverse Events and Survival in Patients with Rectal Cancer Receiving Postoperative Chemoradiotherapy. *Cancer Res. Treat. Off. J. Korean Cancer Assoc.* **2019**, *51*, 1198–1206. [CrossRef]
115. Miao, H.K.; Chen, L.P.; Cai, D.P.; Kong, W.J.; Xiao, L.; Lin, J. MSH3 rs26279 polymorphism increases cancer risk: A meta-analysis. *Int. J. Clin. Exp. Pathol.* **2015**, *8*, 11060–11067. [PubMed]
116. Ma, X.; Zhang, B.; Zheng, W. Genetic variants associated with colorectal cancer risk: Comprehensive research synopsis, meta-analysis, and epidemiological evidence. *Gut* **2014**, *63*, 326–336. [CrossRef] [PubMed]
117. Zhang, B.; Beeghly-Fadiel, A.; Long, J.; Zheng, W. Genetic variants associated with breast-cancer risk: Comprehensive research synopsis, meta-analysis, and epidemiological evidence. *Lancet Oncol.* **2011**, *12*, 477–488. [CrossRef]
118. Li, Z.; Pearlman, A.H.; Hsieh, P. DNA mismatch repair and the DNA damage response. *DNA Repair* **2016**, *38*, 94–101. [CrossRef]
119. Crouse, G.F. Non-canonical actions of mismatch repair. *DNA Repair* **2016**, *38*, 102–109. [CrossRef]
120. Conde, J.; Silva, S.N.; Azevedo, A.P.; Teixeira, V.; Pina, J.E.; Rueff, J.; Gaspar, J.F. Association of common variants in mismatch repair genes and breast cancer susceptibility: A multigene study. *BMC Cancer* **2009**, *9*, 344. [CrossRef]
121. Doherty, J.A.; Sakoda, L.C.; Loomis, M.M.; Barnett, M.J.; Julianto, L.; Thornquist, M.D.; Neuhouser, M.L.; Weiss, N.S.; Goodman, G.E.; Chen, C. DNA repair genotype and lung cancer risk in the beta-carotene and retinol efficacy trial. *Int. J. Mol. Epidemiol. Genet.* **2013**, *4*, 11–34.
122. Kappil, M.; Terry, M.B.; Delgado-Cruzata, L.; Liao, Y.; Santella, R.M. Mismatch Repair Polymorphisms as Markers of Breast Cancer Prevalence in the Breast Cancer Family Registry. *Anticancer Res.* **2016**, *36*, 4437–4441. [CrossRef]
123. Clark, N.; Wu, X.; Her, C. MutS Homologues hMSH4 and hMSH5: Genetic Variations, Functions, and Implications in Human Diseases. *Curr. Genom.* **2013**, *14*, 81–90. [CrossRef]
124. Chu, Y.L.; Wu, X.; Xu, J.; Watts, J.L.; Her, C. DNA damage induced MutS homologue hMSH4 acetylation. *Int. J. Mol. Sci.* **2013**, *14*, 20966–20982. [CrossRef]
125. He, Y.Z.; Chi, X.S.; Zhang, Y.C.; Deng, X.B.; Wang, J.R.; Lv, W.Y.; Zhou, Y.H.; Wang, Z.Q. NBS1 Glu185Gln polymorphism and cancer risk: Update on current evidence. *Tumour Biol. J. Int. Soc. Oncodev. Biol. Med.* **2014**, *35*, 675–687. [CrossRef] [PubMed]
126. Gao, P.; Ma, N.; Li, M.; Tian, Q.B.; Liu, D.W. Functional variants in NBS1 and cancer risk: Evidence from a meta-analysis of 60 publications with 111 individual studies. *Mutagenesis* **2013**, *28*, 683–697. [CrossRef] [PubMed]
127. Yao, F.; Fang, Y.; Chen, B.; Jin, F.; Wang, S. Association between the NBS1 Glu185Gln polymorphism and breast cancer risk: A meta-analysis. *Tumour Biol. J. Int. Soc. Oncodeve. Biol. Med.* **2013**, *34*, 1255–1262. [CrossRef] [PubMed]
128. Stern, M.C.; Lin, J.; Figueroa, J.D.; Kelsey, K.T.; Kiltie, A.E.; Yuan, J.M.; Matullo, G.; Fletcher, T.; Benhamou, S.; Taylor, J.A.; et al. Polymorphisms in DNA repair genes, smoking, and bladder cancer risk: Findings from the international consortium of bladder cancer. *Cancer Res.* **2009**, *69*, 6857–6864. [CrossRef]
129. Wang, J.; Liu, Q.; Yuan, S.; Xie, W.; Liu, Y.; Xiang, Y.; Wu, N.; Wu, L.; Ma, X.; Cai, T.; et al. Genetic predisposition to lung cancer: Comprehensive literature integration, meta-analysis, and multiple evidence assessment of candidate-gene association studies. *Sci. Rep.* **2017**, *7*, 8371. [CrossRef]
130. Wang, Y.; Sun, Z.; Xu, Y. Carriage of NBN polymorphisms and acute leukemia risk. *Int. J. Clin. Exp. Med.* **2015**, *8*, 3769–3776.
131. Zhang, Y.; Huang, Y.S.; Lin, W.Q.; Zhang, S.D.; Li, Q.W.; Hu, Y.Z.; Zheng, R.L.; Tang, T.; Li, X.Z.; Zheng, X.H. NBS1 Glu185Gln polymorphism and susceptibility to urinary system cancer: A meta-analysis. *Tumour Biol. J. Int. Soc. Oncodeve. Biol. Med.* **2014**, *35*, 10723–10729. [CrossRef]
132. Vineis, P.; Manuguerra, M.; Kavvoura, F.K.; Guarrera, S.; Allione, A.; Rosa, F.; Di Gregorio, A.; Polidoro, S.; Saletta, F.; Ioannidis, J.P.; et al. A field synopsis on low-penetrance variants in DNA repair genes and cancer susceptibility. *J. Natl. Cancer Inst.* **2009**, *101*, 24–36. [CrossRef]
133. Sud, A.; Hemminki, K.; Houlston, R.S. Candidate gene association studies and risk of Hodgkin lymphoma: A systematic review and meta-analysis. *Hematol. Oncol.* **2017**, *35*, 34–50. [CrossRef]

Gene Expression (mRNA) Markers for Differentiating between Malignant and Benign Follicular Thyroid Tumours

Bartosz Wojtas [1,2,†], Aleksandra Pfeifer [1,3,†], Malgorzata Oczko-Wojciechowska [1], Jolanta Krajewska [1], Agnieszka Czarniecka [4], Aleksandra Kukulska [1], Markus Eszlinger [5], Thomas Musholt [6], Tomasz Stokowy [1,3,7], Michal Swierniak [1,8], Ewa Stobiecka [9], Ewa Chmielik [9], Dagmara Rusinek [1], Tomasz Tyszkiewicz [1], Monika Halczok [1], Steffen Hauptmann [10], Dariusz Lange [9], Michal Jarzab [11], Ralf Paschke [12] and Barbara Jarzab [1,*]

1 Department of Nuclear Medicine and Endocrine Oncology, Maria Sklodowska-Curie Institute—Oncology Center, Gliwice Branch, Wybrzeze Armii Krajowej 15, 44-101 Gliwice, Poland; Bartosz.Wojtas@io.gliwice.pl (B.W.); Aleksandra.Pfeifer@io.gliwice.pl (A.P.); Malgorzata.Oczko-Wojciechowska@io.gliwice.pl (M.O.-W.); Jolanta.Krajewska@io.gliwice.pl (J.K.); Aleksandra.Kukulska@io.gliwice.pl (A.K.); tomasz.stokowy@k2.uib.no (T.S.); michal.swierniak@wum.edu.pl (M.S.); Dagmara.Rusinek@io.gliwice.pl (D.R.); Tomasz.Tyszkiewicz@io.gliwice.pl (T.T.); Monika.Kowal@io.gliwice.pl (M.H.)

2 Laboratory of Molecular Neurobiology, Neurobiology Center, Nencki Institute of Experimental Biology, Pasteura 3, 02-093 Warsaw, Poland

3 Faculty of Automatic Control, Electronics and Computer Science, Silesian University of Technology, Akademicka 2A, 44-100 Gliwice, Poland

4 The Oncologic and Reconstructive Surgery Clinic, Maria Sklodowska-Curie Institute—Oncology Center, Gliwice Branch, Wybrzeze Armii Krajowej 15, 44-101 Gliwice, Poland; Agnieszka.Czarniecka@io.gliwice.pl

5 Department of Oncology & Arnie Charbonneau Cancer Institute, Cumming School of Medicine, University of Calgary, Calgary, AB T2N 4N1, Canada; markus.eszlinger1@ucalgary.ca

6 Department of General, Visceral, and Transplantation Surgery, University Medical Center of the Johannes Gutenberg University, D55099 Mainz, Germany; musholt@uni-mainz.de

7 Department of Clinical Science, University of Bergen, 5020 Bergen, Norway

8 Genomic Medicine, Department of General, Transplant, and Liver Surgery, Medical University of Warsaw, Zwirki i Wigury 61, 02-093 Warsaw, Poland

9 Tumor Pathology Department, Maria Sklodowska-Curie Institute—Oncology Center, Gliwice Branch, Wybrzeze Armii Krajowej 15, 44-101 Gliwice, Poland; Ewa.Stobiecka@io.gliwice.pl (E.S.); Ewa.Chmielik@io.gliwice.pl (E.C.); dlange693@gmail.com (D.L.)

10 Department of Pathology, Martin Luther University Halle-Wittenberg, 06108 Halle (Saale), Germany; steffen.hauptmann@patho-ao.de

11 III Department of Radiotherapy and Chemotherapy, Maria Sklodowska-Curie Institute—Oncology Center, Gliwice Branch, Wybrzeze Armii Krajowej 15, 44-101 Gliwice, Poland; Michal.Jarzab@io.gliwice.pl

12 Division of Endocrinology, Departments of Medicine, Pathology, Biochemistry & Molecular Biology, and Oncology, and Arnie Charbonneau Cancer Institute, Cumming School of Medicine, University of Calgary, Calgary, Alberta T2N 4N1, Canada; ralf.paschke@ucalgary.ca

* Correspondence: Barbara.Jarzab@io.gliwice.pl

† These authors contributed equally to this work.

Academic Editor: Daniela Gabriele Grimm

Abstract: Distinguishing between follicular thyroid cancer (FTC) and follicular thyroid adenoma (FTA) constitutes a long-standing diagnostic problem resulting in equivocal histopathological diagnoses. There is therefore a need for additional molecular markers. To identify molecular differences between FTC and FTA, we analyzed the gene expression microarray data of 52 follicular neoplasms. We also performed a meta-analysis involving 14 studies employing high throughput methods (365 follicular neoplasms analyzed). Based on these two analyses, we selected 18 genes differentially expressed between FTA and FTC. We validated them by quantitative real-time polymerase chain reaction (qRT-PCR) in an independent set of 71 follicular neoplasms from formaldehyde-fixed paraffin embedded (FFPE) tissue material. We confirmed differential expression for 7 genes (*CPQ, PLVAP, TFF3, ACVRL1, ZFYVE21, FAM189A2*, and *CLEC3B*). Finally, we created a classifier that distinguished between FTC and FTA with an accuracy of 78%, sensitivity of 76%, and specificity of 80%, based on the expression of 4 genes (*CPQ, PLVAP, TFF3, ACVRL1*). In our study, we have demonstrated that meta-analysis is a valuable method for selecting possible molecular markers. Based on our results, we conclude that there might exist a plausible limit of gene classifier accuracy of approximately 80%, when follicular tumors are discriminated based on formalin-fixed postoperative material.

Keywords: follicular thyroid adenoma; follicular thyroid cancer; gene expression; microarray; meta-analysis

---

1. Introduction

Follicular neoplasms are the most controversial area in the thyroid pathology. According to World Health Organization (WHO) follicular adenoma is a benign, encapsulated tumor of the thyroid showing follicular cell differentiation [1]. This tumor demonstrates no evidence of capsular or vascular invasion. Follicular carcinoma is a malignant tumor showing evidence of follicular cell differentiation. The distinction between follicular adenoma and carcinoma is based on the presence of capsular and/or vascular invasion. Capsular invasion is defined by tumor penetration through the entire thickness of the capsule [1]. The invading tumor nests should present a connection with main tumor mass. The interpretation of capsular invasion may be sometimes problematic. According to the literature data and our experience there is a group of patients with only partial capsular invasion but presenting metastases of follicular carcinoma [2]. Yamashina analyzed entire circumference of tumor capsules of follicular neoplasms and observed that tumors with only capsular invasion in initial sections also presented vascular invasion on additional slices adjacent to tumor capsule [3]. Therefore it would be advisable to evaluate gene expression of follicular adenomas and follicular carcinomas.

Between 2000 and 2014, numerous studies have investigated the gene expression (mRNA) profile that would differentiate follicular thyroid adenoma (FTA) from follicular thyroid cancer (FTC) to improve the diagnostic process and to find features of follicular thyroid tumours important for malignant potential (Table S1) [4–17]. However, reproducibility of results obtained between mentioned publications was rather low. This could be a consequence of slight molecular differences between FTC and FTA [18,19] or the insufficient sample size used in these studies. Genetic alterations, such as *RAS* gene family somatic mutations or *PAX8/PPARG* translocations, although very promising in initial studies, were not found to be specific for follicular carcinoma, as these genetic alterations occurred in both FTCs and FTAs with similar frequencies [20–22]. These doubts stimulated us to carry on a meta-analysis.

In our study, we also raised the problem of oncocytic tumors. WHO involves oncocytic thyroid carcinoma (OTC) to FTC and respectively oncocytic adenoma to FTA. Oncocytic tumors (Hurthle cell tumors) are believed to have a different gene expression profile [23,24]. Ganly et al. demonstrated on the basis of mutational, transcriptional, and copy number profiles that Hurthle cell carcinoma was a unique thyroid cancer distinct from papillary thyroid cancer (PTC) and FTC [24].

In the present study we decided to base on FTC definition, proposed by the WHO. Nevertheless, we tried to check whether an inclusion of oncocytic follicular carcinoma does not influence on molecular markers selection. OTC is composed predominantly of oncocytic cells. These tumors are associated with a higher frequency of extrathyroidal extension, local recurrence, nodal metastases in more than 30% of cases and occasionally distant lung and bone metastases [1]. Compared with conventional follicular carcinomas, oncocytic follicular carcinomas are more aggressive [1]. Therefore, it may be reasonable to involve oncocytic feature in our analysis.

Most recent thyroid studies have focused on identifying molecular markers supporting pre-operative FNAB examination to exclude malignancy [25,26]. In 2010, Chudova et al. published a study focused on determining the general preoperative distinction between benign and malignant thyroid nodules, which appeared promising and resulted in the establishment of the Afirma classifier [25]. Our approach, used in the present study, is different.

In our study, we utilised two different approaches to select new gene-expression markers for differentiating between FTC and FTA tumours. We performed a two-step analysis: first a statistical testing of a large gene expression microarray dataset of FTC and FTA previously generated in our laboratory [18,27], and next, a meta-analysis of all available datasets, to select the most robustly represented markers [4–17] (Figure 1). Such approach allowed us to select independent genes coming from own dataset and from a meta-analysis. Meta-analysis by combining the results of various studies enabled us to draw common conclusions. The results of both analyses were further validated by quantitative real-time polymerase chain reaction (qRT-PCR) using an independent dataset of follicular tumours.

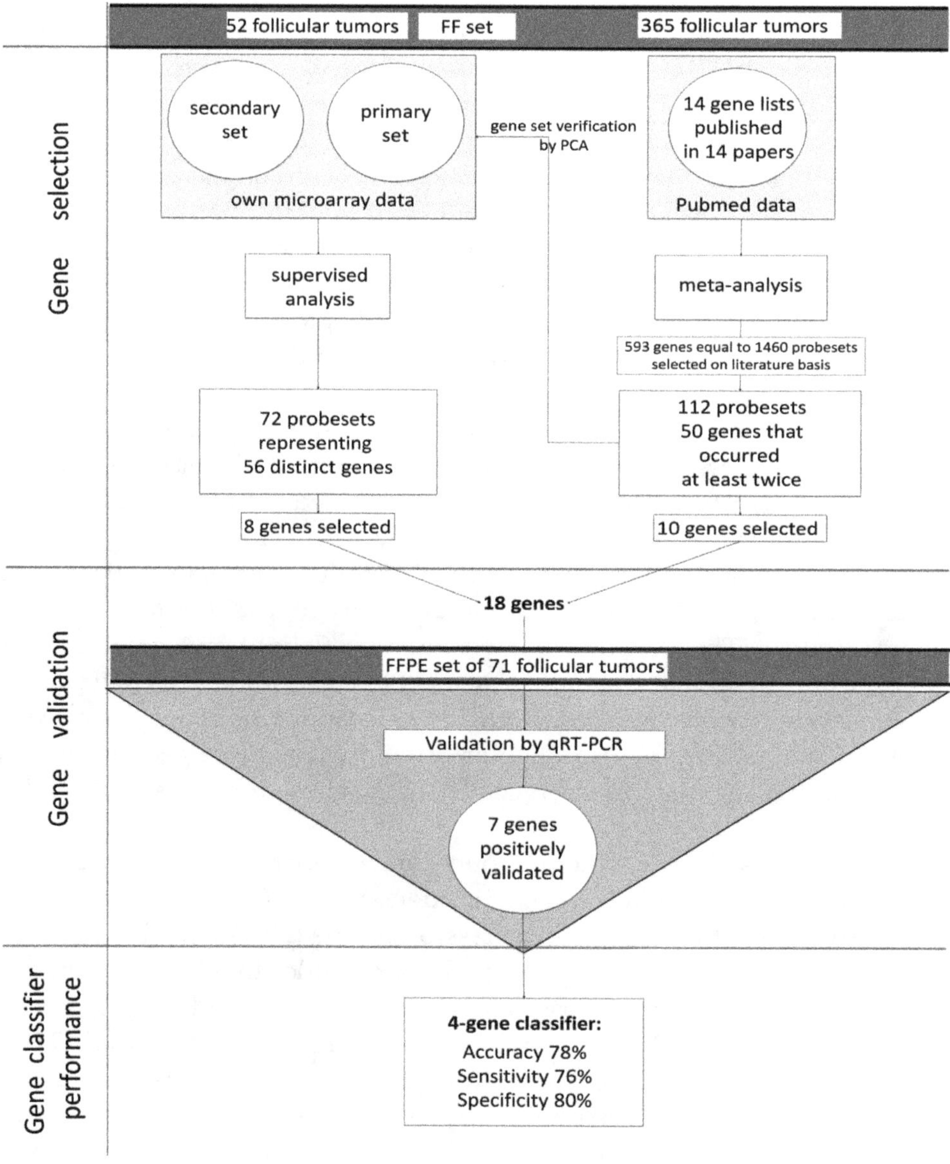

Figure 1. Presentation of a study scheme.

2. Results

2.1. Supervised Analysis of Gene Expression Microarrays

Fresh-frozen (FF) material from 52 tumors (27 FTC, 25 FTA) was used for our gene expression microarray experiment and divided into primary and secondary sets. The primary one was considered as highly reliable dataset and contained all samples that were independently and concordantly diagnosed by two thyroid pathology experts. The secondary set contained samples that were diagnosed by only one expert, equivocal samples diagnosed by two experts and a one sample that was discordantly diagnosed according to malignancy.

To select potential molecular markers useful in the distinction between FTA and FTC, we considered genes that were differentially expressed in the primary and secondary microarray datasets. We compared the lists of genes obtained in the analysis of the primary and the secondary sets and selected only those that were significant in both sets. Our secondary microarray set contained borderline and ambiguous cases, and we established genes as valuable and characteristic when they were also differentially expressed in this set.

There were 72 differentially expressed probe sets (representing 56 distinct genes) and 6 non-annotated probe sets. Eight genes were selected (*ACVRL1, CLEC3B, DIP2B, GABARAPL2, ZFYVE21, LIMK2, ZMYND11,* and *MAFB*) for validation by qRT-PCR (Table 1). Those genes were characterised by low false discovery rate (FDR) value, high fold-change, and from our point of view, they could be biologically interesting. Another selection criterion was that these genes were not previously validated as markers differentiating FTCs from FTAs.

As it has been shown that the oncocytic FTC is a unique thyroid cancer distinct from non-oncocytic FTC [24] we decided to perform an additional analysis. We excluded oncocytic samples from microarray dataset (just for the sake of this particular analysis) and evaluated the significance of eight selected genes in the dataset comprising of non-oncocytic samples only to investigate the differences between FTC and FTA (7 FTC and 11 FTA). All these genes showed significant differential expression between FTC and FTA in this dataset (Table 1).

Table 1. Differentially expressed genes selected based on analysis of our own microarray dataset.

No.	Gene Symbol	Gene Name	Affy ID	Primary Dataset				Primary Dataset—Evaluation of Non-Oncocytic Samples Only
				FDR Corrected p-Value	Mean Expression in FTC	Mean Expression in FTA	Fold-Change	FDR Corrected p-Value
1	*ACVRL1*	activin A receptor type II-like 1	226950_at	0.07	5.52	7.02	0.35	0.12
2	*CLEC3B*	C-type lectin domain family 3, member B	205200_at	0.08	7.54	9.52	0.25	0.13
3	*GABARAPL2*	GABA(A) receptor-associated protein-like 2	209046_s_at	0.08	11.05	11.84	0.58	0.15
4	*ZFYVE21*	zinc finger, FYVE domain containing 21	219929_s_at	0.07	7.39	8.67	0.41	0.04
5	*LIMK2*	LIM domain kinase 2	217475_s_at	0.07	4.32	5.84	0.35	0.12
6	*ZMYND11*	zinc finger, MYND domain containing 11	1554159_a_at	0.10	6.60	8.05	0.37	0.15
7	*DIP2B*	DIP2 disco-interacting protein 2 homolog B (Drosophila)	224872_at	0.11	8.23	7.40	1.78	0.16
8	*MAFB*	v-maf musculoaponeurotic fibrosarcoma oncogene homolog B (avian)	222670_s_at	0.08	8.23	9.78	0.34	0.13

The genes were selected for validation from the genes differentially expressed both in primary and secondary microarray set. Values represented in the table are from analysis of the primary microarray data set.

2.2. Meta-Analysis

We included 14 papers in which the difference in gene expression between FTC and FTA was assessed by a high throughput method (expression microarrays, serial analysis of gene expression (SAGE), high-throughput differential screening by serial analysis of gene expression (HDSS), adapter-tagged competitive polymerase chain reaction (ATAC-PCR)) (Table S1). The papers were published during the years 2000–2014 and in total 365 samples (201 FTA and 164 FTC) were analyzed.

All reported genes differentiating FTC and FTA were extracted from these publications. We identified 600 genes reported in at least one publication, while 57 genes were reported in more than one publication. Fifty out of those 57 genes were reported with concordant direction of change (Table 2). Seven genes (*CA4, EGR2, FAM189A2, KCNAB1, CPQ, SLC26A4, TFF3*) were reported in 3 publications. Two of these genes (*CA4*, and *KCNAB1*) were already evaluated by qRT-PCR as described in our previous study [27].

Among the genes selected based on the meta-analysis, ten genes were chosen for qRT-PCR validation. We chose five down-regulated genes that occurred in three papers (*EGR2, FAM189A2, SLC26A4, TFF3, CPQ*), four up-regulated genes that occurred in two papers (*CKS2, GDF15, ASNS, DDIT3*), and one down-regulated gene that occurred in two papers and simultaneously showed significant differences in expression in our primary microarray dataset (*PLVAP*).

Table 2. The results of a meta-analysis of 14 papers, in which differences in gene expression profile between follicular thyroid cancers (FTC) and follicular thyroid adenomas (FTA) were assessed by a high throughput method. Ten genes (highlighted in bold) were selected for our qRT-PCR validation.

No.	Entrez Gene ID	Symbol	Name	Number of Papers	References	Gene Regulation
1	762	*CA4*	carbonic anhydrase IV	3	[5,9,16]	down
2	**1959**	***EGR2***	**early growth response 2**	**3**	**[5,14,16]**	**down**
3	**9413**	***FAM189A2***	**family with sequence similarity 189, member A2**	**3**	**[5,9,12]**	**down**
4	7881	*KCNAB1*	potassium voltage-gated channel, shaker-related subfamily, beta member 1	3	[6,9,16] Confirmed by us [27]	down
5	**10404**	***CPQ***	**carboxypeptidase Q**	**3**	**[9,11,14]**	**down**
6	**5172**	***SLC26A4***	**solute carrier family 26 (anion exchanger), member 4**	**3**	**[6,14,16]**	**down**
7	**7033**	***TFF3***	**trefoil factor 3 (intestinal)**	**3**	**[5,6,10]**	**down**
8	185	*AGTR1*	angiotensin II receptor, type 1	2	[13,16]	down
9	822	*CAPG*	capping protein (actin filament), gelsolin-like	2	[14,17]	down
10	1306	*COL15A1*	collagen, type XV, alpha 1	2	[5,13]	down
11	1363	*CPE*	carboxypeptidase E	2	[9,17]	down
12	3491	*CYR61*	cysteine-rich, angiogenic inducer, 61	2	[8,16]	down
13	1733	*DIO1*	deiodinase, iodothyronine, type I	2	[6,12]	down
14	11072	*DUSP14*	dual specificity phosphatase 14	2	[5,16]	down
15	129080	*EMID1*	EMI domain containing 1	2	[5,7]	down
16	953	*ENTPD1*	ectonucleoside triphosphate diphosphohydrolase 1	2	[9,14]	down
17	8857	*FCGBP*	Fc fragment of IgG binding protein	2	[5,17]	down
18	2354	*FOSB*	FBJ murine osteosarcoma viral oncogene homolog B	2	[16,17]	down
19	2697	*GJA1*	gap junction protein, alpha 1, 43 kDa	2	[5,11]	down
20	55830	*GLT8D1*	glycosyltransferase 8 domain containing 1	2	[5,11]	down
21	221395	*GPR116*	G protein-coupled receptor 116	2	[5,9]	down
22	3043	*HBB*	hemoglobin, beta	2	[12,15]	down

Table 2. *Cont.*

No.	Entrez Gene ID	Symbol	Name	Number of Papers	References	Gene Regulation
23	3309	*HSPA5*	heat shock 70 kDa protein 5 (glucose-regulated protein, 78 kDa)	2	[9,17]	down
24	3400	*ID4*	inhibitor of DNA binding 4, dominant negative helix-loop-helix protein	2	[5,8]	down
25	3590	*IL11RA*	interleukin 11 receptor, alpha	2	[5,11]	down
26	9452	*ITM2A*	integral membrane protein 2A	2	[9,16]	down
27	3708	*ITPR1*	inositol 1,4,5-trisphosphate receptor, type 1	2	[5,11]	down
28	3725	*JUN*	jun proto-oncogene	2	[5,16]	down
29	3912	*LAMB1*	laminin, beta 1	2	[5,11]	down
30	744	*MPPED2*	metallophosphoesterase domain containing 2	2	[16,17]	down
31	22795	*NID2*	nidogen 2 (osteonidogen)	2	[5,7]	down
32	3164	*NR4A1*	nuclear receptor subfamily 4, group A, member 1	2	[12,16]	down
33	22925	*PLA2R1*	phospholipase A2 receptor 1, 180 kDa	2	[12,16]	down
34	**83483**	***PLVAP***	**plasmalemma vesicle associated protein**	**2**	**[9,13]**	**down**
35	5583	*PRKCH*	protein kinase C, eta	2	[9,14]	down
36	23180	*RFTN1*	raftlin, lipid raft linker 1	2	[5,9]	down
37	8490	*RGS5*	regulator of G-protein signaling 5	2	[9,13]	down
38	6414	*SEPP1*	selenoprotein P, plasma, 1	2	[5,14]	down
39	7038	*TG*	Thyroglobulin	2	[10,17]	down
40	4982	*TNFRSF11B*	tumor necrosis factor receptor superfamily, member 11b	2	[5,11]	down
41	7173	*TPO*	thyroid peroxidase	2	[10,17]	down
42	**440**	***ASNS***	**asparagine synthetase (glutamine-hydrolyzing)**	**2**	**[5,9]**	**up**
43	771	*CA12*	carbonic anhydrase XII	2	[5,12]	up
44	**1164**	***CKS2***	**CDC28 protein kinase regulatory subunit 2**	**2**	**[16,17]**	**up**
45	**1649**	***DDIT3***	**DNA-damage-inducible transcript 3**	**2**	**[5,7]**	**up**
46	2358	*FPR2*	formyl peptide receptor 2	2	[5,11]	up
47	**9518**	***GDF15***	**growth differentiation factor 15**	**2**	**[9,17]**	**up**
48	2896	*GRN*	Granulin	2	[4,8]	up
49	3486	*IGFBP3*	insulin-like growth factor binding protein 3	2	[5,10]	up
50	23089	*PEG10*	paternally expressed 10	2	[5,11]	up

Table 2 shows the Entrez ID, gene symbol, gene name, number of papers in which a particular gene occurs, references to the papers, regulation direction (up–up-regulated in FTC; down–down-regulated in FTC).

2.3. Principal Component Analysis

We selected 593 genes that occurred at least once in the meta-analysis (excluding seven genes with discordant direction of change). We identified HG-U133 PLUS 2 Affymetrix microarray probe sets for these genes. There were 1460 such probe sets (for some genes there was more than one probe set). Next, we performed PCA of our own microarray samples (combined primary and secondary dataset) based on these 1460 probe sets (Figure 2, upper plot). Similarly, we selected 50 genes that occurred at least twice in investigated papers (excluding the genes with discordant direction of change). We identified HG-U133 PLUS 2 Affymetrix microarray probe sets for these genes. There were 112 such probe sets. We performed PCA based on these 112 probe sets (Figure 2, lower plot). Although gene selection was independent of the microarray dataset, we achieved good discrimination of benign and malignant tumors in both analyses. However, the discrimination was not perfect, because a few FTA samples clustered with the FTC group, and a few FTC samples clustered with the FTA group.

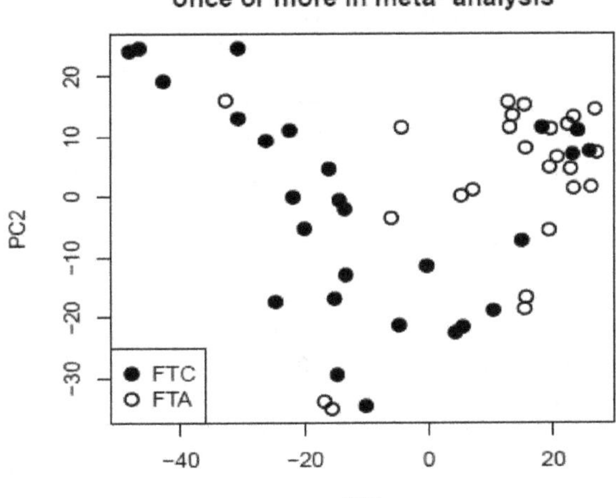

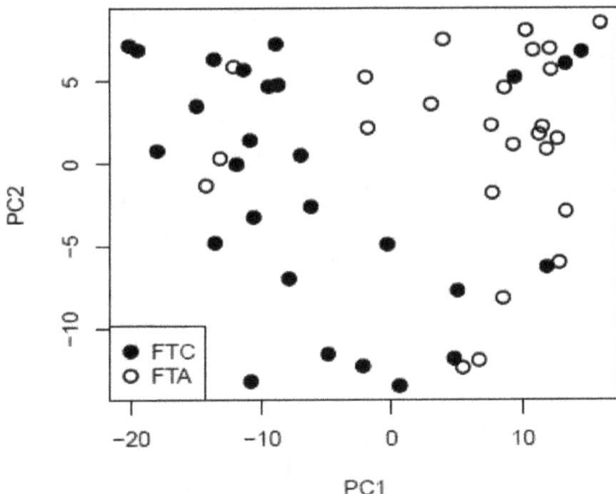

Figure 2. Principal component analysis (PCA) results. PCA plots of samples from our own microarray dataset, based on genes selected in the meta-analysis that occurred in at least one paper (**upper** plot) or at least two papers (**lower** plot).

2.4. *qRT-PCR Validation*

qRT-PCR was used to validate 18 genes selected based on the analysis of our own microarray dataset and the meta-analysis (Table 3). *GABARAPL2, DDIT3,* and *SLC26A4* amplification was not possible in the FFPE samples (probably due to low endogenous expression), and therefore, it was excluded from validation.

Log-transformed expression levels of the remaining 15 genes were analysed using the Student's *t*-test (Table 3). Two FTC samples were extreme outliers (the expression was higher than third quartile (Q3) + 6 × interquartile range (IQR)) in two distinct genes. These samples were excluded from further analysis. Differential expression of *CPQ, PLVAP, TFF3, ACVRL1, ZFYVE21, FAM189A2,* and *CLEC3B* was confirmed by qRT-PCR contrary to the expression of *ZMYND11, LIMK2, DIP2B, MAFB, CKS2, ASNS, EGR2,* and *GDF15*. All confirmed genes were downregulated in FTC and the direction of change agreed between qRT-PCR data and microarray/meta-analysis data. Boxplots of qRT-PCR results for significantly differentially expressed genes are shown on Figure 3. Based on our results, the following genes that most significantly differentiated between FTC/FTA were selected by a meta-analysis: *CPQ (PGCP), PLVAP,* and *TFF3*.

Table 3. Comparison of gene expression between FTC (29 samples) and FTA (40 samples) in qRT-PCR dataset (*t*-test and two-way ANOVA calculated *p*-values corrected for multiple tests by FDR method). FDR corrected *p*-values below 0.05 are highlighted in bold.

No.	Gene	Gene Selection	*t*-Test—FDR Corrected *p*-Value	Fold Change (FTC/FTA)	Two-Way ANOVA—FDR Corrected *p*-Value
1	*ACVRL1*	Microarrays	**0.0017**	0.58	**0.0036**
2	*ZFYVE21*	Microarrays	**0.0024**	0.69	**0.0036**
3	*CLEC3B*	Microarrays	**0.027**	0.75	**0.045**
4	*ZMYND11*	Microarrays	0.068	0.81	0.17
5	*LIMK2*	Microarrays	0.093	0.79	0.17
6	*DIP2B*	Microarrays	0.23	0.86	**0.04**
7	*MAFB*	Microarrays	0.44	0.89	0.56
8	*GABARAPL2*	Microarrays	Amplification not possible in FFPE samples		
9	*CPQ*	Meta-analysis	**0.000001**	0.49	**0.0004**
10	*PLVAP*	Meta-analysis	**0.00001**	0.51	**0.0001**
11	*TFF3*	Meta-analysis	**0.0004**	0.48	**0.0036**
12	*FAM189A2*	Meta-analysis	**0.0094**	0.68	**0.016**
13	*GDF15*	Meta-analysis	0.058	1.49	0.99
14	*CKS2*	Meta-analysis	0.69	1.07	0.94
15	*ASNS*	Meta-analysis	0.90	1.02	0.17
16	*EGR2*	Meta-analysis	0.90	0.97	0.89
17	*DDIT3*	Meta-analysis	Amplification not possible in FFPE samples		
18	*SLC26A4*	Meta-analysis	Amplification not possible in FFPE samples		

Two-way analysis of variance (ANOVA) was used in order to adjust for oncocytic feature and the results are shown in column "two-way ANOVA—FDR corrected *p*-value".

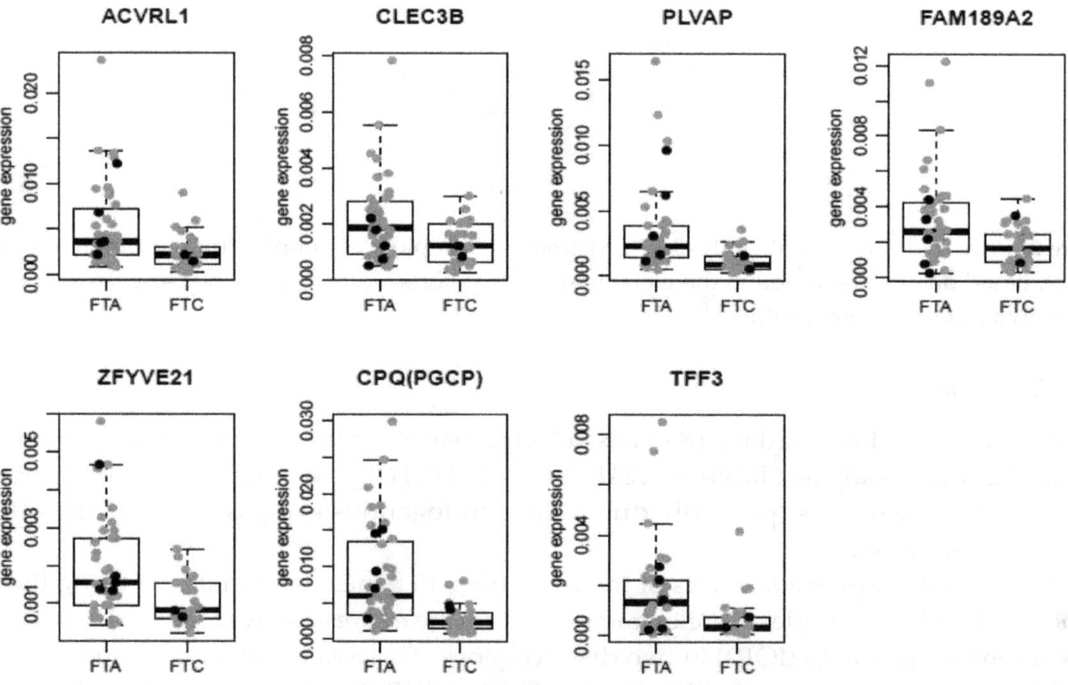

Figure 3. The normalized relative expression levels of positively validated genes in the FFPE dataset of 69 samples. Boxplots superimposed with scatterplots are shown. The line inside each box corresponds to median. Upper and lower edges of boxes correspond to first (Q1) and third (Q3) quartiles, respectively. The whiskers extend to smallest and largest observations within 1.5 times interquartile range (IQR) from the box. Black dots represent *RAS* mutation carrying samples, and grey dots represent samples without *RAS* mutation.

A multivariate ANOVA with two factors: malignancy and oncocytic feature was also performed, in order to evaluate the differential expression between FTC and FTA after adjusting for the effect of oncocytic feature. All seven genes significant in the Student's *t*-test were also significant in this ANOVA analysis (Table 3). Adding the additional variables such as age, gender, and *RAS* mutation status did not substantially modify the ANOVA results.

2.5. Classifier Performance

To evaluate the usefulness of selected genes as diagnostic support, we performed sample classification based on the FFPE dataset. Log-transformation of the gene expression values and a leave-one-out cross-validation of the classifier was performed. In each iteration, the samples were divided into two independent sets: all but one sample were used for significance threshold tuning, gene selection, and classifier training, and the remaining sample was used for testing. Diagonal linear discrimination analysis (DLDA) algorithm was used for the classifier training. After performing all iterations, the classifier's performance was calculated. The accuracy, sensitivity, and specificity were 78% (95% confidence interval (CI): 67–87%), 76% (95% CI: 56–90%), and 80% (95% CI: 64–91%), respectively. The classifier involved 4 genes with p-value below 0.0005 in the Student's *t*-test, namely *CPQ, PLVAP, TFF3*, and *ACVRL1*. When accuracy was calculated for non-oncocytic (45 tumors) and oncocytic (24 tumors) tumors separately it was 84% (95% CI: 71–94%) and 67% (95% CI: 45–84%), respectively.

A receiver operating characteristic (ROC) curve was also created in order to assess the diagnostic efficacy of the classifier (Figure 4). The area under the ROC curve (AUC) equals 0.84.

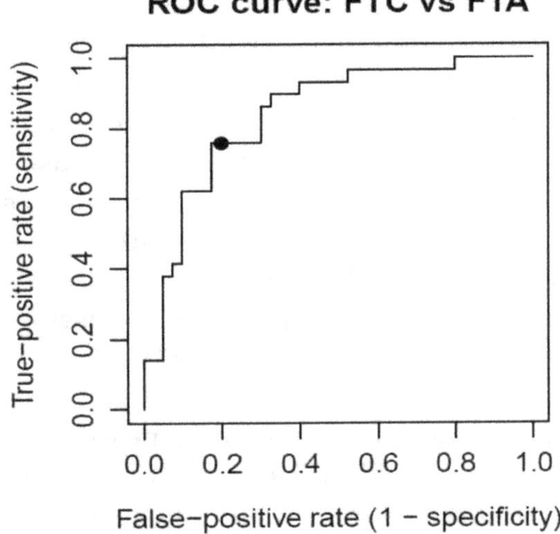

Figure 4. Receiver operating characteristc (ROC) curve analysis for the predictive power of 4-gene classifier, estimated in qRT-PCR dataset. Using a cutoff probability of 50% (marked with black dot), we obtained sensitivity of 76% and specificity of 80%. The calculated area under the ROC curve was 0.84.

2.6. RAS Mutation Status

The presence of the *RAS* gene mutation was investigated in freshly frozen FTC (27) and FTA (25) samples. We identified 3 FTC samples with *NRAS* codon 61 mutation and 1 with *KRAS* codon 61 mutation (in total 14.8%). In the FTA samples, we identified only 1 mutated sample with *NRAS* codon 61 mutation (4%) (Table S2). The frequencies of *RAS* gene mutations in malignant and benign samples did not differ significantly.

The status of the *RAS* gene mutations was also analysed in FFPE specimens, however due to limitations related to sample quantity, 14 samples were not fully profiled (only *NRAS* codon 61 was analysed and mutations were excluded in these samples). Among 31 FFPE FTC specimens, 2 samples with *NRAS* codon 61 mutation and 1 with *HRAS* codon 12 mutation were identified (9.7%) (Table S3). More *RAS* mutations were observed in FFPE FTA samples; however, the difference was not significant. Among 40 FFPE FTA specimens, 3 samples with *NRAS* codon 61 mutations, 1 sample with *KRAS* codon 12 mutation, and 1 with *HRAS* codon 61 mutation were detected (12.5%) (Table S3). However, analysis of the total prevalence of *RAS* mutations in FTC and FTA, regardless of the method used for tissue preservation (FF vs. FFPE) demonstrated that there was no difference in the occurrence of *RAS* mutations between FTC and FTA: 12% and 9.3%, respectively.

3. Discussion

The differential diagnostics between FTC and FTA is still challenging, particularly because in a molecular sense these lesions lie on a continuum, with similar molecular profiles. Perhaps the 2nd or 3rd molecular hit converts adenoma to carcinoma [28,29] In our study, we performed a meta-analysis of markers differentiating FTC and FTA to summarise the results obtained over a 15-year period (2000–2014), and described in multiple papers.

We obtained a list of 50 genes that were significantly differentially expressed in concordant direction in two or more such papers. We selected 10 genes from the meta-analysis and positively validated 4 of them: *CPQ*, *PLVAP*, *TFF3*, and *FAM189A2*. While, of the 8 genes selected from our own gene expression microarray dataset, three genes: *ACVRL1*, *CLEC3B*, and *ZFYVE21*, were positively validated by qRT-PCR (Table 3).

Due to small number of *RAS* mutation positive samples, we were not able to establish its influence on the expression of genes selected for qRT-PCR validation (Figures S1 and S2).

Finally, we created a gene classifier involving 4 genes (*CPQ*, *PLVAP*, *TFF3*, and *ACVRL1*) that showed a diagnostic accuracy of 78%, sensitivity of 76%, and specificity of 80% for FTC and FTA differentiation. We are aware that our set of genes requires confirmation by an independent clinical study, similar to the study by Alexander et al. [30], which positively verified the clinical utility of a gene classifier proposed by Chudova et al. [25]. However, there are some important differences between Afirma and our approach. While FNAB-based Afirma classifier, used in a preoperative diagnostics, considered all malignant tumors and differed them from benign ones, our classifier was devoted to discriminate only between FTC and FTA on the basis of postoperative material. We did not consider the results of fine-needle aspiration biopsy (FNAB) at any time during our analyses as well as did not link our results to Bethesda Categories. We hope that our classifier may help in such cases where there is a dilemma in a post-operative diagnostics in FTA/FTC distinction. Thus, our work may not be considered as a kind of confirmation of Afirma results.

Transcription profiling, as a method for selection of gene expression markers for distinguishing follicular neoplasms, has been used for over a decade. However, to date, no powerful molecular markers have been established. Similarly, our previous study did not fully accomplish this goal [27]. Therefore, we decided to strengthen our results by performing a meta-analysis of all available studies related to FTC and FTA differentiation [4–17].

The analysis of genes differentially expressed in FTC and FTA in our own gene expression microarray dataset revealed 56 genes. Genes with higher fold-changes and lower p values (Table S4), as well as those related to other types of cancer or tumour aggressiveness were preferably selected for qRT-PCR validation. One of these genes, *ACVRL1* correlated with tumour progression in patients with head and neck cancers [31]; whereas two other genes: *ZFYVE21*, and *CLEC3B* were related to cancer invasiveness [32,33]. Four genes, obtained from the meta-analysis were subsequently positively validated *CPQ*, *PLVAP*, *TFF3*, and *FAM189A2*.

Based on the meta-analysis, it appears that building an accurate classifier to differentiate FTCs from FTAs is impossible, even using a large dataset of follicular tumour samples (365 samples in meta-analysis). Therefore, we propose that an accuracy of approximately 80% constitutes a plausible limit of FTC vs. FTA gene classifier performance when analysis is performed in postoperative formalin-fixed material [27].

Possible reason for not satisfying classifier accuracy is that follicular tumours are too similar at the gene expression level. Another hypothetic possible reason is that FTC and FTA classes may have been incorrectly assigned prior to the microarray experiments. Histopathological diagnosis in case of follicular tumours can be influenced by intraobserver variability [34]. To circumvent this, we involved two experienced pathologists in the diagnostic process. It is possible however, that some minimally invasive FTCs did not yet demonstrate any signs of vascular or capsular invasion, and were classified as FTAs.

We assume that FTCs and FTAs are biologically different as they have different clinical outcomes. We are however aware that to date, histopathology constitutes the best option in differential diagnostics of follicular tumours, but a gene-classifier may provide more information in difficult cases. Therefore, we may try to use classifiers ([27], current classifier) to distinguish FTCs and FTAs without histopathological data (unsupervised approach). The results from an unsupervised approach can then be compared to histopathological evaluation, with focus on cases showing discrepancy between the histopathology and classifier data.

It is possible, that we may not reach better classifier performance because of over-simplification that we applied in our analysis. We assumed that both FTC and FTA tumours are internally homogenous, but quite often they are not and they may encompass different zones of differentiation or different histopathological features [35]. Neither FTA nor FTC are completely similar. Considering diversity of biology we cannot expect to cover the whole biological variance with four genes only.

In the present study we decided not to include PTC, because it demonstrated its own, characteristic gene expression profile [36] and the differences between PTC and FTC were quite intense [37]. We believe that an inclusion of PTC to malignant samples may lead to inadequate conclusions, whereas without PTC the study is much cleaner.

The low number of *RAS*-positive samples did not allow an evaluation of the impact of the *RAS* gene mutations on the gene expression profile. However, *RAS*-positive samples did not cluster differentially compared to samples not carrying mutations based on the unsupervised PCA analysis, which suggests small biological differences (Figures S3 and S4). Interestingly, the prevalence of *RAS* somatic mutations in our own FF FTC dataset was 12%, while other studies show the prevalence of *RAS* mutation at 60% [38]. This result might be attributable to the population in the studied region of Europe. Unfortunately, we were not able to analyse of the *RAS* gene mutations in 14 samples due to limited amount of material.

We are aware that our findings would be more robust if we use a single technique of tissue preservation but to a much larger group and the using of FFPE material for validation had a possible limitation. Performing gene expression on FFPE is very challenging and these results could even improve when using cryopreserved samples instead. However, malignant follicular thyroid neoplasms are rare and we had to base on the available material. We did our best to collect as large group as it was possible. We used qRT-PCR with multiple reference genes, to assure that we can amplify sequences coming from reference genes in our tumor samples. Moreover, the results obtained in our study were validated on the independent set of samples. We believe that our results constitute an essential input into the better understanding of molecular biology of follicular thyroid neoplasms.

4. Materials and Methods

4.1. Material

4.1.1. Clinical Materials for Gene Expression Microarray Analysis Using Our Own Thyroid Samples

Fresh-frozen (FF) material from 52 tumours (27 FTC, 25 FTA) was used for our gene expression microarray experiments. The samples and microarray data have been already used in our previous studies and are reused in the current study [18,27]. Surgical procedures on patients were conducted in Polish and German centres, at the MSC Institute—Oncology Center in Gliwice, University of Leipzig, University of Halle, and Mainz University Hospital. Samples collected in hospitals were subsequently sent to our laboratory in Gliwice for microarray molecular profiling. Because the diagnosis of follicular thyroid tumours may be often equivocal [34], we attempted to obtain the evaluation of each pathology slide by two pathologists. However, we had access to the paraffin slides in only a part of the samples. If the slide was available for us, the sample was evaluated by two highly qualified pathologists. If the slide was not available for us, we based on the primary diagnosis, stated in the origin hospital by a single pathologist.

Next, the clinical material was divided into primary and secondary sets of tumors, depending on the concordance in histopathological diagnosis. The primary set contained all samples that were independently and concordantly diagnosed by two thyroid pathology experts (Dariusz Lange, Gliwice, and Steffen Hauptmann, Halle (Saale)). The secondary set contained samples that were diagnosed by only one expert, equivocal samples diagnosed by two experts and one sample that was discordantly diagnosed according to malignancy. A description of the material and the frequency of oncocytic tumors is shown in Table 4 (detailed description is given in Table S2).

The study was approved by the local ethics committees (Bioethics Committee of MSC Institute—Oncology Center in Gliwice; approvals: DK/ZMN-493-1-10/09, 20 November 2002 and KB/492-17/11, 9 February 2011), and informed consent was obtained from all patients.

Table 4. Fresh-frozen material used for microarray analysis.

Set	Histotype	Samples	% of Men	Median Age (Years)	Frequency of Oncocytic Tumours	Concordance of Pathologic Diagnosis by 2 Experts
Primary set	FTC	13	38.5%	66	46.2%	100%
	FTA	13	0%	42	15.4%	100%
Secondary set	FTC	14	21.4%	69	7.1%	28.6%
	FTA	12	25%	49.5	0%	75%
Total	-	52	21.2%	60.5	17.3%	75%

4.1.2. Clinical Materials for Validation Studies

FFPE tissue was used for validation in qRT-PCR experiments. The FFPE tissue consisted of 40 FTA and 31 FTC samples from patients treated in the MSC Institute—Oncology Center in Gliwice. The same set of samples was used in our previous study [27]. Diagnosis of FFPE tumours was based on the independent diagnoses of two pathologists. Material description and frequency of oncocytic tumours is presented in Table 5 (detailed description is given in Table S3 in Supplementary Material). Fresh frozen and FFPE datasets were independent datasets; there was no patient overlap between them.

Table 5. FFPE material used for qRT-PCR validation.

Histopathological Diagnosis	Number of Samples	% of Men	Median Age (Years)	Frequency of Oncocytic Tumours
FTC	31	32.3%	59	61.3%
FTA	40	12.5%	45	15%
Total	71	21.1%	52	35.2%

4.1.3. *RAS* Mutation Screening

All 123 samples of thyroid follicular tumour used for gene expression microarray (52 samples) and qRT-PCR experiments (71 samples) were screened for *RAS* mutations using the Sanger sequencing method with the ABI 3130*xl* Genetic Analyzer. Three *RAS* genes (*H-*, *K-*, *N-RAS*) sequences in commonly mutated codon sites (12, 13, and 61) were analysed. Different primer sets (different size of amplicon) for FF and FFPE samples were used due to sample degradation in FFPE samples (details Table S5).

4.2. *Gene Expression Microarray-Based Analysis of Our Own Follicular Tumours*

4.2.1. Gene Expression Microarray Experiment

FF materials from 52 follicular thyroid tumours (27 FTC, 25 FTA) were used for microarray analysis. RNA was isolated using the RNeasy Mini kit (Qiagen, Hilden, Germany). The RNA quality was assessed with capillary electrophoresis (Bioanalyzer 2100) and all the samples had the RNA integrity number (RIN) higher than 7. An Affymetrix (Santa Clara, CA, USA) HG-U133 PLUS 2 array experiment was performed as described previously [27].

4.2.2. Gene Expression Microarray Data Preprocessing

All microarray data analyses were performed in an R/Bioconductor environment. The microarray data preprocessing was performed in the same way as described in our previous study [27]. The quality of the microarray data was analysed using arrayMvout 1.12.0 library [39]. The raw data were preprocessed using the GCRMA method [40]. The microarray data discussed in this publication have been deposited in NCBI's Gene Expression Omnibus [41], and are accessible through GEO Series accession number GSE82208 (available online: https://www.ncbi.nlm.nih.gov/geo/query/acc.cgi?acc=GSE82208).

4.2.3. Supervised Analysis of Our Own Gene Expression Microarray Data

The selection of differentially expressed genes was performed independently on the primary and secondary microarray dataset (FF material) (Figure 1), in order to take into account the different levels of diagnosis certainty in the two sets. The following criteria were used for the primary dataset: normalized mean expression of the gene above 4.5, the variance of the gene above the 20th percentile, p-value in Student's t-test below 0.001, a fold-change above 1.5 in either direction of the change. The following, less strict criterion was used for the secondary dataset: p-value in Student's t-test < 0.05.

For genes selected for validation study, an additional analysis was performed in order to assess the significance of difference between FTC and FTA in microarray dataset comprised of non-oncocytic samples only. The genes were considered significant if the unadjusted p-value in the Student's t-test was below 0.005 in primary dataset and below 0.05 in secondary dataset.

In order to adjust p-values for multiple comparisons, false discovery rate (FDR) was estimated by Benjamini and Hochberg procedure [42].

4.3. *Meta-Analysis of All Published Papers*

The meta-analysis included all 14 papers in which the difference in gene expression between FTC and FTA was assessed by a high throughput method (gene expression microarrays, SAGE, HDSS, ATAC-PCR); which were published during 2000–2014; and found in PubMed, Google Scholar, or by screening the reference lists of selected papers (Table S1). The following criteria were used for the selection of papers: "follicular thyroid carcinoma/cancer/tumour/adenoma AND microarray/gene expression".

The lists of genes that were reported by the authors as differentially expressed between FTC and FTA, were extracted from each paper. Different types of gene identifiers were used in each study, such as gene symbols, gene names, GenBank accession numbers, cDNA sequences, Affymetrix identifiers, RefSeq accession numbers, and UniGene accession numbers. All gene identifiers were converted to EntrezID, the lists of genes were compared, and common genes were extracted. Finally, ten genes among the most frequently occurring ones were chosen for qRT-PCR validation (Figure 1).

Principal Component Analysis of Microarrays Based on the Meta-Analysis Identified Genes

To visually inspect whether the genes selected in the meta-analysis are able to separate FTC and FTA on an independent dataset, Principal Component Analysis (PCA) was conducted. We performed

PCA on our own microarray samples, based on genes that occurred at least once in the meta-analysis (Figure 2 upper plot). We also performed PCA on these samples, based on the genes that occurred at least twice in the meta-analysis (Figure 2 lower plot).

4.4. qRT-PCR Validation

4.4.1. qRT-PCR Experiment

FFPE materials from 71 follicular thyroid tumours (31 FTC, 40 FTA) were used for qRT-PCR analysis. RNA was isolated using the FFPE RNeasy Mini Kit (Qiagen) from 5 slices of paraffin blocks selected by a histopathologist. qRT-PCR was carried out for 18 genes (gene names given in Table S6, primer probe design given in Table S7). This experiment was performed with the 7900HT Fast Real-Time PCR (Life Technologies, Carlsbad, CA, USA) using Universal Probe Library fluorescent probes (Roche, Basel, Switzerland) and the 5′-nuclease assay, starting from 200 ng of total RNA. All experiments were performed twice. Results were normalised using the Pfaffl method [43] and the GeNorm application [44] with a combination of 3 normalisation genes: *EIF3A* (eukaryotic translation initiation factor 3, subunit A), *EIF5* (eukaryotic translation initiation factor 5), and *HADHA* (hydroxyacyl-CoA dehydrogenase/3-ketoacyl-CoA thiolase/enoyl-CoA hydratase (trifunctional protein), alpha subunit). Obtained normalised relative expression levels were further log-transformed (Figure S5).

Differences between FTC and FTA were tested using the Student's *t*-test. In addition, two-way analysis of variance (ANOVA) was used in order to adjust for oncocytic feature. False Discovery Rate (FDR) correction was applied and genes with FDR < 0.05 in both analyses were considered as significant.

4.4.2. Classifier Performance

The classifier was created and validated on the FFPE dataset using CMA package [45] in R/Bioconductor environment. The DLDA was used as a classification algorithm. Student's *t*-test was used for gene selection with significance level threshold tuned over a grid of significance levels. The performance of the classifier was evaluated by the doubly nested leave-one-out cross validation (LOOCV) approach in order to obtain an unbiased estimate of the accuracy [46]. The outer loop was used for estimating the classifier accuracy, and the inner loop was used for optimising the significance level threshold.

The ROC curve was also created to assess the diagnostic efficacy of the classifier (Figure 4). In the outer leave-one-out loop, for each sample, the probability that the sample belongs to the FTC class was calculated, based on DLDA algorithm. Varying the threshold for the probability, the ROC curve was plotted.

5. Conclusions

In our study, we have demonstrated that meta-analysis is a valuable method for selecting possible molecular markers. We showed that genes *CPQ, PLVAP, TFF3, ACVRL1, ZFYVE21, FAM189A2*, and *CLEC3B* are differentially expressed between FTC and FTA. Furthermore, we propose a 4-gene classifier, which discriminates between benign and malignant follicular neoplasms with the accuracy of 78%. Based on our results, we conclude that there might exist a plausible limit of gene classifier accuracy of approximately 80%, when follicular tumors are discriminated based on postoperative formalin-fixed material.

Acknowledgments: This study was supported by the Ministry of Science and Higher Education (grant number N N401 072637); Polish National Science Center (decision number DEC-2011/03/N/NZ5/05623); Foundation for Polish Science (MPD Program "Molecular Genomics, Transcriptomics and Bioinformatics in Cancer"); Postgraduate School of Molecular Medicine (fellowships to Bartosz Wojtas and Tomasz Stokowy); National Center for Research and Development project under the program "Prevention practices and treatment of civilisation diseases" STRATEGMED (MILESTONE, project number STRATEGMED2/267398/4/NCBR/2015);

and DFG (grant number ES162/4-1 to Markus Eszlinger). The costs to publish in open access were covered by Maria Sklodowska-Curie Institute—Oncology Center, Gliwice Branch.

Author Contributions: Bartosz Wojtas, Aleksandra Pfeifer, Jolanta Krajewska, Michal Jarzab and Ewa Chmielik contributed to the writing of the manuscript; Michal Jarzab, Markus Eszlinger, Ralf Paschke, and Barbara Jarzab designed and coordinated the study; Agnieszka Czarniecka and Thomas Musholt collected the tissue material; Aleksandra Kukulska and Jolanta Krajewska analyzed patient data; Ewa Stobiecka, Ewa Chmielik, Steffen Hauptmann, and Dariusz Lange performed the histopathological examination of the samples; Bartosz Wojtas, Malgorzata Oczko-Wojciechowska, Dagmara Rusinek, Tomasz Tyszkiewicz and Monika Halczok performed the experiments described in this study; Aleksandra Pfeifer, Tomasz Stokowy and Michal Swierniak performed the bioinformatics analysis.

Abbreviations

ANOVA	Analysis of variance
ATAC-PCR	Adapter-tagged competitive polymerase chain reaction
AUC	Area under the ROC curve
DLDA	Diagonal linear discrimination analysis
FDR	False discovery rate
FF	Fresh-frozen
FFPE	Formaldehyde-fixed paraffin embedded
FNAB	Fine needle aspiration biopsy
FTA	Follicular thyroid adenoma
FTC	Follicular thyroid cancer
HDSS	High-throughput differential screening by serial analysis of gene expression
IQR	Interquartile range
LOOCV	Leave-one-out cross validation
OTC	Oncocytic thyroid carcinoma
PCA	Principal component analysis
Q1	First quartile
Q3	Third quartile
qRT-PCR	Quantitative real-time polymerase chain reaction
RIN	RNA integrity number
ROC	Receiver operating characteristc
SAGE	Serial analysis of gene expression
WHO	World Health Organization

References

1. DeLellis, R.; Lloyd, R.; Heitz, P.; Eng, C. *WHO Pathology and Genetics. Tumours of Endocrine Organs*; IARC Press: Lyon, France, 2004.
2. LiVolsi, V.A.; Baloch, Z.W. Follicular-patterned tumors of the thyroid: The battle of benign vs. malignant vs. so-called uncertain. *Endocr. Pathol.* **2011**, *22*, 184–189. [CrossRef] [PubMed]
3. Yamashina, M. Follicular neoplasms of the thyroid. Total circumferential evaluation of the fibrous capsule. *Am. J. Surg. Pathol.* **1992**, *16*, 392–400. [CrossRef] [PubMed]
4. Takano, T.; Hasegawa, Y.; Matsuzuka, F.; Miyauchi, A.; Yoshida, H.; Higashiyama, T.; Kuma, K.; Amino, N. Gene expression profiles in thyroid carcinomas. *Br. J. Cancer* **2000**, *83*, 1495–1502. [CrossRef] [PubMed]
5. Barden, C.B.; Shister, K.W.; Zhu, B.; Guiter, G.; Greenblatt, D.Y.; Zeiger, M.A.; Fahey, T.J., III. Classification of follicular thyroid tumors by molecular signature: Results of gene profiling. *Clin. Cancer Res.* **2003**, *9*, 1792–1800. [PubMed]
6. Takano, T.; Miyauchi, A.; Yoshida, H.; Kuma, K.; Amino, N. High-throughput differential screening of mRNAs by serial analysis of gene expression: Decreased expression of trefoil factor 3 mRNA in thyroid follicular carcinomas. *Br. J. Cancer* **2004**, *90*, 1600–1605. [CrossRef] [PubMed]
7. Cerutti, J.M.; Delcelo, R.; Amadei, M.J.; Nakabashi, C.; Maciel, R.M.; Peterson, B.; Shoemaker, J.; Riggins, G.J. A preoperative diagnostic test that distinguishes benign from malignant thyroid carcinoma based on gene expression. *J. Clin. Investig.* **2004**, *113*, 1234–1242. [CrossRef] [PubMed]

8. Chevillard, S.; Ugolin, N.; Vielh, P.; Ory, K.; Levalois, C.; Elliott, D.; Clayman, G.L.; El-Naggar, A.K. Gene expression profiling of differentiated thyroid neoplasms: Diagnostic and clinical implications. *Clin. Cancer Res.* **2004**, *10*, 6586–6597. [CrossRef] [PubMed]
9. Weber, F.; Shen, L.; Aldred, M.A.; Morrison, C.D.; Frilling, A.; Saji, M.; Schuppert, F.; Broelsch, C.E.; Ringel, M.D.; Eng, C. Genetic classification of benign and malignant thyroid follicular neoplasia based on a three-gene combination. *J. Clin. Endocrinol. Metab.* **2005**, *90*, 2512–2521. [CrossRef] [PubMed]
10. Taniguchi, K.; Takano, T.; Miyauchi, A.; Koizumi, K.; Ito, Y.; Takamura, Y.; Ishitobi, M.; Miyoshi, Y.; Taguchi, T.; Tamaki, Y.; et al. Differentiation of follicular thyroid adenoma from carcinoma by means of gene expression profiling with adapter-tagged competitive polymerase chain reaction. *Oncology* **2005**, *69*, 428–435. [CrossRef] [PubMed]
11. Lubitz, C.C.; Gallagher, L.A.; Finley, D.J.; Zhu, B.; Fahey, T.J., III. Molecular analysis of minimally invasive follicular carcinomas by gene profiling. *Surgery* **2005**, *138*, 1042–1048. [CrossRef] [PubMed]
12. Fryknas, M.; Wickenberg-Bolin, U.; Goransson, H.; Gustafsson, M.G.; Foukakis, T.; Lee, J.J.; Landegren, U.; Hoog, A.; Larsson, C.; Grimelius, L.; et al. Molecular markers for discrimination of benign and malignant follicular thyroid tumors. *Tumour Biol.* **2006**, *27*, 211–220. [PubMed]
13. Stolf, B.S.; Santos, M.M.; Simao, D.F.; Diaz, J.P.; Cristo, E.B.; Hirata, R., Jr.; Curado, M.P.; Neves, E.J.; Kowalski, L.P.; Carvalho, A.F. Class distinction between follicular adenomas and follicular carcinomas of the thyroid gland on the basis of their signature expression. *Cancer* **2006**, *106*, 1891–1900. [CrossRef] [PubMed]
14. Zhao, J.; Leonard, C.; Gemsenjager, E.; Heitz, P.U.; Moch, H.; Odermatt, B. Differentiation of human follicular thyroid adenomas from carcinomas by gene expression profiling. *Oncol. Rep.* **2008**, *19*, 329–337. [CrossRef]
15. Hinsch, N.; Frank, M.; Doring, C.; Vorlander, C.; Hansmann, M.L. QPRT: A potential marker for follicular thyroid carcinoma including minimal invasive variant; a gene expression, RNA and immunohistochemical study. *BMC Cancer* **2009**, *9*, 93. [CrossRef] [PubMed]
16. Borup, R.; Rossing, M.; Henao, R.; Yamamoto, Y.; Krogdahl, A.; Godballe, C.; Winther, O.; Kiss, K.; Christensen, L.; Hogdall, E.; et al. Molecular signatures of thyroid follicular neoplasia. *Endocr. Relat. Cancer* **2010**, *17*, 691–708. [CrossRef] [PubMed]
17. Williams, M.D.; Zhang, L.; Elliott, D.D.; Perrier, N.D.; Lozano, G.; Clayman, G.L.; El-Naggar, A.K. Differential gene expression profiling of aggressive and nonaggressive follicular carcinomas. *Hum. Pathol.* **2011**, *42*, 1213–1220. [CrossRef] [PubMed]
18. Wojtas, B.; Pfeifer, A.; Jarzab, M.; Czarniecka, A.; Krajewska, J.; Swierniak, M.; Stokowy, T.; Rusinek, D.; Kowal, M.; Zebracka-Gala, J.; et al. Unsupervised analysis of follicular thyroid tumours transcriptome by oligonucleotide microarray gene expression profiling. *Endokrynol. Pol.* **2013**, *64*, 328–334. [CrossRef]
19. Swierniak, M.; Pfeifer, A.; Stokowy, T.; Rusinek, D.; Chekan, M.; Lange, D.; Krajewska, J.; Oczko-Wojciechowska, M.; Czarniecka, A.; Jarzab, M.; et al. Somatic mutation profiling of follicular thyroid cancer by next generation sequencing. *Mol. Cell. Endocrinol.* **2016**, *433*, 130–137. [CrossRef] [PubMed]
20. Cheung, L.; Messina, M.; Gill, A.; Clarkson, A.; Learoyd, D.; Delbridge, L.; Wentworth, J.; Philips, J.; Clifton-Bligh, R.; Robinson, B.G. Detection of the PAX8-PPARγ fusion oncogene in both follicular thyroid carcinomas and adenomas. *J. Clin. Endocrinol. Metab.* **2003**, *88*, 354–357. [CrossRef] [PubMed]
21. Sahin, M.; Allard, B.L.; Yates, M.; Powell, J.G.; Wang, X.L.; Hay, I.D.; Zhao, Y.; Goellner, J.R.; Sebo, T.J.; Grebe, S.K.; et al. PPARγ staining as a surrogate for PAX8/PPARγ fusion oncogene expression in follicular neoplasms: Clinicopathological correlation and histopathological diagnostic value. *J. Clin. Endocrinol. Metab.* **2005**, *90*, 463–468. [CrossRef] [PubMed]
22. Kloos, R.T.; Reynolds, J.D.; Walsh, P.S.; Wilde, J.I.; Tom, E.Y.; Pagan, M.; Barbacioru, C.; Chudova, D.I.; Wong, M.; Friedman, L.; et al. Does addition of BRAF V600E mutation testing modify sensitivity or specificity of the Afirma Gene Expression Classifier in cytologically indeterminate thyroid nodules? *J. Clin. Endocrinol. Metab.* **2013**, *98*, 761–768. [CrossRef] [PubMed]
23. Baris, O.; Savagner, F.; Nasser, V.; Loriod, B.; Granjeaud, S.; Guyetant, S.; Franc, B.; Rodien, P.; Rohmer, V.; Bertucci, F.; et al. Transcriptional profiling reveals coordinated up-regulation of oxidative metabolism genes in thyroid oncocytic tumors. *J. Clin. Endocrinol. Metab.* **2004**, *89*, 994–1005. [CrossRef] [PubMed]
24. Ganly, I.; Ricarte Filho, J.; Eng, S.; Ghossein, R.; Morris, L.G.; Liang, Y.; Socci, N.; Kannan, K.; Mo, Q.; Fagin, J.A.; et al. Genomic dissection of Hurthle cell carcinoma reveals a unique class of thyroid malignancy. *J. Clin. Endocrinol. Metab.* **2013**, *98*, 962–972. [CrossRef] [PubMed]

25. Chudova, D.; Wilde, J.I.; Wang, E.T.; Wang, H.; Rabbee, N.; Egidio, C.M.; Reynolds, J.; Tom, E.; Pagan, M.; Rigl, C.T.; et al. Molecular classification of thyroid nodules using high-dimensionality genomic data. *J. Clin. Endocrinol. Metab.* **2010**, *95*, 5296–5304. [CrossRef] [PubMed]
26. Keutgen, X.M.; Filicori, F.; Crowley, M.J.; Wang, Y.; Scognamiglio, T.; Hoda, R.; Buitrago, D.; Cooper, D.; Zeiger, M.A.; Zarnegar, R.; et al. A panel of four miRNAs accurately differentiates malignant from benign indeterminate thyroid lesions on fine needle aspiration. *Clin. Cancer Res.* **2012**, *18*, 2032–2038. [CrossRef] [PubMed]
27. Pfeifer, A.; Wojtas, B.; Oczko-Wojciechowska, M.; Kukulska, A.; Czarniecka, A.; Eszlinger, M.; Musholt, T.; Stokowy, T.; Swierniak, M.; Stobiecka, E.; et al. Molecular differential diagnosis of follicular thyroid carcinoma and adenoma based on gene expression profiling by using formalin-fixed paraffin-embedded tissues. *BMC Med. Genom.* **2013**, *6*, 38. [CrossRef] [PubMed]
28. Evans, H.L.; Vassilopoulou-Sellin, R. Follicular and Hurthle cell carcinomas of the thyroid: A comparative study. *Am. J. Surg. Pathol.* **1998**, *22*, 1512–1520. [CrossRef] [PubMed]
29. Parameswaran, R.; Brooks, S.; Sadler, G.P. Molecular pathogenesis of follicular cell derived thyroid cancers. *Int. J. Surg.* **2010**, *8*, 186–193. [CrossRef] [PubMed]
30. Alexander, E.K.; Kennedy, G.C.; Baloch, Z.W.; Cibas, E.S.; Chudova, D.; Diggans, J.; Friedman, L.; Kloos, R.T.; LiVolsi, V.A.; Mandel, S.J.; et al. Preoperative diagnosis of benign thyroid nodules with indeterminate cytology. *N. Engl. J. Med.* **2012**, *367*, 705–715. [CrossRef] [PubMed]
31. Chien, C.Y.; Chuang, H.C.; Chen, C.H.; Fang, F.M.; Chen, W.C.; Huang, C.C.; Huang, H.Y. The expression of activin receptor-like kinase 1 among patients with head and neck cancer. *Otolaryngol. Head Neck Surg.* **2013**, *148*, 965–973. [CrossRef] [PubMed]
32. Arvanitis, D.L.; Kamper, E.F.; Kopeikina, L.; Stavridou, A.; Sgantzos, M.N.; Kallioras, V.; Athanasiou, E.; Kanavaros, P. Tetranectin expression in gastric adenocarcinomas. *Histol. Histopathol.* **2002**, *17*, 471–475. [PubMed]
33. Hoshino, D.; Nagano, M.; Saitoh, A.; Koshikawa, N.; Suzuki, T.; Seiki, M. The phosphoinositide-binding protein ZF21 regulates ECM degradation by invadopodia. *PLoS ONE* **2013**, *8*, e50825. [CrossRef] [PubMed]
34. Franc, B.; de la Salmonière, P.; Lange, F.; Hoang, C.; Louvel, A.; de Roquancourt, A.; Vilde, F.; Hejblum, G.; Chevret, S.; Chastang, C. Interobserver and intraobserver reproducibility in the histopathology of follicular thyroid carcinoma. *Hum. Pathol.* **2003**, *34*, 1092–1100. [CrossRef]
35. Da, S.L.; James, D.; Simpson, P.T.; Walker, D.; Vargas, A.C.; Jayanthan, J.; Lakhani, S.R.; McNicol, A.M. Tumor heterogeneity in a follicular carcinoma of thyroid: A study by comparative genomic hybridization. *Endocr. Pathol.* **2011**, *22*, 103–107.
36. Jarzab, B.; Wiench, M.; Fujarewicz, K.; Simek, K.; Jarzab, M.; Oczko-Wojciechowska, M.; Wloch, J.; Czarniecka, A.; Chmielik, E.; Lange, D.; et al. Gene expression profile of papillary thyroid cancer: Sources of variability and diagnostic implications. *Cancer Res.* **2005**, *65*, 1587–1597. [CrossRef] [PubMed]
37. Aldred, M.A.; Huang, Y.; Liyanarachchi, S.; Pellegata, N.S.; Gimm, O.; Jhiang, S.; Davuluri, R.V.; de la Chapelle, A.; Eng, C. Papillary and follicular thyroid carcinomas show distinctly different microarray expression profiles and can be distinguished by a minimum of five genes. *J. Clin. Oncol.* **2004**, *22*, 3531–3539. [CrossRef] [PubMed]
38. Rodrigues, H.G.; de Pontes, A.A.; Adan, L.F. Use of molecular markers in samples obtained from preoperative aspiration of thyroid. *Endocr. J.* **2012**, *59*, 417–424. [CrossRef] [PubMed]
39. Asare, A.L.; Gao, Z.; Carey, V.J.; Wang, R.; Seyfert-Margolis, V. Power enhancement via multivariate outlier testing with gene expression arrays. *Bioinformatics* **2009**, *25*, 48–53. [CrossRef] [PubMed]
40. Wu, Z.J.; Irizarry, R.A.; Gentleman, R.; Martinez-Murillo, F.; Spencer, F. A model-based background adjustment for oligonucleotide expression arrays. *J. Am. Stat. Assoc.* **2004**, *99*, 909–917. [CrossRef]
41. Edgar, R.; Domrachev, M.; Lash, A.E. Gene expression omnibus: NCBI gene expression and hybridization array data repository. *Nucleic Acids Res.* **2002**, *30*, 207–210. [CrossRef] [PubMed]
42. Benjamini, Y.; Hochberg, Y. Controlling the false discovery rate: A practical and powerful approach to multiple testing. *J. R. Stat. Soc. Ser. B* **1995**, *57*, 289–300.
43. Pfaffl, M.W. A new mathematical model for relative quantification in real-time RT-PCR. *Nucleic Acids Res.* **2001**, *29*, e45. [CrossRef] [PubMed]

44. Vandesompele, J.; de Preter, K.; Pattyn, F.; Poppe, B.; van Roy, N.; de Paepe, A.; Speleman, F. Accurate normalization of real-time quantitative RT-PCR data by geometric averaging of multiple internal control genes. *Genome Biol.* **2002**, *3*, 1–11. [CrossRef]
45. Slawski, M.; Daumer, M.; Boulesteix, A.L. CMA: A comprehensive bioconductor package for supervised classification with high dimensional data. *BMC Bioinform.* **2008**, *9*, 439. [CrossRef] [PubMed]
46. Varma, S.; Simon, R. Bias in error estimation when using cross-validation for model selection. *BMC Bioinform.* **2006**, *7*. [CrossRef] [PubMed]

12

A Comprehensive Characterization of Mitochondrial Genome in Papillary Thyroid Cancer

Xingyun Su [1], Weibin Wang [1], Guodong Ruan [2], Min Liang [3], Jing Zheng [3], Ye Chen [3], Huiling Wu [4], Thomas J. Fahey III [5], Minxin Guan [3,*] and Lisong Teng [1,*]

1 Department of Surgical Oncology, First Affiliated Hospital, School of Medicine, Zhejiang University, Hangzhou 310003, China; luckymaimai@sina.cn (X.S.); wbwang@zju.edu.cn (W.W.)
2 Department of Oncology, the Second Hospital of Shaoxing, Shaoxing 312000, China; recardos@163.com
3 Institute of Genetics, School of Medicine, Zhejiang University, Hangzhou 310058, China; liangmin85685@126.com (M.L.); candy88zj@zju.edu.cn (J.Z.); yechency@zju.edu.cn (Y.C.)
4 Department of Plastic Surgery, First Affiliated Hospital, School of Medicine, Zhejiang University, Hangzhou 310003, China; whl1616@126.com
5 Department of Surgery, New York Presbyterian Hospital and Weill Medical College of Cornell University, New York, NY 10021, USA; tjfahey@med.cornell.edu
* Correspondence: gminxin88@zju.edu.cn (M.G.); lsteng@zju.edu.cn (L.T.)

Academic Editor: Daniela Gabriele Grimm

Abstract: Nuclear genetic alterations have been widely investigated in papillary thyroid cancer (PTC), however, the characteristics of the mitochondrial genome remain uncertain. We sequenced the entire mitochondrial genome of 66 PTCs, 16 normal thyroid tissues and 376 blood samples of healthy individuals. There were 2508 variations (543 sites) detected in PTCs, among which 33 variations were novel. Nearly half of the PTCs (31/66) had heteroplasmic variations. Among the 31 PTCs, 28 specimens harbored a total of 52 somatic mutations distributed in 44 sites. Thirty-three variations including seven nonsense, 11 frameshift and 15 non-synonymous variations selected by bioinformatic software were regarded as pathogenic. These 33 pathogenic mutations were associated with older age ($p = 0.0176$) and advanced tumor stage ($p = 0.0218$). In addition, they tended to be novel ($p = 0.0003$), heteroplasmic ($p = 0.0343$) and somatic ($p = 0.0018$). The mtDNA copy number increased in more than two-third (46/66) of PTCs, and the average content in tumors was nearly four times higher than that in adjacent normal tissues ($p < 0.0001$). Three sub-haplogroups of N (A4, B4a and B4g) and eight single-nucleotide polymorphisms (mtSNPs) (A16164G, C16266T, G5460A, T6680C, G9123A, A14587G, T16362C, and G709A) were associated with the occurrence of PTC. Here we report a comprehensive characterization of the mitochondrial genome and demonstrate its significance in pathogenesis and progression of PTC. This can help to clarify the molecular mechanisms underlying PTC and offer potential biomarkers or therapeutic targets for future clinical practice.

Keywords: mitochondrial DNA; mitochondrial DNA copy number; haplogroup; papillary thyroid cancer

1. Introduction

Mitochondria are semiautonomous organelles responsible for bioenergetic metabolism, aging and apoptosis [1]. Otto Warburg et al. first proposed that metabolic reprogramming occurred in cancer cells evidenced by highly activated glycolysis even in the presence of oxygen, and this was regarded as a hallmark of cancer [2]. This phenomenon, called the Warburg effect, is probably triggered by insufficient energy supply that is the result of the combination of mitochondrial defects and activated cellular proliferation [3]. Mitochondrial DNA (mtDNA) is a 16,569 bp, double-stranded circular molecule encoding 13 polypeptides, two ribosomal RNAs (rRNAs) and 22 transfer RNAs (tRNAs) for mitochondrial respiration. The replicative origins and transcriptive promoters are located in the non-coding displacement-loop (D-loop) region [4]. Accumulated evidence demonstrates that mtDNA variations and copy number alterations are common in human cancers [5]. Pathogenic mtDNA mutations can severely affect mitochondrial respiration and overproduce endogenous reactive oxygen species (ROS) contributing to anti-apoptosis, proliferation and metastasis of cancer [5,6].

Papillary thyroid cancer (PTC) is the main histological type of thyroid cancer. Most PTC patients have favorable outcome with the 30-year survival rate more than 90% after routine treatment by thyroidectomy with or without radioiodine ablation [7]. However, a small group of PTC patients suffer from tumor persistence, recurrence and even death [8]. Investigating the underlying molecular mechanisms of PTC can provide promising biomarkers and therapeutic targets for early diagnosis and treatment, thus improving prognosis and survival quality of patients, especially those with aggressive tumor behavior and adverse outcomes. The malignant transformation and progression of thyroid cancer is driven by accumulated genetic alterations. Among them, the $BRAF^{V600E}$ mutation is the most significant factor for PTC and is associated with high-risk clinicopathological features and unfavorable outcomes [9]. Therefore, many researchers suggest that $BRAF^{V600E}$ mutation can be a valuable biomarker and therapeutic target for diagnosis, risk stratification, prognostic prediction and treatment of PTC [9].

In spite of the research achievements in understanding the nuclear genome, the role of mitochondrial genome in pathogenesis and progression of thyroid cancer is still incompletely characterized. Previous researchers have found abnormally excessive mitochondria and prevalent mtDNA alterations in thyroid cancer. However, the majority of these studies are restricted to the oncocytic subtype of thyroid cancer and only focused on mutation hotspots of mtDNA [10–12]. Here we comprehensively characterized the mitochondrial genome in papillary thyroid cancer by sequencing the entire mtDNA of 66 PTCs, 16 normal thyroid tissues and 376 blood samples of healthy individuals. The mtDNA variation distribution, haplogroup and copy number were further analyzed.

2. Results

2.1. Distribution of mtDNA Variations

A total of 2508 variations in 543 sites were identified in 66 PTC cases, and the D-loop region was the hotspot of mtDNA (Figure S1a,b). Single-base substitution was the main component of mtDNA variations, in addition to 76 deletions (13 sites) and 112 insertions (10 sites) (Figure S1c). About 30.9% (101/327) transitions and 60% (12/20) transversions were non-synonymous, suggesting that transversion was more likely to alter the encoded amino-acid and affect the structure or function of protein (Figure S1d). In the protein-coding region, most variations were synonymous (Figure S1e). ATPase6 (14/22, 63.6%), Cytb (20/45, 44.4%), ND4L (3/8, 37.5%) and ND5 (25/71, 35.2%) genes harbored relatively high ratio of nonsynonymous variation (Figure S1e,f). A total of 33 variations—including 11 non-synonymous, seven nonsense and eight frameshift variations—in 25 PTC patients were novel, and all of them were singular (Table 1). Heteroplasmy was one of the most important characteristics of mitochondrial genome, presenting in nearly half of the 66 PTCs (31/66). Among the heteroplasmic variations, 52 somatic mutations (44 sites) in 28 PTC patients and 28 germline variations (20 sites) in 16 patients were detected (Table S1).

Table 1. Novel mtDNA variations in the entire mitochondrial genome.

Position	Gene	Replacement	Amino-Acid Change or Watson-Crick Base-Pairing [a]	Conservation Index (%) [b]	Number of 66 PTC Patients (%)	Number of 376 Healthy Controls (%)	Heter/Homo [c]
RNA Region							
1629	$tRNA^{Val}$	A–T	A–U↓	24.4%	1 (1.52%)	0 (0.00%)	Homo
2274	16S rRNA	A–G		100%	1 (1.52%)	0 (0.00%)	Heter
3275–3276	$tRNA^{Leu(UUR)}$	Del CA		-	1 (1.52%)	0 (0.00%)	Heter
4272	$tRNA^{Ile}$	T–C	A–U↓	100%	1 (1.52%)	0 (0.00%)	Homo
5835	$tRNA^{Tyr}$	Ins T		-	1 (1.52%)	0 (0.00%)	Homo
5881	$tRNA^{Tyr}$	G–C	C–G↓	100%	1 (1.52%)	0 (0.00%)	Homo
10040	$tRNA^{Gly}$	C–A		43.9%	1 (1.52%)	0 (0.00%)	Homo
Protein-Coding Region							
4520–4521	ND2	Del AC	-	-	1 (1.52%)	0 (0.00%)	Homo
4875	ND2	C–T	Leu -> Leu	100%	1 (1.52%)	0 (0.00%)	Homo
4969	ND2	G–A	No: Trp -> Ter [d]	100%	1 (1.52%)	0 (0.00%)	Homo
4971	ND2	G–A	No: Gly -> Ser	100%	1 (1.52%)	0 (0.00%)	Homo
5977	COI	G–A	No: Trp -> Ter	100%	1 (1.52%)	0 (0.00%)	Heter
6238	COI	T–C	No: Leu -> Pro	100%	1 (1.52%)	0 (0.00%)	Heter
7104	COI	T–C	No: Ser -> Pro	100%	1 (1.52%)	0 (0.00%)	Heter
7750	COII	C–A	No: Ile -> Met	58.5%	1 (1.52%)	0 (0.00%)	Homo
7928	COII	G–A	No: Gly -> Ter	56.1%	1 (1.52%)	0 (0.00%)	Homo
9253	COIII	G–A	No: Trp -> Ter	100%	1 (1.52%)	0 (0.00%)	Heter
10521	ND4L	G–A	No: Gly -> Ter	100%	1 (1.52%)	0 (0.00%)	Homo
10622	ND4L	C–T	Thr -> Thr	36.6%	1 (1.52%)	0 (0.00%)	Homo
11646	ND4	Ins T	-	-	1 (1.52%)	0 (0.00%)	Homo
11673–11677	ND4	C5–C4	-	-	1 (1.52%)	0 (0.00%)	Heter
11673–11677	ND4	C5–C6	-	-	1 (1.52%)	0 (0.00%)	Homo
12794	ND5	T–A	No: Leu -> Ter	100%	1 (1.52%)	0 (0.00%)	Heter
12858	ND5	Ins T	-	-	1 (1.52%)	0 (0.00%)	Heter
12943	ND5	C–T	No: Leu -> Phe	24.4%	1 (1.52%)	0 (0.00%)	Heter
13128–13132	ND5	C5–4	-	-	1 (1.52%)	0 (0.00%)	Homo
13170	ND5	Del A	-	-	1 (1.52%)	0 (0.00%)	Homo
13621	ND5	C–T	No: Leu -> Phe	51.2%	1 (1.52%)	0 (0.00%)	Homo
13825	ND5	G–A	No: Gly -> Ter	100%	1 (1.52%)	0 (0.00%)	Homo
14310	ND6	C–A	No: Gly -> Trp	70.7%	1 (1.52%)	0 (0.00%)	Heter
14495–14502	ND6	(AAAT)2–1	-	-	1 (1.52%)	0 (0.00%)	Homo
14774	Cytb	C–A	No: Leu -> Ile	63.4%	1 (1.52%)	0 (0.00%)	Heter
15018	Cytb	T–A	No: Phe -> Tyr	100%	1 (1.52%)	0 (0.00%)	Heter

[a] Watson–Crick base-pairing: abolished (↓); [b] Conservation index denotes the conservative properties of amino-acid or nucleotides in 41 primate species; [c] Heter: Heteroplasmy; Homo: Homoplasmy; [d] Ter: Terminator.

2.2. *The mtDNA Variations in Non-Coding Region*

There were 103 substitutions and 10 frameshift alterations in D-loop region. Nearly all the insertions and deletions were located in mitochondrial microsatellite instability (mtMSI) regions, such as poly-C in np 303–315 or np 16184–16193 and poly-CA stretch in np 514–523. In the RNA region, 20, 21 and 29 variations were, respectively, identified in 12S rRNA, 16S rRNA and tRNAs. The published secondary structures of RNAs were used to localize the alterations in the stem and loop structure [13]. A total of seven variations in 12S rRNA, one alteration in 16S rRNA and 13 alterations in tRNAs changed the Waston–Crick base-pairing. According to their frequencies in control groups and conservation of the altered nucleotides, 13 variations were identified as potentially deleterious and five of them had been reported in diseases (Table S2, Figure 1).

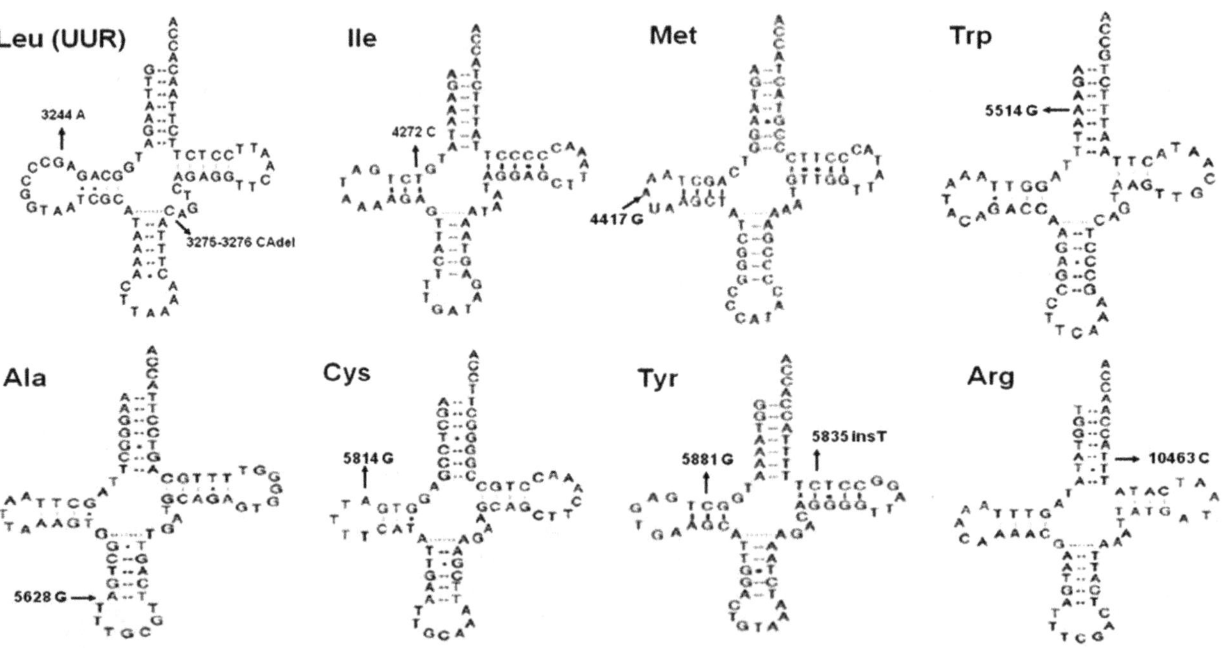

Figure 1. Potential pathogenic tRNA variations in PTC Schematic structures of eight mitochondrial tRNAs are shown. Arrows point out the position of tRNA variation.

2.3. *The mtDNA Variations in Protein-Coding Region*

A total of 234 synonymous, 113 non-synonymous, seven nonsense and 11 frameshift variations were detected in protein-coding region. All the nonsense and frameshift variations brought in advanced stop-codon (UAG, UGA) and leaded to premature termination of protein synthesis (Table 2, Figure 2). Among the 113 non-synonymous alterations, 26 variations were selected as potentially pathogenic based on their frequencies in control groups and conservation of the altered amino-acid (Table 3). These 26 selected variations were further evaluated by seven bioinformatic programs, and 15 of them were predicted as deleterious by more than half of the programs (Table 3). Therefore, these 33 mutations in 32 patients, including 15 nonsynonymous, seven nonsense and 11 frameshift mutations, were classified as pathogenic mutations. These pathogenic mtDNA mutations were associated with patients' older age ($p = 0.018$) and advanced tumor stage ($p = 0.022$), and tended to be novel ($p < 0.001$), heteroplasmic ($p = 0.034$) and somatic ($p = 0.002$) (Table S3).

Table 2. Nonsense and frameshift mutations identified in protein-coding region.

Position	Gene	Change	Reported [a]	Number of 66 PTC Patients (%)	Number of 16 Normal Thyroid Tissues (%)	Number of 376 Healthy Controls (%)	Heter/Homo [b]
Nonsense Mutation							
4969	ND2	G–A	N	1 (1.52%)	0 (0.00%)	0 (0.00%)	Homo
5977	COI	G–A	N	1 (1.52%)	0 (0.00%)	0 (0.00%)	Heter
7928	COII	G–A	N	1 (1.52%)	0 (0.00%)	0 (0.00%)	Homo
9253	COIII	G–A	N	1 (1.52%)	0 (0.00%)	0 (0.00%)	Heter
10521	ND4L	G–A	N	1 (1.52%)	0 (0.00%)	0 (0.00%)	Homo
12794	ND5	T–A	N	1 (1.52%)	0 (0.00%)	0 (0.00%)	Heter
13825	ND5	G–A	N	1 (1.52%)	0 (0.00%)	0 (0.00%)	Homo
Frameshift Mutation							
4520–4521	ND2	Del AC	N	1 (1.52%)	0 (0.00%)	0 (0.00%)	Homo
10952	ND4	Ins C	Y	1 (1.52%)	0 (0.00%)	0 (0.00%)	Homo
11032–11038	ND4	A7–6	Y	4 (6.06%)	0 (0.00%)	0 (0.00%)	Homo + Heter
11646	ND4	Ins T	N	1 (1.52%)	0 (0.00%)	0 (0.00%)	Homo
11673–11677	ND4	C5–C4	N	1 (1.52%)	0 (0.00%)	0 (0.00%)	Heter
11673–11677	ND4	C5–C6	N	1 (1.52%)	0 (0.00%)	0 (0.00%)	Homo
12418–12425	ND5	Del A	Y	1 (1.52%)	0 (0.00%)	0 (0.00%)	Heter
12858	ND5	Ins T	N	1 (1.52%)	0 (0.00%)	0 (0.00%)	Heter
13128–13132	ND5	C5–4	N	1 (1.52%)	0 (0.00%)	0 (0.00%)	Homo
13170	ND5	Del A	N	1 (1.52%)	0 (0.00%)	0 (0.00%)	Homo
14495–14502	ND6	(AAAT)2–1	N	1 (1.52%)	0 (0.00%)	0 (0.00%)	Homo

[a] According to Mitomap (http://www.mitomap.org); [b] Heter: Heteroplasmy; Homo: Homoplasmy.

Table 3. Potential pathogenic mtDNA variations identified in protein-coding region.

Position	Gene	Change	Amino-Acid Change	Conservation Index (%) [a]	Reported [b]	Number of 66 PTC Patients (%)	Number of 16 Normal Thyroid Tissues (%)	Number of 376 Healthy Controls (%)	Polyphen-2 [c]	SIFT	Mutation Assesor	Provean	SNP&GO	Align GVGD [d]	PANTHER (Pdeleterious) [e]
3392 [f]	ND1	G-A	No: Gly -> Asp	100.00%	Y	1 (1.52%)	0 (0.00%)	0 (0.00%)	Probably	Not Tolerated	High	Deleterious	Disease	C65	NA [g]
3644	ND1	T-C	No: Val -> Ala	97.60%	Y	1 (1.52%)	0 (0.00%)	2 (0.53%)	Benign	Not Tolerated	Medium	Deleterious	Neutral	C65	0.29125
3679	ND1	T-C	No: Ser -> Pro	100.00%	Y	1 (1.52%)	0 (0.00%)	0 (0.00%)	Probably	Not Tolerated	High	Deleterious	Disease	C65	0.74261
3745	ND1	G-A	No: Ala -> Thr	92.70%	Y	1 (1.52%)	0 (0.00%)	0 (0.00%)	Benign	Not Tolerated	Low	Neutral	Neutral	C55	0.21113
4971	ND2	G-A	No: Gly -> Ser	100.00%	N	1 (1.52%)	0 (0.00%)	0 (0.00%)	Probably	Not Tolerated	Medium	Deleterious	Neutral	C55	0.36251
6238	COI	T-C	No: Leu -> Pro	100.00%	N	1 (1.52%)	0 (0.00%)	0 (0.00%)	Probably	Not Tolerated	High	Deleterious	Disease	C65	0.87509
6340	COI	C-T	No: Thr -> Ile	82.90%	Y	1 (1.52%)	0 (0.00%)	0 (0.00%)	Benign	Not Tolerated	Medium	Neutral	Neutral	C65	0.21096
6681	COI	T-C	No: Tyr -> His	85.40%	Y	1 (1.52%)	0 (0.00%)	0 (0.00%)	Benign	Tolerated	Neutral	Neutral	Neutral	C65	0.32881
7104	COI	T-C	No: Ser -> Pro	100.00%	N	1 (1.52%)	0 (0.00%)	0 (0.00%)	Possibly	Not Tolerated	Neutral	Neutral	Disease	C65	0.5134
7329	COI	T-C	No: Phe ->Leu	100.00%	N	1 (1.52%)	0 (0.00%)	0 (0.00%)	Benign	Tolerated	Low	Neutral	Neutral	C15	0.16379
8156	COII	G-A	No: Val -> Met	75.61%	N	1 (1.52%)	0 (0.00%)	0 (0.00%)	Probably	Not Tolerated	Medium	Neutral	Neutral	C15	0.53442
8989	ATP6	G-A	No: Ala -> Thr	100.00%	Y	1 (1.52%)	0 (0.00%)	0 (0.00%)	Probably	Not Tolerated	Low	Deleterious	Neutral	C55	0.47286
9187	ATP6	T-C	No: Tyr -> His	100.00%	Y	1 (1.52%)	0 (0.00%)	0 (0.00%)	Probably	Not Tolerated	High	Deleterious	Disease	C65	NA
9355	COIII	A-G	No: Asn -> Ser	82.90%	Y	1 (1.52%)	0 (0.00%)	0 (0.00%)	Benign	Tolerated	Neutral	Neutral	Neutral	C45	0.14014
10573	ND4L	G-A	No: Gly -> Glu	97.60%	Y	1 (1.52%)	0 (0.00%)	0 (0.00%)	Probably	Not Tolerated	High	Deleterious	Neutral	C65	0.40946
12850	ND5	A-G	No: Ile -> Val	90.20%	Y	1 (1.52%)	0 (0.00%)	0 (0.00%)	Possibly	Tolerated	Neutral	Neutral	Neutral	C25	0.50297
13535	ND5	A-G	No: Asn -> Ser	87.80%	Y	1 (1.52%)	0 (0.00%)	0 (0.00%)	Benign	Not Tolerated	Low	Deleterious	Neutral	C45	NA
13748	ND5	A-G	No: Asn -> Ser	85.40%	Y	1 (1.52%)	0 (0.00%)	0 (0.00%)	Benign	Tolerated	Neutral	Neutral	Neutral	C45	0.5082
14310	ND6	C-A	No: Gly -> Trp	78.05%	N	1 (1.52%)	0 (0.00%)	0 (0.00%)	Probably	Not Tolerated	Medium	Deleterious	Disease	C65	0.71527
14463	ND6	T-C	No: Thr -> Ala	90.20%	Y	1 (1.52%)	0 (0.00%)	0 (0.00%)	Benign	Tolerated	Neutral	Deleterious	Neutral	C55	0.15283
15018	Cytb	T-A	No: Phe -> Tyr	100.00%	N	1 (1.52%)	0 (0.00%)	0 (0.00%)	Possibly	Not Tolerated	High	Deleterious	Disease	C15	0.68543
15045	Cytb	G-A	No: Arg -> Gln	100.00%	Y	1 (1.52%)	0 (0.00%)	0 (0.00%)	Probably	Not Tolerated	High	Deleterious	Disease	C35	0.59378
15090	Cytb	T-C	No: Ile -> Thr	85.40%	Y	1 (1.52%)	0 (0.00%)	1 (0.27%)	Possibly	Tolerated	Low	Deleterious	Neutral	C65	0.42865
15479	Cytb	T-C	No: Phe -> Leu	80.50%	Y	1 (1.52%)	0 (0.00%)	0 (0.00%)	Benign	Tolerated	Low	Deleterious	Neutral	C15	0.39962
15483	Cytb	C-T	No: Ser -> Leu	80.50%	Y	1 (1.52%)	0 (0.00%)	0 (0.00%)	Possibly	Tolerated	Low	Deleterious	Neutral	C65	0.45816

[a] Conservation index denotes the conservative properties of amino-acid or nucleotides in 41 primate species; [b] According to Mitomap (http://www.mitomap.org); [c] Polyphen-2 classified the variations as probably damaging, possibly damaging and benign according to their pathogenic potential; [d] Align GVGD classified the variations as C65, C55, C45, C35, C25, C15 and C0 according to the risk estimates, and here we regarded the C65 as pathogenic; [e] PANTHER predicted the pathogenicity of variations by values of Pdeleterious, and we regarded Pdeleterious >0.5 as deleterious; [f] The variants predicted as by more than half of the bioinformatic software packagess were classified as PTC-associated mutations which were highlighted by bold and italic; [g] NA, not available.

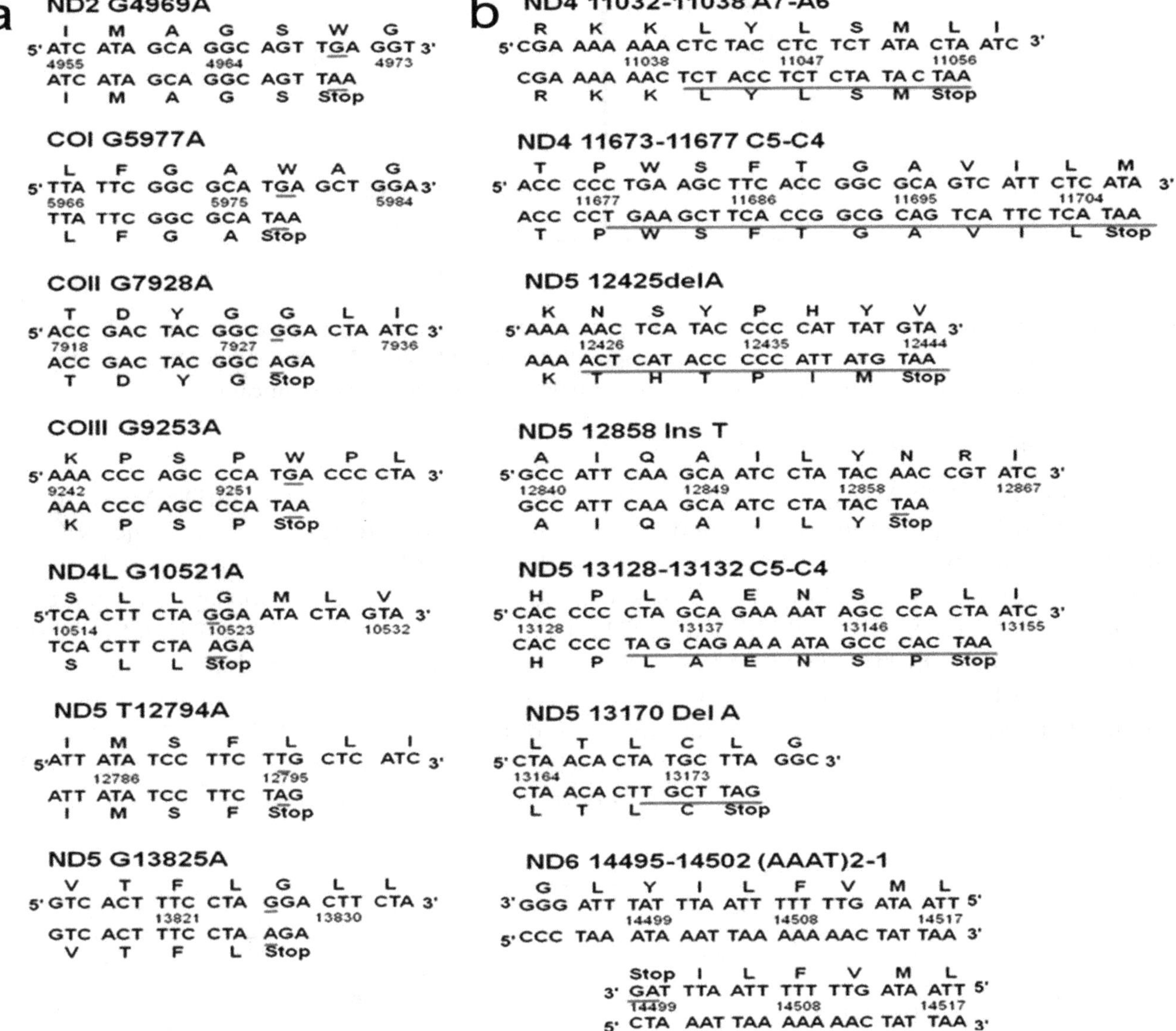

Figure 2. The nonsense and framshift mutations: (**a**) Seven nonsense mutations directly introduce stop-codon and thus create premature termination of protein synthesis immediately; and (**b**) Seven frameshift alterations bring stop-codon in the following transcription and induce truncated polypeptide.

2.4. The Alteration of mtDNA Copy Number

In comparison with corresponding normal tissues, more than two-thirds (46/66) of the PTCs had increased mtDNA copy number. The average mtDNA content in tumors was nearly four times higher than that in adjacent normal tissues ($p < 0.0001$) (Figure 3). Interestingly, mtDNA content in the tumor of patient No. 48 was more than 38 times higher than the corresponding normal tissue. However, our analysis showed that increased mtDNA content had no significant association with clinicopathological features. No obvious association was observed between mtDNA content with novel or heteroplasmic mtDNA variations, PTC-associated mutations or mtMSIs (309insC/CC and 523del/insCA).

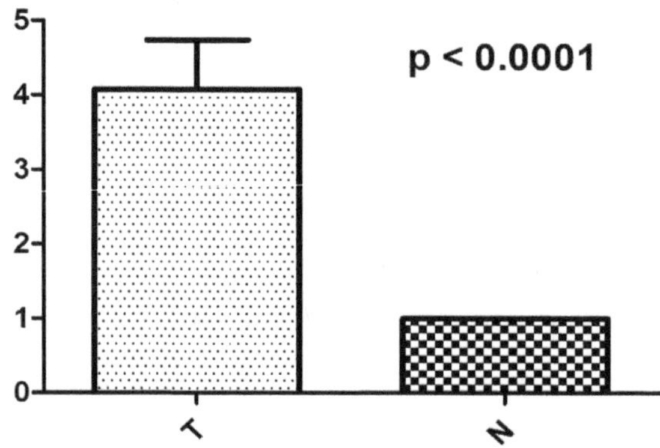

Figure 3. Copy number analysis of mtDNA in thyroid cancer: comparison of the average mtDNA copy number between PTC cases (T) and their corresponding normal tissues (N). Two-sided Mann–Whitney *U* test was used to analysis the difference, and $p < 0.05$ was considered as significant.

2.5. Analysis of Haplogroup and mtSNP

The entire mtDNA sequences of 66 PTCs were assigned to Asian mtDNA lineage and classified into 11 haplogroups distributed between macro-haplogroups M (n = 30) and N (n = 36). Sub-haplogroups were descended from macro-haplogroups M (C, D, G and Z) and N (A, B, F, N, R and Y) (Figure 4). Although no statistical significance was found in haplogroup M or N, the sub-haplogroups A4 (OR 3.903, 95% CI 1.070–14.23, p = 0.027), B4a (OR 3.903, 95% CI 1.070–14.23, p = 0.027) and B4g (OR 11.5, 95% CI 1.027–128.8, p = 0.013) descending from haplogroup N tended to be associated with the occurrence of PTC (Table S4). Frequencies of 15 mtSNPs were statistically different between PTC and healthy groups, and eight of them (A16164G, T16362C, C16266T, G5460A, T6680C, G9123A, A14587G, and G709A) may be associated with a predisposition to developing PTC according to their frequencies between PTC and normal thyroid groups (Table S5).

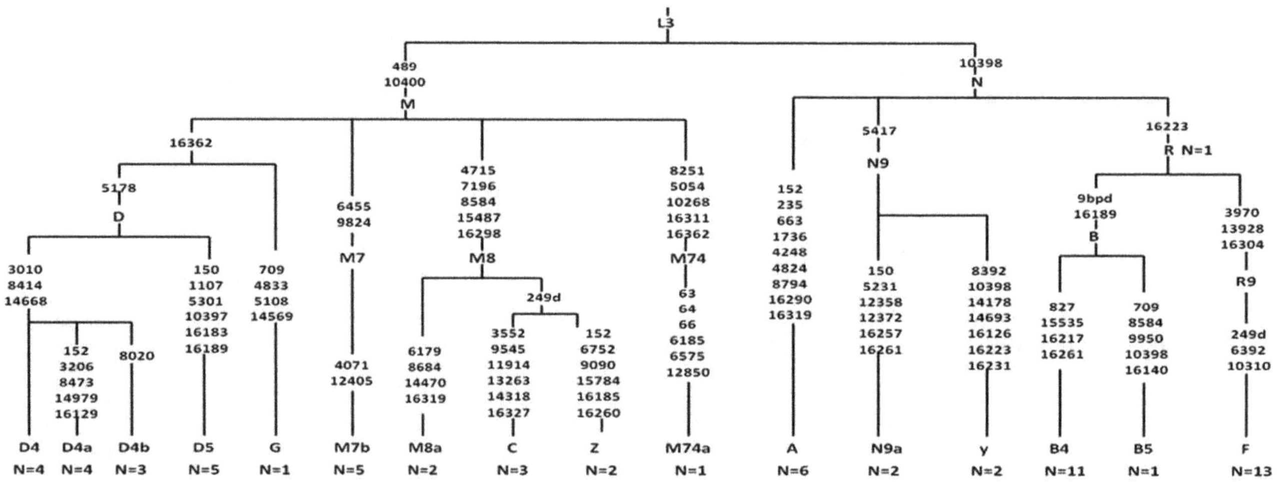

Figure 4. Phylogenetic tree was constructed to reveal the underlying lineages of 16 mtDNA haplogroups in 66 PTC cases.

3. Discussion

In spite of generally indolent behavior and favorable prognosis associated with papillary thyroid cancer, tumor recurrence and distant metastasis are intractable issues in the clinical treatment of a subset of PTC patients [8]. Identifying high-risk patients and offering appropriate, more aggressive therapy in the early stages has been an important goal for clinical researchers. Considering the crucial role of mitochondria in carcinogenesis, investigation of mitochondrial genome may provide potential biomarkers and therapeutic targets for clinical practice. Here we identified 33 pathogenic mtDNA mutations in the protein-coding region, and found three sub-haplogroups and eight mtSNPs that were associated with PTC predisposition. In addition, the average mtDNA copy number in PTCs was significantly higher than that in corresponding normal tissues.

The mutation load of mtDNA is 10–20 times higher than nuclear DNA, probably because the protect and repair system in mitochondria is insufficient and mtDNA is more vulnerable to oxidative stress generated by oxidative phosphorylation [14]. The D-loop region is a mutation hotspot of mtDNA due to the unique triple-stranded DNA structure [15]. The mtMSIs in the D-loop region can modify the binding affinity of transacting elements and direct the formation of persistent RNA-DNA hybrids regulating the efficiency of replication and transcription, which are probably produced by direct oxidative attack, slippage or mis-incorporation during replication and inefficient repair of polymerase. The mtDNA copy number varies in different cell types and microenvironments, and is precisely modulated by alterations in the D-loop region. The content of mtDNA is important for functional maintenance of mitochondria, but alterations in mtDNA and their significance in different types of cancer are still discrepant [16]. Our analysis found excessive replication of mtDNA in PTCs. However, no significant association was presented between mtDNA content and clinicopathological features, and no obvious association was observed between mtDNA content with novel or heteroplasmic mtDNA variations, PTC-associated mutations or mtMSIs. Probably, other factors also take part in the increased copy number of mtDNA. Corver et al. demonstrated that the presence of near-homozygous genome (NHG), rather than damaging or disruptive mtDNA mutations, was correlated with oncocytic phenotype which showed a strikingly mitochondrial proliferation [10]. Interestingly, mtDNA content in tumor of No. 48, a conventional variant PTC, was more than 38 times higher than corresponding normal tissue. In this specimen, we identified a novel frameshift alteration 14495–14502 del (AAAT) in the ND6 gene, which directly resulted in a premature stop-codon (UAG) being introduced and truncated the polypeptide from 175 amino-acid to 58 amino-acid. Thus we speculate that the highly increased mtDNA copy number may have been triggered by defective mitochondrial function caused by this novel deletion [10,16].

Heteroplasmy is a unique characteristic of mitochondrial genome, and also a typical feature of pathogenicity [17]. Once the pathogenic threshold is surpassed, the heteroplasmic level can affect the biochemical and clinical phenotype from mild functional deficiency to complete disassembly of the mitochondrial complex [18]. In our study, nearly half of the PTC cases harbored heteroplasmic variations. Among these heteroplasmic variations, 52 variations were somatic and the majority of them were novel—which dramatically increases their likelihood of being cancer-specific [19]. These somatic variations may confer a neoplastic advantage for tumor cells, and their successive introduction within a developing tumor may provide necessary genetic diversity to satisfy the adaptive evolution and drive tumor progression [20].

Cybrid models have demonstrated that the mitochondrion, but not nuclei, is the master contributor to mitochondrial dysfunction [21]. Pathogenic mtDNA mutations can hamper the electron transport chain (ETC) and generate excessive electrons, which triggers cancer-associated pathways and in turn produces more mutations aggravating the respiratory deficiency. It is reported that more than half of the pathogenic mutations are located in tRNAs which comprise only 10% coding capacity of mitochondrial genome, while the protein-coding region occupying about 70% mtDNA accounts for 40% disease-related mutations. The two rRNAs harbor only about 2% of the pathogenic mutations [20]. In the RNA genes, we identified 13 possibly detrimental variations and five of them had been previously reported in diseases according to the Mitomap database. For example, G3244A in $tRNA^{Leu(UUR)}$, next to the famous pathogenic mutation A3243G, was first detected in mitochondrial myopathy, encephalopathy, lactic acidosis, and stroke-like episodes (MELAS) and later found in several cancers including oncocytic thyroid tumors [22,23]. The A5514G in $tRNA^{Trp}$ damaging an A–U base-pair in ACC-stem was identified in neonatal onset mito-disease and analyzed to be damaging by clinicopathology and biochemistry [24]. The T5628C in $tRNA^{Ala}$ disrupted an extremely conserved

A–U base-pair in the anti-codon stem and resulted in nine unmatched nucleotides (rather than the seven in normal cells) which decreased the energetic stability of $tRNA^{Ala}$ [25].

In the coding region, seven nonsense and 11 frameshift mutations introduced premature stop-codons (UAG, UGA) in protein synthesis and resulted in loss-of-function or even disassembly of the complex. Among them, both 10952insC and 11032–11038delA have been detected in renal oncocytoma [26], and 11032-11038delA was also found in prostate cancer [27]. The 12425delA has been previously identified in a girl having chronic renal failure, persistent lactic acidosis and myopathy [28]. A similar variation 12425insA has been reported in several cancers in a heteroplasmic status [29,30]. These nonsense and frameshift mutations, together with 15 non-synonymous mutations selected by bioinformatics programs, were regarded as pathogenic, and may interfere the OXPHOS system of mitochondrial respiration and contribute to the molecular pathogenesis of thyroid cancer. The association between these pathogenic mtDNA mutations and advanced tumor stage suggests the possible involvement of mtDNA mutations in malignant transformation and progression. Apart from pathogenic mutations, "non-pathologic" mtSNPs can also affect carcinogenesis and progression of cancer in multifactorial manners. Haplotypes, classified by specific combinations of tightly linked mtSNPs, are also correlated with the predisposition to specific cancers [31]. For example, haplogroup U increased the risk of prostate cancer and renal cancer in white North American individuals [32], but decreased the risk of breast cancer in European-American women [33].

The application value of mtDNA variations in early diagnosis, risk stratification, prognostic prediction and disease monitoring of cancer have been widely investigated and discussed. Since mtDNA is a small size and close-circular molecular entity and does not undergo recombination, mtDNA variations are more fixed and persistent than nuclear alterations. Due to the high copy number of mtDNA, detecting mtDNA biomarkers can be more sensitive and powerful than nuclear ones. Therefore, mtDNA biomarkers may have special advantage in samples of limited cellularity including fine-needle aspiration or core-needle aspiration of thyroid nodule. Furthermore, mitochondria are potential therapeutic targets for cancer treatment and can be specifically targeted by antioxidant compounds, selective gene-therapy or approaches changing the mtDNA variation load. Dai et al. demonstrated that mitophagy induced by rapamycin can eliminate pathogenic mtDNA mutations and increase ATP restoration [34]. Recently, several researchers reported that resistance to BRAF inhibition was partly caused by increased mitochondrial biogenesis and oxidative respiration, and therapies inhibiting this metabolic reprogramming restored the function of the BRAF inhibitor and improved treatment efficiency [35,36].

The major limitation of our study is that we do not analyze the mitochondrial genome in anaplastic thyroid cancer (ATC), which has more aggressive behaviors and worse prognosis than PTC. We plan to analyze the mitochondrial characteristics in ATC and evaluate their clinical and prognostic significance. Furthermore, we can compare the role of mitochondrial genome in different histological types of thyroid cancer.

4. Materials and Methods

4.1. Sample Collection

A total of 66 PTC patients underwent primary surgery in the First Affiliated Hospital, Zhejiang University School of Medicine (Hangzhou, China) were enrolled. None of them had a history of cancer or radiotherapy before surgery. Histopathology of tumor specimens was independently evaluated by two experienced pathologists according to the World Health Organization (WHO) classification [37]. Among the 66 PTCs, two were follicular variant and the others were classical variant. Tumors and adjacent normal tissues were immediately frozen in -80 °C after resection. The 16 normal thyroid tissues were used to distinguish tissue-specific variations, and 376 blood samples of healthy individuals from the same geographic region were collected to identify polymorphisms in this population. All the samples were obtained with informed consent. The study was conducted in accordance with the Declaration of Helsinki, and the protocol was approved by the Ethics Committee of the First Affiliated Hospital, College of Medicine, Zhejiang University (2015-443, 30 December 2015).

4.2. Sequencing of the Mitochondrial Genome

Genomic DNA was isolated from frozen tissues and blood samples using a commercial kit (QIAamp DNA Mini Kit from QIAGEN, Hilden, Germany). Concentration and purity of DNA were analyzed by spectrometry. The entire mitochondrial genome was PCR-amplified by 24 pairs of overlapping primer as described previously [38]. The PCR products were detected by electrophoresis in 1% agarose gel and then sequencing by the ABI 3700 automated DNA sequencer (Applied BioSystems, Foster City, CA, USA) using BigDye Terminator v3.1 Cycle Sequencing Kit (Applied BioSystems).

4.3. Sequence Analysis and Haplogroup Classification

The sequences of mtDNA were aligned to the revised Cambridge Reference Sequence (rCRS) (GeneBank accession number: NC_012920) to identify mtDNA variations [39]. The variation load referred to the percentage of variations per gene or complex, which was calculated as follows: total number of altered nucleotides per gene or complex/total number of nucleotides per gene or complex ×100. Variations not recorded in the Mitomap database (http://www.mitomap.org) were regarded as novel. All the heteroplasmic variations were confirmed by repeat analysis of the other strand and compared with the corresponding positions in adjacent normal tissues. The mtDNA haplogroups were classified according to the updated phylogenetic tree of mtDNA (mtDNA tree Built 16) provided by PhyloTree (http://www.phylotree.org) [31].

4.4. Phylogenetic Conservation Analysis and Pathogenic Prediction

Inter-species conservation of the altered amino acids or nucleotides was evaluated by mitochondrial sequences of 41 primates (Table S6). The conservation index (CI) was defined as the percentage of species having wild-type amino-acid or nucleotide by comparing the amino-acid or nucleotide of human with the other 40 species. The higher the conservation of the altered amino-acid or nucleotide was, the greater the pathogenic possibility will be. The variations with potential pathogenicity were selected based on the following criteria: (1) presented in less than 1% of 376 healthy individuals—those variations existed in more than 1% healthy controls were regarded as polymorphisms; (2) were absent in normal thyroid samples, and those variations also identified in normal thyroid samples were regarded as tissue-specific variations; and (3) the altered amino-acids or nucleotides had high conservation (CI > 75%), which indicated the high possibility of functional consequence. Furthermore, the potentially pathogenic variations in protein-coding region were evaluated by 7 bioinformatic programs including PolyPhen-2 (http://genetics.bwh.harvard.edu/pph2/), SIFT (http://sift.jcvi.org/), MutationAssessor (http://mutationassessor.org/), Provean (http://provean.jcvi.org/index.php), SNP & GO (http://snps-and-go.biocomp.unibo.it/), Align GVGD (https://www.biostars.org/) and PANTHER (http://fathmm.biocompute.org.uk/). The variations that were predicted as deleterious by more than half of these 7 programs had high possibility to be "pathogenic" for mitochondrial function and associated with PTC.

4.5. Determination of mtDNA Copy Number

The mtDNA content relative to nuclear encoded 18s RNA was determined by quantitative real-time PCR in ABI Prim 7900HT system using FastStart Universal SYBR Green Master Mix (Roche Diagnostics GmbH, Mannheim, Germany). The primers used for amplification of mtDNA copy number were: the forward primer 5′ CACCCAAGAACAGGGTTTGT 3′ and the reverse primer 5′ TGGCCATGGGTATGTTGTTAA 3′. Another pair of primers was designed to amplify 18s RNA: the forward primer 5′ TAGAGGGACAAGTGGCGTTC 3′ and the reverse primer 5′ CGCTGAGCCAGTCAGTGT 3′. The total volume of PCR mixture was 10 μL including 2 μL DNA (2 ng/μL), 3 μL primers (10 μM) and 5 μL SYBR Green Master Mix. The action was conducted as follows: 50 °C for 2 min, 95 °C for 10 min and followed by 45 cycles of 95 °C for 5 s, 58 °C for 30 s and 72 °C for 1 min. All the reactions were repeated 3 times. Non-template control and a serial dilution of reference DNA were used in each reaction.

4.6. Statistical Analysis

All the statistical analyses were conducted by SPSS software (version 21.0) (SPSS Inc., Chicago, IL, USA). The Pearson chi-square test was performed to analyze the clinicopathological significance of mitochondrial characteristics. Two-sided Mann–Whitney *U* test was used to analyze the difference of the average mtDNA copy number between PTC cases and their corresponding normal tissues. The odds ratios (ORs) with 95% confidence intervals (CIs) were calculated to clarify the association of haplogroups and single-nucleotide polymorphisms (mtSNPs) with PTC occurrence. For all analyses, $p < 0.05$ was regarded as statistically significant.

5. Conclusions

Here, we have reported a comprehensive characterization of the mitochondrial genome in PTC, and demonstrated that pathogenic mtDNA mutations, as well as some specific mtSNPs and haplogroups, may be involved in the pathogenesis and progression of PTC. These results provide an alternative dimension to clarify the molecular mechanisms underlying PTC carcinogenesis, and present possible novel biomarkers and therapeutic targets for the diagnosis, risk stratification, prognostic prediction and treatment of papillary thyroid cancer.

Acknowledgments: This study is supported by Grants from National Natural Science Foundation of China (No. 81202141, and 81272676), the Key Project of Scientific and Technological Innovation of Zhejiang Province (No. 2015C03G2010206), National Science and Technology Major Project of the Ministry of Science and Technology of China (No. 2013ZX09506015), Medical Science and Technology Project of Zhejiang Province (No. 2011ZDA009), and Natural Science Foundation of Zhejiang Province (No. Y2110414).

Author Contributions: Lisong Teng and Minxin Guan conceived and designed the study; Xingyun Su performed the experiment; Weibin Wang and Guodong Ruan contributed the specimens; Min Liang, Jing Zheng, Ye Chen and Huiling Wu contributed reagents/materials/analysis tools; Xingyun Su analyzed the data and wrote the paper; and Thomas J. Fahey III helped to modify the manuscript.

References

1. Chan, D.C. Mitochondria: Dynamic organelles in disease, aging, and development. *Cell* **2006**, *125*, 1241–1252. [CrossRef] [PubMed]
2. Warburg, O. On the origin of cancer cells. *Science* **1956**, *123*, 309–314. [CrossRef] [PubMed]
3. Kroemer, G. Mitochondria in cancer. *Oncogene* **2006**, *25*, 4630–4632. [CrossRef] [PubMed]
4. Wallace, D.C.; Fan, W. Energetics, epigenetics, mitochondrial genetics. *Mitochondrion* **2010**, *10*, 12–31. [CrossRef] [PubMed]
5. Larman, T.C.; DePalma, S.R.; Hadjipanayis, A.G.; Protopopov, A.; Zhang, J.; Gabriel, S.B.; Chin, L.; Seidman, C.E.; Kucherlapati, R.; Seidman, J.G. Spectrum of somatic mitochondrial mutations in five cancers. *Proc. Natl. Acad. Sci. USA* **2012**, *109*, 14087–14091. [CrossRef] [PubMed]
6. Ishikawa, K.; Imanishi, H.; Takenaga, K.; Hayashi, J. Regulation of metastasis; mitochondrial DNA mutations have appeared on stage. *J. Bioenerg. Biomembr.* **2012**, *44*, 639–644. [CrossRef] [PubMed]
7. Markovina, S.; Grigsby, P.W.; Schwarz, J.K.; DeWees, T.; Moley, J.F.; Siegel, B.A.; Perkins, S.M. Treatment approach, surveillance, and outcome of well-differentiated thyroid cancer in childhood and adolescence. *Thyroid* **2014**, *24*, 1121–1126. [CrossRef] [PubMed]
8. Ito, Y.; Miyauchi, A.; Ito, M.; Yabuta, T.; Masuoka, H.; Higashiyama, T.; Fukushima, M.; Kobayashi, K.; Kihara, M.; Miya, A. Prognosis and prognostic factors of differentiated thyroid carcinoma after the appearance of metastasis refractory to radioactive iodine therapy. *Endocr. J.* **2014**, *61*, 821–824. [CrossRef] [PubMed]

9. Xing, M. Molecular pathogenesis and mechanisms of thyroid cancer. *Nat. Rev. Cancer* **2013**, *13*, 184–199. [CrossRef] [PubMed]
10. Corver, W.E.; van Wezel, T.; Molenaar, K.; Schrumpf, M.; van den Akker, B.; van Eijk, R.; Ruano Neto, D.; Oosting, J.; Morreau, H. Near-haploidization significantly associates with oncocytic adrenocortical, thyroid, and parathyroid tumors but not with mitochondrial DNA mutations. *Genes Chromosomes Cancer* **2014**, *53*, 833–844. [CrossRef] [PubMed]
11. Ding, Z.; Ji, J.; Chen, G.; Fang, H.; Yan, S.; Shen, L.; Wei, J.; Yang, K.; Lu, J.; Bai, Y. Analysis of mitochondrial DNA mutations in D-loop region in thyroid lesions. *Biochim. Biophys. Acta* **2010**, *1800*, 271–274. [CrossRef] [PubMed]
12. Gasparre, G.; Porcelli, A.M.; Bonora, E.; Pennisi, L.F.; Toller, M.; Iommarini, L.; Ghelli, A.; Moretti, M.; Betts, C.M.; Martinelli, G.N.; et al. Disruptive mitochondrial DNA mutations in complex I subunits are markers of oncocytic phenotype in thyroid tumors. *Proc. Natl. Acad. Sci. USA* **2007**, *104*, 9001–9006. [CrossRef] [PubMed]
13. Ruiz-Pesini, E.; Wallace, D.C. Evidence for adaptive selection acting on the tRNA and rRNA genes of human mitochondrial DNA. *Hum. Mutat.* **2006**, *27*, 1072–1081. [CrossRef] [PubMed]
14. Cui, H.; Kong, Y.; Zhang, H. Oxidative stress, mitochondrial dysfunction, and aging. *J. Signal Transduct.* **2012**, *2011*. [CrossRef] [PubMed]
15. Kwok, C.S.N.; Quah, T.C.; Ariffin, H.; Tay, S.K.H.; Yeoh, A.E.J. Mitochondrial D-loop polymorphisms and mitochondrial DNA content in childhood acute lymphoblastic leukemia. *J. Pediatr. Hematol. Oncol.* **2011**, *33*, e239–e244. [CrossRef] [PubMed]
16. Yu, M. Generation, function and diagnostic value of mitochondrial DNA copy number alterations in human cancers. *Life Sci.* **2011**, *89*, 65–71. [CrossRef] [PubMed]
17. Chinnery, P.F.; Hudson, G. Mitochondrial genetics. *Br. Med. Bull.* **2013**, *106*, 135–159. [CrossRef] [PubMed]
18. Picard, M.; Zhang, J.; Hancock, S.; Derbeneva, O.; Golhar, R.; Golik, P.; O'Hearn, S.; Levy, S.; Potluri, P.; Lvova, M.; et al. Progressive increase in mtDNA 3243A>G heteroplasmy causes abrupt transcriptional reprogramming. *Proc. Natl. Acad. Sci. USA* **2014**, *111*, E4033–E4042. [CrossRef] [PubMed]
19. He, Y.; Wu, J.; Dressman, D.C.; Iacobuzio-Donahue, C.; Markowitz, S.D.; Velculescu, V.E.; Diaz, L.A., Jr.; Kinzler, K.W.; Vogelstein, B.; Papadopoulos, N. Heteroplasmic mitochondrial DNA mutations in normal and tumour cells. *Nature* **2010**, *464*, 610–614. [CrossRef] [PubMed]
20. Schon, E.A.; DiMauro, S.; Hirano, M. Human mitochondrial DNA: Roles of inherited and somatic mutations. *Nat. Rev. Genet.* **2012**, *13*, 878–890. [CrossRef] [PubMed]
21. Bonora, E.; Porcelli, A.M.; Gasparre, G.; Biondi, A.; Ghelli, A.; Carelli, V.; Baracca, A.; Tallini, G.; Martinuzzi, A.; Lenaz, G.; et al. Defective oxidative phosphorylation in thyroid oncocytic carcinoma is associated with pathogenic mitochondrial DNA mutations affecting complexes I and III. *Cancer Res.* **2006**, *66*, 6087–6096. [CrossRef] [PubMed]
22. Lorenc, A.; Bryk, J.; Golik, P.; Kupryjanczyk, J.; Ostrowski, J.; Pronicki, M.; Semczuk, A.; Szolkowska, M.; Bartnik, E. Homoplasmic melas A3243G mtDNA mutation in a colon cancer sample. *Mitochondrion* **2003**, *3*, 119–124. [CrossRef]
23. Mimaki, M.; Hatakeyama, H.; Ichiyama, T.; Isumi, H.; Furukawa, S.; Akasaka, M.; Kamei, A.; Komaki, H.; Nishino, I.; Nonaka, I.; et al. Different effects of novel mtDNA G3242A and G3244A base changes adjacent to a common A3243G mutation in patients with mitochondrial disorders. *Mitochondrion* **2009**, *9*, 115–122. [CrossRef] [PubMed]
24. Del Mar O'Callaghan, M.; Emperador, S.; López-Gallardo, E.; Jou, C.; Buján, N.; Montero, R.; Garcia-Cazorla, A.; Gonzaga, D.; Ferrer, I.; Briones, P.; et al. New mitochondrial DNA mutations in tRNA associated with three severe encephalopamyopathic phenotypes: Neonatal, infantile, and childhood onset. *Neurogenetics* **2012**, *13*, 245–250. [CrossRef] [PubMed]
25. Spagnolo, M.; Tomelleri, G.; Vattemi, G.; Filosto, M.; Rizzuto, N.; Tonin, P. A new mutation in the mitochondrial tRNAAla gene in a patient with ophthalmoplegia and dysphagia. *Neuromuscul. Disord.* **2001**, *11*, 481–484. [CrossRef]
26. Mayr, J.A.; Meierhofer, D.; Zimmermann, F.; Feichtinger, R.; Kogler, C.; Ratschek, M.; Schmeller, N.; Sperl, W.; Kofler, B. Loss of complex I due to mitochondrial DNA mutations in renal oncocytoma. *Clin. Cancer Res.* **2008**, *14*, 2270–2275. [CrossRef] [PubMed]

27. Jeronimo, C.; Nomoto, S.; Caballero, O.L.; Usadel, H.; Henrique, R.; Varzim, G.; Oliveira, J.; Lopes, C.; Fliss, M.S.; Sidransky, D. Mitochondrial mutations in early stage prostate cancer and bodily fluids. *Oncogene* **2001**, *20*, 5195–5198. [CrossRef] [PubMed]
28. Alston, C.L.; Morak, M.; Reid, C.; Hargreaves, I.P.; Pope, S.A.; Land, J.M.; Heales, S.J.; Horvath, R.; Mundy, H.; Taylor, R.W. A novel mitochondrial MTND5 frameshift mutation causing isolated complex I deficiency, renal failure and myopathy. *Neuromuscul. Disord.* **2010**, *20*, 131–135. [CrossRef] [PubMed]
29. Tseng, L.M.; Yin, P.H.; Yang, C.W.; Tsai, Y.F.; Hsu, C.Y.; Chi, C.W.; Lee, H.C. Somatic mutations of the mitochondrial genome in human breast cancers. *Genes Chromosomes Cancer* **2011**, *50*, 800–811. [CrossRef] [PubMed]
30. Yin, P.H.; Wu, C.C.; Lin, J.C.; Chi, C.W.; Wei, Y.H.; Lee, H.C. Somatic mutations of mitochondrial genome in hepatocellular carcinoma. *Mitochondrion* **2010**, *10*, 174–182. [CrossRef] [PubMed]
31. Van Oven, M.; Kayser, M. Updated comprehensive phylogenetic tree of global human mitochondrial DNA variation. *Hum. Mutat.* **2009**, *30*, E386–E394. [CrossRef] [PubMed]
32. Booker, L.M.; Habermacher, G.M.; Jessie, B.C.; Sun, Q.C.; Baumann, A.K.; Amin, M.; Lim, S.D.; Fernandez-Golarz, C.; Lyles, R.H.; Brown, M.D.; et al. North american white mitochondrial haplogroups in prostate and renal cancer. *J. Urol.* **2006**, *175*, 468–472. [CrossRef]
33. Bai, R.K.; Leal, S.M.; Covarrubias, D.; Liu, A.; Wong, L.J. Mitochondrial genetic background modifies breast cancer risk. *Cancer Res.* **2007**, *67*, 4687–4694. [CrossRef] [PubMed]
34. Dai, Y.; Zheng, K.; Clark, J.; Swerdlow, R.H.; Pulst, S.M.; Sutton, J.P.; Shinobu, L.A.; Simon, D.K. Rapamycin drives selection against a pathogenic heteroplasmic mitochondrial DNA mutation. *Hum. Mol. Genet.* **2014**, *23*, 637–647. [CrossRef] [PubMed]
35. Livingstone, E.; Swann, S.; Lilla, C.; Schadendorf, D.; Roesch, A. Combining BRAF V 600E inhibition with modulators of the mitochondrial bioenergy metabolism to overcome drug resistance in metastatic melanoma. *Exp. Dermatol.* **2015**, *24*, 709–710. [CrossRef] [PubMed]
36. Spagnolo, F.; Ghiorzo, P.; Queirolo, P. Overcoming resistance to BRAF inhibition in BRAF-mutated metastatic melanoma. *Oncotarget* **2014**, *5*, 10206–10221. [CrossRef] [PubMed]
37. Hedinger, C.; Williams, E.D.; Sobin, L.H. The who histological classification of thyroid tumors: A commentary on the second edition. *Cancer* **1989**, *63*, 908–911. [CrossRef]
38. Rieder, M.J.; Taylor, S.L.; Tobe, V.O.; Nickerson, D.A. Automating the identification of DNA variations using quality-based fluorescence re-sequencing: Analysis of the human mitochondrial genome. *Nucleic Acids Res.* **1998**, *26*, 967–973. [CrossRef] [PubMed]
39. Andrews, R.M.; Kubacka, I.; Chinnery, P.F.; Lightowlers, R.N.; Turnbull, D.M.; Howell, N. Reanalysis and revision of the Cambridge Reference Sequence for human mitochondrial DNA. *Nat. Genet.* **1999**, *23*. [CrossRef]

Diagnostic Limitation of Fine-Needle Aspiration (FNA) on Indeterminate Thyroid Nodules can be Partially Overcome by Preoperative Molecular Analysis: Assessment of *RET/PTC1* Rearrangement in *BRAF* and *RAS* Wild-Type Routine Air-Dried FNA Specimens

Young Sin Ko [1,2], Tae Sook Hwang [2,3,*], Ja Yeon Kim [3], Yoon-La Choi [4], Seung Eun Lee [5], Hye Seung Han [2,3], Wan Seop Kim [2,3], Suk Kyeong Kim [6] and Kyoung Sik Park [7]

1 Diagnostic Pathology Center, Seegene Medical Foundation, Seoul KS013, Korea; noteasy@mf.seegene.com
2 Molecular Genetics and Pathology, Department of Medicine, Graduate School of Konkuk University, Seoul KS013, Korea; aphsh@kuh.ac.kr (H.S.H.); wskim@kuh.ac.kr (W.S.K.)
3 Department of Pathology, Konkuk University School of Medicine, Seoul KS013, Korea; 78jykim@hanmail.net
4 Department of Pathology and Translational Genomics, Samsung Medical Center, Sungkyunkwan University School of Medicine, Seoul KS013, Korea; yla.choi@samsung.com
5 Department of Pathology, Konkuk University Medical Center, Seoul KS013, Korea; 20150063@kuh.ac.kr
6 Department of Internal Medicine, Konkuk University School of Medicine, Seoul KS013, Korea; endolife@kuh.ac.kr
7 Department of Surgery, Konkuk University School of Medicine, Seoul KS013, Korea; kspark@kuh.ac.kr
* Correspondence: tshwang@kuh.ac.kr

Academic Editor: Daniela Gabriele Grimm

Abstract: Molecular markers are helpful diagnostic tools, particularly for cytologically indeterminate thyroid nodules. Preoperative *RET/PTC1* rearrangement analysis in *BRAF* and *RAS* wild-type indeterminate thyroid nodules would permit the formulation of an unambiguous surgical plan. Cycle threshold values according to the cell count for detection of the *RET/PTC1* rearrangement by real-time reverse transcription-polymerase chain reaction (RT-PCR) using fresh and routine air-dried TPC1 cells were evaluated. The correlation of *RET/PTC1* rearrangement between fine-needle aspiration (FNA) and paired formalin-fixed paraffin-embedded (FFPE) specimens was analyzed. *RET/PTC1* rearrangements of 76 resected *BRAF* and *RAS* wild-type classical PTCs were also analyzed. Results of RT-PCR and the Nanostring were compared. When 100 fresh and air-dried TPC1 cells were used, expression of *RET/PTC1* rearrangement was detectable after 35 and 33 PCR cycles, respectively. The results of *RET/PTC1* rearrangement in 10 FNA and paired FFPE papillary thyroid carcinoma (PTC) specimens showed complete correlation. Twenty-nine (38.2%) of 76 *BRAF* and *RAS* wild-type classical PTCs had *RET/PTC1* rearrangement. Comparison of *RET/PTC1* rearrangement analysis between RT-PCR and the Nanostring showed moderate agreement with a κ value of 0.56 ($p = 0.002$). The *RET/PTC1* rearrangement analysis by RT-PCR using routine air-dried FNA specimen was confirmed to be technically applicable. A significant proportion (38.2%) of the *BRAF* and *RAS* wild-type PTCs harbored *RET/PTC1* rearrangements.

Keywords: *RET/PTC* gene rearrangement; air-dried FNA specimen; RT-PCR; Nanostring

1. Introduction

The evaluation of a thyroid nodule is a very common clinical problem. Epidemiologic studies have shown the prevalence of palpable thyroid nodules to be approximately 5% in women and 1% in men living in iodine-sufficient parts of the world [1,2]. In contrast, high-resolution ultrasound (US) can detect thyroid nodules in 19–68% of randomly selected individuals, with higher frequencies in women and the elderly [3,4]. The clinical importance of thyroid nodules rests with the need to exclude thyroid cancer, which occurs in 7–15% of cases depending on age, sex, radiation exposure history, family history, and other factors [5,6]. Differentiated thyroid cancer (DTC) includes papillary and follicular cancer, and comprises the vast majority (>90%) of all thyroid cancers [7]. In the United States, approximately 63,000 new cases of thyroid cancer were predicted to be diagnosed in 2014 [8] compared with 37,200 in 2009 when the last ATA guidelines were published. The yearly incidence has nearly tripled from 4.9 per 100,000 in 1975 to 14.3 per 100,000 in 2009 [9].

The most prevalent type of thyroid malignancy in Korea is papillary thyroid carcinoma (PTC), which constitutes more than 97% of the cases, followed by follicular thyroid carcinoma (FTC), comprising 1.5% of the thyroid cancer [10]. Compared to Western countries, the prevalence of PTC is much higher. Therefore, the evaluation of a thyroid nodule in Korea is primarily a search for PTC.

Fine-needle aspiration (FNA) is the safest and most reliable test that can provide a definitive preoperative diagnosis of malignancy [11]. The sensitivity and specificity of FNA are reported to be 68–98% and 56–100%, respectively [12]. However, 15–30% of thyroid FNA diagnoses are "atypia of undetermined significance (AUS)/follicular lesion of undetermined significance (FLUS)", "follicular neoplasm or suspicious for follicular neoplasm (FN/SFN)", and "suspicious for malignancy" [13]. This leads to an increased rate of unnecessary surgery, as only about 25% of the indeterminate cases will receive a postoperative malignant diagnosis by histological examination [11]. Moreover, patients with a diagnosis of indeterminate category usually undergo hemithyroidectomy, and about 25% of the patients need to have a second stage completion thyroidectomy in most centers [12]. Two-stage surgery has higher morbidity than initial total thyroidectomy undertaken with a definitive malignant diagnosis on FNA. Preoperative molecular analysis using a panel of genetic alterations would overcome the limitation of FNA diagnosis. The most common genetic alteration in thyroid cancer is the activation of the mitogen-activated protein kinase pathway. Activation of this pathway occurs through mutually exclusive mutations of the *BRAF* and *RAS* genes and rearrangements of the *RET/PTC* and *NTRK*. The overall prevalence of the *BRAF* mutations is approximately 45% (range, 27.3–87.1%) [14,15], with a significantly higher prevalence in Asia—especially Korea—relative to Western countries [15–17]. The mutations of the *RAS* genes are the second most common genetic alterations in thyroid tumors, and are mostly present in follicular-patterned lesions. The prevalence of *RAS* mutations in follicular variant of papillary thyroid carcinoma (FVPTC) varies from 26.5% to 33.3% in Korea, where most of the follicular patterned thyroid malignancy is FVPTC [18,19].

RET proto-oncogene rearrangements are commonly seen in PTC. These rearrangements play a role in pathogenesis of PTC, and derive from the fusion of the *RET* tyrosine kinase domain sequence with 50 sequences of heterologous genes. The resulting chimeric oncogenes are termed *RET/PTCs* [20–24]. *RET/PTC* rearrangements are typically common in tumors from patients with a history of radiation exposure (50–80%) and PTC of children and young adults (40–70%) [25,26]. The distribution of *RET/PTC* rearrangements within this tumor is quite heterogeneous, and varies from the involvement of almost all neoplastic cells to presence in only a small fraction of the tumor cells [27,28]. To date, 13 different types of *RET/PTC* rearrangements have been reported; *RET/PTC1* and *RET/PTC3* account for more than 90% of all rearrangements.

The prevalence of the *RET/PTC* rearrangements in PTC varies widely in different populations (range, 0–86.8%) [29–31], with significant variability in mutational frequency—even within the same geographical regions. Rates of 0–54.5% have been reported in Asia [30–32], 2.4–72.0% in the United States [17,33], and 8.1–42.9% in Europe [34,35]. The marked variations may reflect the small size of the studies, geographic variability, or different sensitivities of the detection methods [36,37].

When this variability is considered, the prevalence of *RET/PTC* rearrangements in Asia is generally low [29–32,38,39]. The subclonal occurrence of *RET/PTC* rearrangement in PTC can influence the sensitivity of some methods, and might explain why the reported prevalence of *RET/PTC* rearrangements in PTCs varies in different studies. Very recent studies demonstrated that *RET/PTC* rearrangements in benign thyroid nodules are not an uncommon occurrence, and suggested that its presence could be associated with a faster nodular enlargement [40–42]. A variety of methods have been used to identify *RET/PTC* rearrangements. These include real-time reverse transcription-polymerase chain reaction (RT-PCR), Southern blot analysis, fluorescence in situ hybridization, and NanoString nCounter Gene Expression Assay.

Most preoperative detection of these rearrangements has been performed in fresh FNA material. Recently, detection of the *PAX8/PPARG* and *RET/PTC* rearrangements in routine air-dried FNA samples was reported [43–48]. The FNA approach suffers from the limitation that indeterminate FNA specimens usually contain small numbers of atypical cells, and these cells are often mixed with many inflammatory cells, benign follicular cells, and stromal cells. Therefore, harvesting the cells of interest is the key step in molecular analysis of the FNA specimen.

Preoperative *RET/PTC1* rearrangement analysis in *BRAF* and *RAS* wild-type indeterminate thyroid nodules would permit the formulation of an unambiguous surgical plan, while foregoing the need for other less-specific diagnostic tests like repeat FNA and intraoperative frozen section evaluation. We have previously reported the value of the preoperative *BRAF* and *RAS* mutation analysis in diagnosing PTC in routine air-dried FNA specimens [18,49–51]. In our institution, we recommend surgery for *BRAF* or *RAS*-positive thyroid nodules with preoperative cytological diagnosis of AUS/FLUS and FN/SFN categories, and have been able to detect considerable numbers of PTCs in cytologically-indeterminate nodules [50]. Considering that 88% of the PTCs harbor either a *BRAF* or a *RAS* mutation (Thyroid, 2017, Epub ahead of time), we hypothesized that detection of *RET/PTC* rearrangements on *BRAF* and *RAS* mutation wild-type FNA specimens of the indeterminate thyroid nodules will improve the diagnostic yield of PTC. An algorithmic approach is cost-effective and efficient—especially in *BRAF* mutation-prevalent populations.

In this study, we investigated the clinical feasibility of preoperative *RET/PTC1* rearrangement analysis as an ancillary diagnostic tool in routine air-dried FNA samples. We also evaluated the *RET/PTC1* rearrangement status for 76 *BRAF* and *RAS* wild-type classical PTC cases.

2. Results

2.1. Detection of the RET/PTC1 Rearrangement in a Fresh TPC1 Cell Line

The C_t value was increased when the cell numbers used for analysis were decreased and showed an inverse correlation (Table 1 and Figure 1). *RET/PTC1* rearrangement was detectable after 35 PCR cycles when 100 TPC1 cells were used.

Table 1. C_t values and cell counts of *RET/PTC1* rearrangement analysis by RT-PCR using fresh cultured TPC1 cells.

Cell Number	*RET/PTC1* (C_t)	*GAPDH* (C_t)
1000	30.3	23.1
500	31.2	24.2
250	34.1	27.1
100	35.6	29.4
50	36.7	30.6

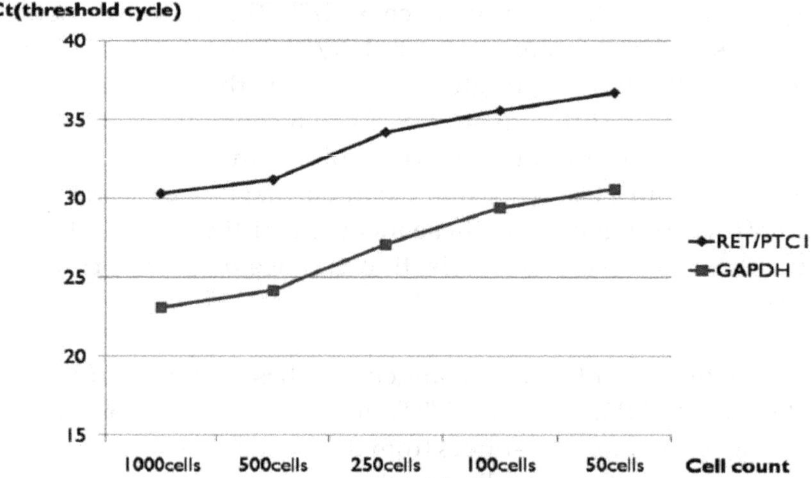

Figure 1. Threshold cycle (C_t) values and cell counts of *RET/PTC1* rearrangement analysis by real-time reverse transcription-polymerase chain reaction (RT-PCR) using fresh cultured TPC1 cells. *GAPDH*: glyceraldehyde-3-phosphate dehydrogenase.

2.2. Detection of the RET/PTC1 Rearrangement in Routine Air-Dried TPC1 Cell Line

When *RET/PTC1* rearrangement was analyzed using various numbers of smeared, alcohol-fixed, and Papanicolaou-stained PTC1 cells, the cell number and the threshold cycle (C_t) value also showed an inverse correlation (Table 2 and Figure 2). The expression of *RET/PTC1* rearrangement was detectable after 33 PCR cycles when 100 cells were used.

Table 2. C_t values and cell counts of *RET/PTC1* rearrangement analysis by RT-PCR using RNA extracted from routine air-dried and Papanicolaou-stained TPC1 cells.

Cell Number	*RET/PTC1* (C_t)	*GAPDH* (C_t)
1000	32.3	29.4
500	33.9	31.1
250	34.2	32.8
100	33.3	31.1
50	34.6	33.3

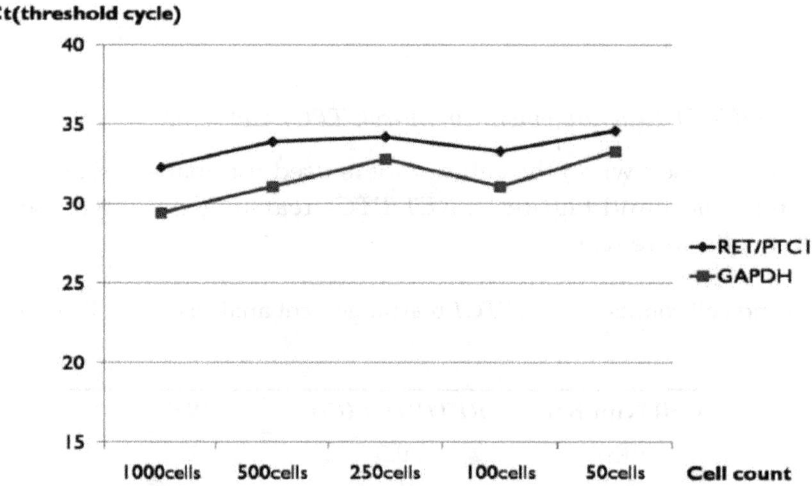

Figure 2. C_t values and cell counts of *RET/PTC1* rearrangement analysis by RT-PCR using RNA extracted from routine air-dried and Papanicolaou-stained TPC1 cells.

2.3. Correlation of the RET/PTC1 Rearrangement between Routine Air-Dried FNA and Paired FFPE PTC Tissue Specimens

When *RET/PTC1* rearrangement was analyzed using PTC cells from archival air-dried FNA slides aspirated from the patients proven to have a histopathological diagnosis of PTC, *RET/PTC1* rearrangement was detected in all 6 cases even though the C_t values of the archival specimen were higher than those of formalin-fixed paraffin-embedded (FFPE) PTC tissue specimens (Table 3). Four cases lacking *RET/PTC1* rearrangement in tissue specimen also failed to reveal rearrangement in FNA samples. These results confirmed that *RET/PTC1* rearrangement analysis by RT-PCR can be applied in preoperative FNA samples as an ancillary diagnostic tool.

Table 3. Correlation of *RET/PTC1* rearrangement status between routine air-dried fine-needle aspiration (FNA) and paired formalin-fixed paraffin-embedded (FFPE) specimens.

C_t of FFPE Specimen			C_t of FNA Specimen		
Case	***RET/PTC1***	***GAPDH***	**Case**	***RET/PTC1***	***GAPDH***
1	26.15	27.40	1	35.05	35.86
2	26.15	29.23	2	36.41	37.54
3	26.32	28.96	3	37.03	34.79
4	40	34.67	4	>50	36.74
5	24.64	28.84	5	37.66	35.86
6	31.71	29.92	6	34.26	35.47
7	24.71	26.98	7	36.62	36.78
8	>50.00	28.64	8	>50.00	31.69
9	>50.00	27.55	9	>50.00	30.34
10	>50.00	29.31	10	>50.00	30.01

2.4. Detection of the RET/PTC1 Rearrangement in Resected BRAF and RAS Wild-Type PTC Cases Using FFPE Tissue Specimen

Of 600 surgically resected FFPE specimens histologically diagnosed as PTC, classical type, 518 had *BRAF* mutations and 6 had *RAS* mutations. Among 76 *BRAF* and *RAS* wild-type PTCs, 29 (38.2%) cases turned out to have *RET/PTC1* rearrangement. Considering that alteration of *BRAF*, *RAS*, and *RET* genes are mutually exclusive, 29 (4.8%) of 600 classical PTC cases harbored *RET/PTC1* rearrangement.

2.5. Comparative Analysis of RT-PCR with the NanoString nCounter Gene Expression Assay for Detecting RET/PTC1 Rearrangement in FFPE PTC Tissue Specimen

Twenty-six cases showed correlation on both methods (5 positives and 21 negatives), whereas five cases showed discrepancy between the two methods (three cases positive for Nanostring but not for RT-PCR, two cases positive for RT-PCR but not for Nanostring). Two different analysis methods showed moderate agreement with a κ value of 0.56 ($p = 0.002$).

3. Discussion

The value of molecular markers on preoperative FNA specimens has been described in various thyroid nodules [18,47,49–53]. *RET/PTC* rearrangements are commonly found in adult sporadic PTCs with a marked variable prevalence in different studies owing to geographic variability or different sensitivity of the detection methods [17,29–37]. The reported prevalence rates of *RET/PTC* rearrangements varied largely among studies. While geographical factors and radiation exposure can partially account for this wide range of prevalence, the methodology applied appears to be the most important factor to explain this variability. Searching for *RET/PTC* rearrangements by a less sensitive method may have the drawback of leaving some PTCs undiagnosed, but has the advantage of reducing false positive findings. Indeed, while sporadic cells harboring *RET/PTC* rearrangements can be present in benign nodules, its clonal occurrence is exclusive to PTC. Hence, the less sensitive

RT-PCR seems to be more suitable for diagnostic purposes. *RET/PTC* rearrangements analysis on thyroid tumor has not been extensively performed in Korea, given the prevalence of the *BRAF* V600E mutation in PTC in Korea.

In this report, we assessed the clinical usability of preoperative *RET/PTC1* rearrangement analysis as an ancillary diagnostic tool for *BRAF* and *RAS* wild-type indeterminate thyroid nodules, and explored the *RET/PTC1* rearrangement status in a large number of PTC cases. These explorations have never been done in Korea, to our knowledge. We routinely use atypical follicular cells marked by the cytopathologists and dissected from routine air-dried FNA samples to increase the sensitivity. Since clinical FNA samples contain limited numbers of cells to perform several steps required for deciding optimum number of cells for successful analysis and cutoff values, we performed same analysis using fresh TPC1 cells which are equivalent to the fresh FNA samples in step 1 and air-dried Papanicolaou-stained TPC1 cells equivalent to the archival FNA slides in step 2.

The C_t values in Table 2 tend to decrease when the cell numbers were increased; however, both C_t values of the *RET/PTC1* and *GAPDH* expression using 250 cells are greater than those using 100 cells. Since C_t values of the housekeeping gene expression also showed the same phenomenon, we assumed that a considerable amount of RNA in 250-cell groups might have been deteriorated. At any rate, we found that *RET/PTC1* expression could be measured when 50–100 air-dried Papanicolaou-stained TPC1 cells were used.

When we compared the C_t values of fresh and air-dried Papanicolaou-stained TPC1 cells according to the cell numbers, the C_t values were slightly decreased when air-dried Papanicolaou-stained cells were used. We assumed that this finding might have resulted from the imprecise cell count in step 2. Fresh cells were counted using a hemocytometer, whereas air-dried and Papanicolaou-stained cells were counted on a slide using a square micrometer under the microscope. The expression of *RET/PTC1* rearrangement detectable after 33 PCR cycles when routine air-dried 100 TPC1 cells were used suggests that *RET/PTC1* expression could be detected in routine air-dried FNA samples containing 100 cells.

When *RET/PTC1* rearrangement status from ten FNA and paired FFPE samples were compared, the results showed complete agreement. The higher C_t value of FNA samples compared to the matched FFPE samples could be attributed to the much smaller numbers of cells in FNA samples. The other reason might be the different RNA extraction method used for the two different samples.

Since *BRAF* mutations, *RAS* mutations, and *RET/PTC* rearrangements are mutually exclusive, we analyzed the *RET/PTC1* rearrangement status on both *BRAF* (V600E and K601E) and *RAS* (*NRAS* codons 12, 13, 61; *HRAS* codons 12, 13, 61; *KRAS* codons 12, 13, 61) wild-type PTC cases to save cost and effort. The main limitation of our experiment is that we only performed *RET/PTC1* rearrangement, even though the prevalence for *RET/PTC3* arrangement in previous Korean report was 0%. Another reason for analyzing *RET/PTC1* is that we were able to secure a cell line harboring only the *RET/PTC1* rearrangement.

Among 76 surgically resected both *BRAF* and *RAS* wild-type FFPE specimens histopathologically diagnosed as PTC, classical type, 29 (38.2%) cases turned out to have *RET/PTC1* rearrangement; this means that *RET/PTC1* rearrangement was detected in 29 (4.8%) of 600 classical-type PTCs. Two previous studies reported *REP/PTC* rearrangements in Korea. One study failed to identify any *RET/PTC1, 2, 3* rearrangements in 24 cases of PTC by RT-PCR [31]. The other study detected 2 (6.5%) *RET/PTC1*, 2 (6.5%) *RET/PTC2*, and no (0%) *RET/PTC3* rearrangements in 31 PTCs by RT-PCR [38]. Both studies used fresh frozen tumor tissue. The slight discrepancy could be explained by the difference of the sample size. The slightly lower prevalence of *RET/PTC1* rearrangement compared to the second study might also be attributed to the poor RNA preservation in the FFPE specimens.

The NanoString nCounter Gene Expression Assay is a robust and highly reproducible method for detecting the expression of up to 800 genes in a single reaction with high sensitivity and linearity across a broad range of expression levels. The methodology serves to bridge the gap between genome-wide (microarrays) and targeted (real-time quantitative PCR) expression profiling. The nCounter assay is based on direct digital detection of mRNA molecules of interest using target-specific, color-coded probe pairs. It does not require the conversion of mRNA to cDNA by reverse transcription or the amplification of the resulting cDNA by PCR. The expression level of a gene is measured by counting the number of times the color-coded barcode for that gene is detected, and the barcode counts are then tabulated [54]. Comparative analysis of RT-PCR with the Nanostring method for detecting *RET/PTC1* rearrangement in FFPE PTC tissue showed moderate agreement with a k value of 0.56 (p = 0.002). There is a discrepancy between these two methods (three cases positive for Nanostring but not for RT-PCR, two cases positive for RT-PCR but not for Nanostring). The discrepancy might be attributed to the different RNA extraction methods and cut-off values of each method. In three cases with discrepancy, the results were near to the cut-off value. Another reason might be attributed to the difference of tumor portion used in two different methods. Since we did not initially plan to compare RT-PCR with Nanostring, we made the tumor sections only for RT-PCR analysis. Therefore, the tumor portions which were used for Nanostring might have been slightly different from the initial tumor portion. Next generation sequencing (NGS) is being used to study genetic alterations in institutions worldwide. However, it may be a long time until NGS becomes a routine part of thyroid cancer practice in Korea, since only NGS panels relevant for the therapeutic modality have been approved by the Korean government. Furthermore, only large institutions like university hospitals can adopt NGS in practice. Therefore, algorithmic approach of *BRAF* mutation analysis followed by *RAS* mutation and *RET/PTC1* rearrangement may be of more practical help to refine FNA diagnosis of indeterminate thyroid nodules.

We confirmed the technical applicability of *RET/PTC1* rearrangement analysis using routine air-dried FNA samples as an ancillary diagnostic tool through several steps of the experiment. The presence of *RET/TPC1* rearrangement in a significant proportion (38.2%) of the patients with *BRAF* and *RAS* wild-type PTCs can be used to diagnose and manage patients with *BRAF* and *RAS* wild-type indeterminate thyroid nodules. Since the *BRAF* V600E mutation, *NRAS* codon 61 mutation, and *RET/PTC1* rearrangement comprise more than 90%, 75%, and 50% of the *BRAF* mutations, *RAS* mutations, and *RET/PTC* rearrangements [18,50], an algorithmic approach of *BRAF* V600E mutation analysis followed by *NRAS* 61 mutation and *RET/PTC1* rearrangement analysis would cost-effectively and efficiently overcome a diagnostic limitation of the thyroid FNA by triaging considerable numbers of PTCs in cytologically indeterminate nodules.

4. Materials and Methods

4.1. Total RNA Extraction and First-Strand Synthesis

Total RNA from fresh and fixed TPC1 cells (derived from human thyroid papillary carcinoma, classic type and harboring *RET/PTC1* rearrangement) was extracted using MasterPure Complete DNA and RNA Purification Kit (Epicentre, Madison, WI, USA). Total RNA from formalin-fixed paraffin-embedded (FFPE) specimen was extracted using a High Pure FFPE RNA isolation kit (Roche Diagnostics, Mannheim, Germany). First-strand synthesis was performed on 2 μg of total RNA using a Tetro cDNA synthesis kit (Bioline, London, UK). Tetro reverse transcriptase with diethyl pyrocarbonate water and cDNA reverse transcribed product from the TPC1 cells were used as negative and positive controls, respectively.

4.2. RT-PCR

Amplification was performed by RT-PCR using a LightCycler 480 Instrument (Roche Diagnostics), and measurement was performed using LightCycler quantification software version 1.5 (Roche Diagnostics). The RT-PCR reaction mixture was prepared in a Light Cycler® 480 Multiwell Plate 96 containing 0.5 μM of each primer set (*RET/PTC1* and *glyceraldehyde-3-phosphate isomerase, GAPDH*), 0.25 μM of the probes, 2X of LightCycler 480 Probes Master (Roche Diagnostics), and 1–2 μg (1 μg for the cell and 2 μg for the FFPE tissue) of cDNA template in a final reaction volume of 20 μL (Table 4).

Table 4. Primers and probes sequences for RT-PCR.

RET/PTC1	Primers and Probes Sequences
Forward primer (5′–3′)	CGC GAC CTG CGC AAA
Reverse primer (5′–3′)	CAA GTT CTT CCG AGG GAA TTC C
TaqMan Probe (5′–3′)	FAM-CCA GCG TTA CCA TCG AGG ATC CAA AGT-BHQ1
GAPDH	
Forward primer (5′–3′)	GTT CGA CAG TCA GCC GCA TC
Reverse primer (5′–3′)	GGA ATT TGC CAT GGG TGG A
TaqMan Probe (5′–3′)	FAM-ACC AGG CGC CCA ATA CGA CCA A-BHQ1

4.3. NanoString nCounter Gene Expression Assay

Tumor portion on the hematoxylin and eosin-stained FFPE tissue slides was marked by the pathologist, and total RNA was isolated from two to three FFPE tissue sections (10 μm thick) using an miRNeasy FFPE Kit (Qiagen, Hilden, Germany) according to the manufacturer's instructions. The probe sets were custom designed and synthesized by NanoString Technologies (Seattle, WA, USA), and nCounter assays were performed according to the manufacturer's protocol. Briefly, 500 ng of total RNA was hybridized to nCounter probe sets for 16 hours at 65 °C. Samples were then processed using an automated nCounter Sample Prep Station (NanoString Technologies, Inc., Seattle, WA, USA). Cartridges containing immobilized and aligned reporter complexes were subsequently imaged on an nCounter Digital Analyzer (NanoString Technologies, Inc.). Reporter counts were collected using the NanoString's nSolver analysis software version 1, normalized, and analyzed. A total of eight expression probes were designed, four (5′-1 to 5′-4) proximal and four distal (3′-1 to 3′-4) to most commonly-known junction sites for *RET* fusions. An imbalance between 5′ and 3′ probe signals was indicative of the presence of a *RET* fusion transcript. We used a cutoff of three-fold for 3′/5′ ratio. Therefore, a case was considered positive for rearrangement if 3′/5′ imbalance was three-fold or more.

We used Cohen's κ coefficient to measure agreement between RT-PCR and Nanostring method.

4.4. Detection of the RET/PTC1 Rearrangement in Fresh TPC1 Cell Line

Total RNA was extracted by Master Pure Complete DNA and RNA Purification Kit (Epicentre) using a fresh cell colony formed from 1000 cultured TPC1 cells (provided by Nagataki, Nakasaki University, Japan). RT-PCR was performed and the minimum number of cycles (C_t value) needed to detect the expression of *RET/PTC1* rearrangement and *GAPDH* was determined. Similarly, the number of the cells was reduced to 500, 250, 100, and 50, and RT-PCR was performed to evaluate C_t values according to cell count. The whole procedure was performed in triplicate after TPC1 cells were harvested

4.5. Detection of RET/PTC1 Rearrangement in Routine Air-Dried TPC1 Cell Line

To make a condition identical to that in the routine air-dried FNA preparation, cultured TPC1 cells were smeared on a slide and fixed with 95% ethanol according to the routine FNA preparation in our cytology laboratory. The fixed cells were stained by the routine Papanicolaou procedure. After the coverslips were removed from the smeared slides, the atypical cells of interest were dissected with a 26-gauge needle under the light microscope. Approximately 50, 100, 250, 500, and 1000 cells were dissected using a square micrometer under the microscope. A needle tip was carefully submerged in a tube containing extraction buffer supplied by MasterPure Complete DNA and RNA Purification Kit (Epicentre), and total RNA was extracted. RT-PCR was performed, and C_t values for the expression of *RET/PTC1* rearrangement and *GAPDH* were evaluated using 50, 100, 250, 500, and 1000 air-dried and alcohol fixed TPC1 cells, respectively. The whole procedure was performed in triplicate after TPC1 cells were harvested.

4.6. Correlation of RET/PTC1 Rearrangement between Routine Air-Dried FNA and Paired FFPE PTC Tissue Specimens

PTC cells from the archival FNA slides from the Department of Pathology, Konkuk University Medical Center were used. The slides that were selected were from samples aspirated from ten thyroid nodules with histopathological diagnosis of classical-type PTC. Study approval was obtained from the Institutional Review Board (KUH1210043). After the coverslips were removed from the slides, approximately 100 atypical follicular cells were dissected with a 26-gauge needle under the light microscope, and total RNA was extracted using MasterPure Complete DNA and RNA Purification Kit (Epicentre). RT-PCR was performed, and C_t values of the *RET/PTC1* rearrangement and *GAPDH* expression were evaluated. Tumor portion on the hematoxylin and eosin-stained FFPE tissue slides was marked by the pathologist, and total RNA was isolated from two-to-three FFPE tissue sections (10 μm thick) using High Pure FFPE RNA isolation kit (Roche Diagnostics). RT-PCR was performed and C_t values of the *RET/PTC1* rearrangement and *GAPDH* expression were evaluated. The C_t values defining the analysis as positive is greater than 40 cycles.

4.7. Detection of the RET/PTC1 Rearrangement in Resected BRAF and RAS Wild-Type PTC Cases Using FFPE Tissue Specimen

Archival thyroid neoplasm that had been surgically removed between 2010 and 2014 at Konkuk University Medical Center were blindly re-evaluated according to the 2004 World Health Organization classification of thyroid neoplasm by the two pathologists (Tae Sook Hwang, who is an endocrine pathologist, and Young Sin Ko). In case of a disagreement and to reach a consensus, another endocrine pathologist (Chan-Kwon Jung) independently reviewed the cases. Of the 600 classical PTC cases selected, 518 had *BRAF* mutation and 6 had *RAS* mutation. Finally, 76 *BRAF* and *RAS* wild-type classical PTC cases were selected. Tumor portion on the hematoxylin and eosin-stained FFPE tissue slides was marked by the pathologist, and total RNA was isolated from two-to-three FFPE tissue sections (10 μm thick) using High Pure FFPE RNA isolation kit (Roche Diagnostics). RT-PCR was performed, and C_t values of the *RET/PTC1* rearrangement and *GAPDH* expression were evaluated. The C_t value defining the analysis as positive is greater than 40 cycles.

4.8. Comparison Analysis of RT-PCR with the NanoString nCounter Gene Expression Assay for Detecting RET/PTC1 Rearrangement

RET/PTC1 rearrangement status was also analyzed by the Nanostring method, using 31 cases having sufficient cancer tissue remaining for the comparative analysis.

5. Conclusions

RET/PTC1 rearrangement analysis by RT-PCR using routine air-dried FNA specimen was confirmed to be technically applicable and significant population (38.2%) of the *BRAF* and *RAS* wild type PTCs harbor *RET/PTC1* rearrangement. Preoperative *RET/PTC1* rearrangement analysis in *BRAF* and *RAS* wild type indeterminate thyroid nodules would permit a formulation of unambiguous surgical plan, while foregoing the need for other less specific diagnostic test such as repeat FNA and intraoperative frozen section evaluation. An algorithmic approach is cost-effective and efficient especially in *BRAF* mutation prevalent populations.

Acknowledgments: This paper was supported by Konkuk University. The authors thank Chan-Kwon Jung (Department of Pathology, College of Medicine, The Catholic University, Seoul, Korea) for reviewing thyroid tissue slides.

Author Contributions: Young Sin Ko designed the experiments, conducted the main experiments and prepared the manuscript; Tae Sook Hwang conceived and designed the experiments and revised the manuscript; Ja Yeon Kim also conducted the main experiments and analyzed the data; Seung Eun Lee conducted Nanostring and analyzed the data; Yoon-La Choi, Hye Seung Han, Wan Seop Kim, Suk Kyeong Kim, and Kyoung Sik Park contributed clarifications and guidance on the manuscript. All authors read and approved the manuscript.

Abbreviations

AUS	Atypia of undetermined significance
C_t	Threshold cycle
FFPE	Formalin-fixed paraffin-embedded
FN	Follicular neoplasm;
FNA	Fine needle aspiration
FLUS	Follicular lesion of undetermined significance
FVPTC	Follicular variant of papillary thyroid carcinoma
FTC	Follicular thyroid carcinoma
NGS	Next generation sequencing
RT-PCR	Real-time reverse transcription-polymerase chain reaction
SFN	Suspicious for follicular neoplasm
PTC	Papillary thyroid carcinoma
TPC1	Thyroid papillary carcinoma 1

References

1. Vander, J.B.; Gaston, E.A.; Dawber, T.R. The significance of nontoxic thyroid nodules. Final report of a 15-year study of the incidence of thyroid malignancy. *Ann. Intern. Med.* **1968**, *69*, 537–540. [CrossRef] [PubMed]
2. Tunbridge, W.M.; Evered, D.C.; Hall, R.; Appleton, D.; Brewis, M.; Clark, F.; Evans, J.G.; Young, E.; Bird, T.; Smith, P.A. The spectrum of thyroid disease in a community: The whickham survey. *Clin. Endocrinol.* **1977**, *7*, 481–493. [CrossRef]
3. Tan, G.H.; Gharib, H. Thyroid incidentalomas: Management approaches to nonpalpable nodules discovered incidentally on thyroid imaging. *Ann. Intern. Med.* **1997**, *126*, 226–231. [CrossRef] [PubMed]
4. Guth, S.; Theune, U.; Aberle, J.; Galach, A.; Bamberger, C.M. Very high prevalence of thyroid nodules detected by high frequency (13 MHz) ultrasound examination. *Eur. J. Clin. Investig.* **2009**, *39*, 699–706. [CrossRef] [PubMed]
5. Hegedus, L. Clinical practice. The thyroid nodule. *N. Engl. J. Med.* **2004**, *351*, 1764–1771. [CrossRef] [PubMed]
6. Mandel, S.J. A 64-year-old woman with a thyroid nodule. *JAMA* **2004**, *292*, 2632–2642. [CrossRef] [PubMed]
7. Sherman, S.I. Thyroid carcinoma. *Lancet* **2003**, *361*, 501–511. [CrossRef]
8. Siegel, R.; Ma, J.; Zou, Z.; Jemal, A. Cancer statistics, 2014. *CA Cancer J. Clin.* **2014**, *64*, 9–29. [CrossRef] [PubMed]
9. Davies, L.; Welch, H.G. Current thyroid cancer trends in the United States. *JAMA Otolaryngol. Head Neck Surg.* **2014**, *140*, 317–322. [CrossRef] [PubMed]
10. *National Cancer Registration and Statistics in Korea 2015*; Korea Central Cancer Registry: Goyang, Korea, 2015.
11. Gharib, H.; Goellner, J.R. Fine-needle aspiration biopsy of the thyroid: An appraisal. *Ann. Intern. Med.* **1993**, *118*, 282–289. [CrossRef] [PubMed]
12. Udelsman, R.; Chen, H. The current management of thyroid cancer. *Adv. Surg.* **1999**, *33*, 1–27. [PubMed]
13. Haugen, B.R.; Alexander, E.K.; Bible, K.C.; Doherty, G.M.; Mandel, S.J.; Nikiforov, Y.E.; Pacini, F.; Randolph, G.W.; Sawka, A.M.; Schlumberger, M.; et al. 2015 American thyroid association management guidelines for adult patients with thyroid nodules and differentiated thyroid cancer: The American thyroid association guidelines task force on thyroid nodules and differentiated thyroid cancer. *Thyroid* **2016**, *26*, 1–133. [CrossRef] [PubMed]
14. Goutas, N.; Vlachodimitropoulos, D.; Bouka, M.; Lazaris, A.C.; Nasioulas, G.; Gazouli, M. BRAF and K-RAS mutation in a Greek papillary and medullary thyroid carcinoma cohort. *Anticancer Res.* **2008**, *28*, 305–308. [PubMed]
15. Kim, S.K.; Song, K.H.; Lim, S.D.; Lim, Y.C.; Yoo, Y.B.; Kim, J.S.; Hwang, T.S. Clinical and pathological features and the $BRAF^{V600E}$ mutation in patients with papillary thyroid carcinoma with and without concurrent hashimoto thyroiditis. *Thyroid* **2009**, *19*, 137–141. [CrossRef] [PubMed]

16. Davies, L.; Welch, H.G. Increasing incidence of thyroid cancer in the United States, 1973–2002. *JAMA* **2006**, *295*, 2164–2167. [CrossRef] [PubMed]
17. Jung, C.K.; Little, M.P.; Lubin, J.H.; Brenner, A.V.; Wells, S.A., Jr.; Sigurdson, A.J.; Nikiforov, Y.E. The increase in thyroid cancer incidence during the last four decades is accompanied by a high frequency of BRAF mutations and a sharp increase in RAS mutations. *J. Clin. Endocrinol. Metab.* **2014**, *99*, E276–E285. [CrossRef] [PubMed]
18. Park, J.Y.; Kim, W.Y.; Hwang, T.S.; Lee, S.S.; Kim, H.; Han, H.S.; Lim, S.D.; Kim, W.S.; Yoo, Y.B.; Park, K.S. BRAF and RAS mutations in follicular variants of papillary thyroid carcinoma. *Endocr. Pathol.* **2013**, *24*, 69–76. [CrossRef] [PubMed]
19. Lee, S.R.; Jung, C.K.; Kim, T.E.; Bae, J.S.; Jung, S.L.; Choi, Y.J.; Kang, C.S. Molecular genotyping of follicular variant of papillary thyroid carcinoma correlates with diagnostic category of fine-needle aspiration cytology: Values of RAS mutation testing. *Thyroid* **2013**, *23*, 1416–1422. [CrossRef] [PubMed]
20. Bongarzone, I.; Butti, M.G.; Coronelli, S.; Borrello, M.G.; Santoro, M.; Mondellini, P.; Pilotti, S.; Fusco, A.; Della Porta, G.; Pierotti, M.A. Frequent activation of ret protooncogene by fusion with a new activating gene in papillary thyroid carcinomas. *Cancer Res.* **1994**, *54*, 2979–2985. [PubMed]
21. Bongarzone, I.; Monzini, N.; Borrello, M.G.; Carcano, C.; Ferraresi, G.; Arighi, E.; Mondellini, P.; Della Porta, G.; Pierotti, M.A. Molecular characterization of a thyroid tumor-specific transforming sequence formed by the fusion of ret tyrosine kinase and the regulatory subunit RI α of cyclic AMP-dependent protein kinase A. *Mol. Cell. Biol.* **1993**, *13*, 358–366. [CrossRef] [PubMed]
22. Grieco, M.; Santoro, M.; Berlingieri, M.T.; Melillo, R.M.; Donghi, R.; Bongarzone, I.; Pierotti, M.A.; Della Porta, G.; Fusco, A.; Vecchio, G. PTC is a novel rearranged form of the RET proto-oncogene and is frequently detected in vivo in human thyroid papillary carcinomas. *Cell* **1990**, *60*, 557–563. [CrossRef]
23. Jhiang, S.M.; Smanik, P.A.; Mazzaferri, E.L. Development of a single-step duplex RT-PCR detecting different forms of RET activation, and identification of the third form of in vivo ret activation in human papillary thyroid carcinoma. *Cancer Lett.* **1994**, *78*, 69–76. [CrossRef]
24. Santoro, M.; Dathan, N.A.; Berlingieri, M.T.; Bongarzone, I.; Paulin, C.; Grieco, M.; Pierotti, M.A.; Vecchio, G.; Fusco, A. Molecular characterization of RET/PTC3; a novel rearranged version of the retproto-oncogene in a human thyroid papillary carcinoma. *Oncogene* **1994**, *9*, 509–516. [PubMed]
25. Fenton, C.L.; Lukes, Y.; Nicholson, D.; Dinauer, C.A.; Francis, G.L.; Tuttle, R.M. The RET/PTC mutations are common in sporadic papillary thyroid carcinoma of children and young adults. *J. Clin. Endocrinol. Metab.* **2000**, *85*, 1170–1175. [CrossRef] [PubMed]
26. Rabes, H.M.; Demidchik, E.P.; Sidorow, J.D.; Lengfelder, E.; Beimfohr, C.; Hoelzel, D.; Klugbauer, S. Pattern of radiation-induced ret and NTRK1 rearrangements in 191 post-chernobyl papillary thyroid carcinomas: Biological, phenotypic, and clinical implications. *Clin. Cancer Res.* **2000**, *6*, 1093–1103. [PubMed]
27. Unger, K.; Zitzelsberger, H.; Salvatore, G.; Santoro, M.; Bogdanova, T.; Braselmann, H.; Kastner, P.; Zurnadzhy, L.; Tronko, N.; Hutzler, P.; et al. Heterogeneity in the distribution of RET/PTC rearrangements within individual post-chernobyl papillary thyroid carcinomas. *J. Clin. Endocrinol. Metab.* **2004**, *89*, 4272–4279. [CrossRef] [PubMed]
28. Zhu, Z.; Ciampi, R.; Nikiforova, M.N.; Gandhi, M.; Nikiforov, Y.E. Prevalence of RET/PTC rearrangements in thyroid papillary carcinomas: Effects of the detection methods and genetic heterogeneity. *J. Clin. Endocrinol. Metab.* **2006**, *91*, 3603–3610. [CrossRef] [PubMed]
29. Namba, H.; Yamashita, S.; Pei, H.C.; Ishikawa, N.; Villadolid, M.C.; Tominaga, T.; Kimura, H.; Tsuruta, M.; Yokoyama, N.; Izumi, M.; et al. Lack of *PTC* gene (RET proto-oncogene rearrangement) in human thyroid tumors. *Endocrinol. Jpn.* **1991**, *38*, 627–632. [CrossRef] [PubMed]
30. Nikiforov, Y.E.; Rowland, J.M.; Bove, K.E.; Monforte-Munoz, H.; Fagin, J.A. Distinct pattern of RET oncogene rearrangements in morphological variants of radiation-induced and sporadic thyroid papillary carcinomas in children. *Cancer Res.* **1997**, *57*, 1690–1694. [PubMed]
31. Park, K.Y.; Koh, J.M.; Kim, Y.I.; Park, H.J.; Gong, G.; Hong, S.J.; Ahn, I.M. Prevalences of GS α, ras, p53 mutations and RET/PTC rearrangement in differentiated thyroid tumours in a Korean population. *Clin. Endocrinol.* **1998**, *49*, 317–323. [CrossRef]
32. Lee, C.H.; Hsu, L.S.; Chi, C.W.; Chen, G.D.; Yang, A.H.; Chen, J.Y. High frequency of rearrangement of the ret protooncogene (RET/PTC) in chinese papillary thyroid carcinomas. *J. Clin. Endocrinol. Metab.* **1998**, *83*, 1629–1632. [CrossRef] [PubMed]

33. Rhoden, K.J.; Johnson, C.; Brandao, G.; Howe, J.G.; Smith, B.R.; Tallini, G. Real-time quantitative RT-PCR identifies distinct C-RET, RET/PTC1 and RET/PTC3 expression patterns in papillary thyroid carcinoma. *Lab. Investig.* **2004**, *84*, 1557–1570. [CrossRef] [PubMed]
34. Di Cristofaro, J.; Vasko, V.; Savchenko, V.; Cherenko, S.; Larin, A.; Ringel, M.D.; Saji, M.; Marcy, M.; Henry, J.F.; Carayon, P.; et al. Ret/PTC1 and RET/PTC3 in thyroid tumors from chernobyl liquidators: Comparison with sporadic tumors from ukrainian and french patients. *Endocr. Relat. Cancer* **2005**, *12*, 173–183. [CrossRef] [PubMed]
35. Mayr, B.; Potter, E.; Goretzki, P.; Ruschoff, J.; Dietmaier, W.; Hoang-Vu, C.; Dralle, H.; Brabant, G. Expression of RET/PTC1, -2, -3, -Δ3 and -4 in German papillary thyroid carcinoma. *Br. J. Cancer* **1998**, *77*, 903–906. [CrossRef] [PubMed]
36. Nikiforov, Y.E. RET/PTC rearrangement in thyroid tumors. *Endocr. Pathol.* **2002**, *13*, 3–16. [CrossRef] [PubMed]
37. Tallini, G.; Asa, S.L. Ret oncogene activation in papillary thyroid carcinoma. *Adv. Anat. Pathol.* **2001**, *8*, 345–354. [CrossRef] [PubMed]
38. Chung, J.H.; Hahm, J.R.; Min, Y.K.; Lee, M.S.; Lee, M.K.; Kim, K.W.; Nam, S.J.; Yang, J.H.; Ree, H.J. Detection of RET/PTC oncogene rearrangements in Korean papillary thyroid carcinomas. *Thyroid* **1999**, *9*, 1237–1243. [CrossRef] [PubMed]
39. Motomura, T.; Nikiforov, Y.E.; Namba, H.; Ashizawa, K.; Nagataki, S.; Yamashita, S.; Fagin, J.A. Ret rearrangements in Japanese pediatric and adult papillary thyroid cancers. *Thyroid* **1998**, *8*, 485–489. [CrossRef] [PubMed]
40. Guerra, A.; Sapio, M.R.; Marotta, V.; Campanile, E.; Moretti, M.I.; Deandrea, M.; Motta, M.; Limone, P.P.; Fenzi, G.; Rossi, G.; et al. Prevalence of RET/PTC rearrangement in benign and malignant thyroid nodules and its clinical application. *Endocr. J.* **2011**, *58*, 31–38. [CrossRef] [PubMed]
41. Marotta, V.; Guerra, A.; Sapio, M.R.; Campanile, E.; Motta, M.; Fenzi, G.; Rossi, G.; Vitale, M. Growing thyroid nodules with benign histology and RET rearrangement. *Endocr. J.* **2010**, *57*, 1081–1087. [CrossRef] [PubMed]
42. Sapio, M.R.; Guerra, A.; Marotta, V.; Campanile, E.; Formisano, R.; Deandrea, M.; Motta, M.; Limone, P.P.; Fenzi, G.; Rossi, G.; et al. High growth rate of benign thyroid nodules bearing RET/PTC rearrangements. *J. Clin. Endocrinol. Metab.* **2011**, *96*, E916–E919. [CrossRef] [PubMed]
43. Eszlinger, M.; Krogdahl, A.; Munz, S.; Rehfeld, C.; Precht Jensen, E.M.; Ferraz, C.; Bosenberg, E.; Drieschner, N.; Scholz, M.; Hegedus, L.; et al. Impact of molecular screening for point mutations and rearrangements in routine air-dried fine-needle aspiration samples of thyroid nodules. *Thyroid* **2014**, *24*, 305–313. [CrossRef] [PubMed]
44. Ferraz, C.; Rehfeld, C.; Krogdahl, A.; Precht Jensen, E.M.; Bosenberg, E.; Narz, F.; Hegedus, L.; Paschke, R.; Eszlinger, M. Detection of PAX8/PPARG and RET/PTC rearrangements is feasible in routine air-dried fine needle aspiration smears. *Thyroid* **2012**, *22*, 1025–1030. [CrossRef] [PubMed]
45. Cheung, C.C.; Carydis, B.; Ezzat, S.; Bedard, Y.C.; Asa, S.L. Analysis of RET/PTC gene rearrangements refines the fine needle aspiration diagnosis of thyroid cancer. *J. Clin. Endocrinol. Metab.* **2001**, *86*, 2187–2190. [CrossRef] [PubMed]
46. Musholt, T.J.; Fottner, C.; Weber, M.M.; Eichhorn, W.; Pohlenz, J.; Musholt, P.B.; Springer, E.; Schad, A. Detection of papillary thyroid carcinoma by analysis of BRAF and RET/PTC1 mutations in fine-needle aspiration biopsies of thyroid nodules. *World J. Surg.* **2010**, *34*, 2595–2603. [CrossRef] [PubMed]
47. Nikiforov, Y.E.; Steward, D.L.; Robinson-Smith, T.M.; Haugen, B.R.; Klopper, J.P.; Zhu, Z.; Fagin, J.A.; Falciglia, M.; Weber, K.; Nikiforova, M.N. Molecular testing for mutations in improving the fine-needle aspiration diagnosis of thyroid nodules. *J. Clin. Endocrinol. Metab.* **2009**, *94*, 2092–2098. [CrossRef] [PubMed]
48. Salvatore, G.; Giannini, R.; Faviana, P.; Caleo, A.; Migliaccio, I.; Fagin, J.A.; Nikiforov, Y.E.; Troncone, G.; Palombini, L.; Basolo, F.; et al. Analysis of BRAF point mutation and RET/PTC rearrangement refines the fine-needle aspiration diagnosis of papillary thyroid carcinoma. *J. Clin. Endocrinol. Metab.* **2004**, *89*, 5175–5180. [CrossRef] [PubMed]
49. An, J.H.; Song, K.H.; Kim, S.K.; Park, K.S.; Yoo, Y.B.; Yang, J.H.; Hwang, T.S.; Kim, D.L. Ras mutations in indeterminate thyroid nodules are predictive of the follicular variant of papillary thyroid carcinoma. *Clin. Endocrinol.* **2015**, *82*, 760–766. [CrossRef] [PubMed]

50. Hwang, T.S.; Kim, W.Y.; Han, H.S.; Lim, S.D.; Kim, W.S.; Yoo, Y.B.; Park, K.S.; Oh, S.Y.; Kim, S.K.; Yang, J.H. Preoperative RAS mutational analysis is of great value in predicting follicular variant of papillary thyroid carcinoma. *BioMed Res. Int.* **2015**, *2015*, 697068. [CrossRef] [PubMed]

51. Kim, S.K.; Kim, D.L.; Han, H.S.; Kim, W.S.; Kim, S.J.; Moon, W.J.; Oh, S.Y.; Hwang, T.S. Pyrosequencing analysis for detection of a $BRAF^{V600E}$ mutation in an fnab specimen of thyroid nodules. *Diagn. Mol. Pathol.* **2008**, *17*, 118–125. [CrossRef] [PubMed]

52. Cantara, S.; Capezzone, M.; Marchisotta, S.; Capuano, S.; Busonero, G.; Toti, P.; Di Santo, A.; Caruso, G.; Carli, A.F.; Brilli, L.; et al. Impact of proto-oncogene mutation detection in cytological specimens from thyroid nodules improves the diagnostic accuracy of cytology. *J. Clin. Endocrinol. Metab.* **2010**, *95*, 1365–1369. [CrossRef] [PubMed]

53. Ohori, N.P.; Nikiforova, M.N.; Schoedel, K.E.; LeBeau, S.O.; Hodak, S.P.; Seethala, R.R.; Carty, S.E.; Ogilvie, J.B.; Yip, L.; Nikiforov, Y.E. Contribution of molecular testing to thyroid fine-needle aspiration cytology of "follicular lesion of undetermined significance/atypia of undetermined significance". *Cancer Cytopathol.* **2010**, *118*, 17–23. [CrossRef] [PubMed]

54. Kulkarni, M.M. Digital multiplexed gene expression analysis using the nanostring ncounter system. *Curr. Protoc. Mol. Biol.* **2011**. [CrossRef]

14

Expression of Tenascin C, EGFR, E-Cadherin and TTF-1 in Medullary Thyroid Carcinoma and the Correlation with RET Mutation Status

Florian Steiner [1], Cornelia Hauser-Kronberger [1], Gundula Rendl [2], Margarida Rodrigues [2] and Christian Pirich [2,*]

[1] Department of Pathology, Paracelsus Medical University Salzburg, Müllner Hauptstrasse 48, A-5020 Salzburg, Austria; f.steiner@salk.at (F.S.); c.hauser-kronberger@salk.at (C.H.-K.)

[2] Department of Nuclear Medicine and Endocrinology, Paracelsus Medical University Salzburg, Müllner Hauptstrasse 48, A-5020 Salzburg, Austria; g.rendl@salk.at (G.R.); rodriguesradischat@hotmail.com (M.R.)

* Correspondence: c.pirich@salk.at

Academic Editor: Daniela Gabriele Grimm

Abstract: Tenascin C expression correlates with tumor grade and indicates worse prognosis in several tumors. Epidermal growth factor receptor (EGFR) plays an important role in driving proliferation in many tumors. Loss of E-cadherin function is associated with tumor invasion and metastasis. Thyroid transcription factor-1 (TTF-1) is involved in rearranged during transfection (RET) transcription in Hirschsprung's disease. Tenascin C, EGFR, E-cadherin, TTF-1-expression, and their correlations with RET mutation status were investigated in 30 patients with medullary thyroid carcinoma (MTC) (n = 26) or C-cell hyperplasia (n = 4). Tenascin C was found in all, EGFR in 4/26, E-cadherin in 23/26, and TTF-1 in 25/26 MTC. Tenascin C correlated significantly with tumor proliferation (overall, $r = 0.61$, $p < 0.005$; RET-mutated, $r = 0.81$, $p < 0.01$). E-cadherin showed weak correlation, whereas EGFR and TTF-1 showed no significant correlation with tumor proliferation. EGFR, E-cadherin, and TTF-1 showed weak correlation with proliferation of RET-mutated tumors. Correlation between TTF-1 and tenascin C, E-cadherin, and EGFR was $r = -0.10$, 0.37, and 0.21, respectively. In conclusion, MTC express tenascin C, E-cadherin, and TTF-1. Tenascin C correlates significantly with tumor proliferation, especially in RET-mutated tumors. EGFR is low, and tumors expressing EGFR do not exhibit higher proliferation. TTF-1 does not correlate with RET mutation status and has a weak correlation with tenascin C, E-cadherin, and EGFR expression.

Keywords: tenascin C; epidermal growth factor receptor (EGFR); E-cadherin; thyroid transcription factor-1 (TTF-1); medullary thyroid carcinoma

---

1. Introduction

Medullary thyroid carcinoma (MTC) may arise sporadically in about 75% of cases or as part of multiple endocrine neoplasia type 2 (MEN2) syndrome in 20%–25% of cases [1]. MEN 2 syndromes are caused by activating mutations of the proto-oncogene rearranged during transfection (RET) [2]. On the other hand, a loss of function mutation of RET leads to Hirschsprung's disease [3].

Tenascin C is an extracellular glycoprotein complex expressed by a variety of cells including epithelial, stromal, and tumor cells [4]. It is overexpressed in a wide variety of tumors including gliomas, where it was originally discovered [5]. In most cases, the expression of tenascin C correlates with the tumor grade and is indicative of a worse prognosis [6]. Koperek et al. [7] found tenascin C expression in medullary microcarcinoma and C-cell hyperplasia and suggested that stromal tenascin C expression seems to be an indicator of a further step in carcinogenesis of MTC, irrespective of a RET germ-line mutation.

Mutations of epidermal growth factor receptor (EGFR) have been found in several tumor entities including gliomas, breast cancer, and non-small lung cancer [8]. In the case of MTC, mutations are rarely found, and their significance is unknown [9]. Rodríguez-Antona et al. [9] showed that EGFR overexpression in MTC is seen in as many as 13% of tumors and that metastases show stronger positivity than primary tumors. Furthermore, EGFR overexpression is linked to RET activation. However, in the presence of RET, EGFR does not appear to play an important role in signaling [10].

Loss of function of the molecule E-cadherin in tumors is associated with invasion and metastasis [11,12]. Naito et al. [13] found that expression of E-cadherin was reduced or absent in 50% or more of thyroid cancer cases, and concluded that this loss of E-cadherin expression may be involved in regional lymph node metastasis and in malignant potential of thyroid neoplasms.

Thyroid transcription factor-1 (TTF-1) is involved in gene expression of thyroperoxidase [14] and thyreoglobulin [15]. TTF-1 expression is seen in follicular cell neoplasms [16] as well as in MTC [17]. In the parafollicular cells of MTC, TTF-1 modulates the activity of genes involved in calcium homeostasis [18]. It was recently shown that TTF-1 is also involved in the transcription of human RET in Hirschsprung's disease [19].

In MTC, the Ki-67 index correlates with the stage of the disease [20]. Primary tumors that had metastasized were found to have higher Ki-67 indices than primary tumors that had not metastasized. Recurrent lymph node metastases were shown to have higher Ki-67 indices than the primary tumors. The Ki-67 index can therefore be used as a prognostic marker in MTC.

In this study, we investigated the expression of tenascin C, EGFR, E-cadherin, and TTF-1 in MTC, and their correlation with RET mutation status. Furthermore, EGFR mutation status in MTC was evaluated.

2. Results

Tenascin C showed positive staining results in all the 26 tumors (Figure 1). In contrast, all four cases of C-cell hyperplasia stained negative for tenascin C. The tumor-staining pattern was homogeneously located in all areas of the tumor. However, 14 out of 26 tumors showed expression in the whole tumor field, with the remaining 12 tumors showing partial expression. Except for one case that showed much stronger staining in the periphery, no predominance for tumor center or invasion front could be detected.

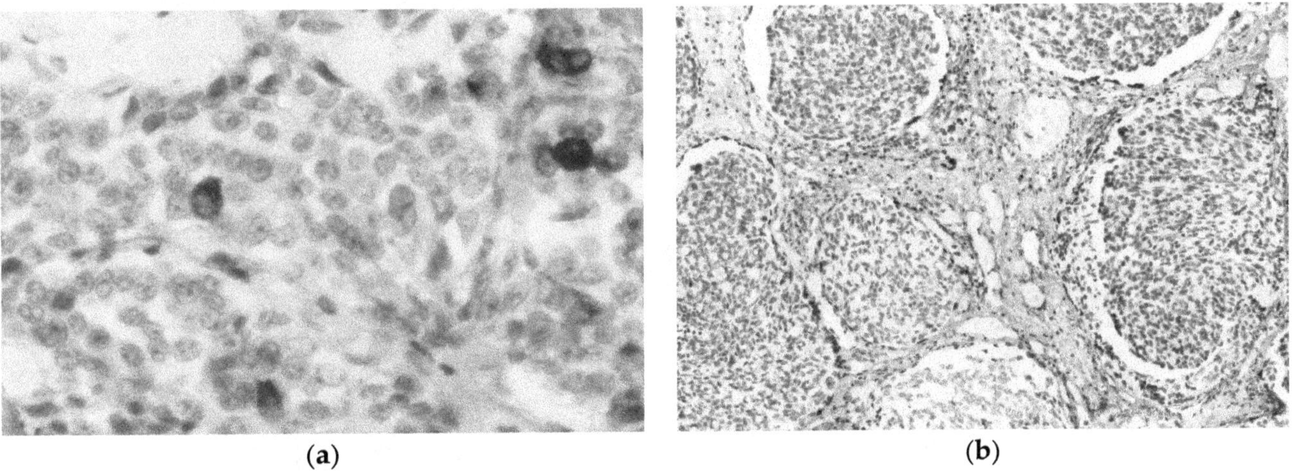

(a) (b)

Figure 1. Staining results of tenascin C: (**a**) 40× magnification, showing cytoplasmic staining; (**b**) 10× magnification, depicting staining of the extracellular matrix and the lymph follicle-like accumulation of tumor cells.

Expression of tenascin C was primarily located in the extracellular matrix but also in the plasma membrane and the cytoplasm of parafollicular cells. In areas of lymphocyte infiltration expression levels of tenascin C were particularly high. In non-pathological areas, staining was observed in endothelial cells of blood vessels. The average immunoreactivity score for tenascin C staining was 4.69 ± 2.18. The score ranged from 0 (all negative stained samples) to a maximum score of 7.5.

Staining with E-cadherin showed positive expression in 27 out of 30 cases. However, highest expression was observed in three cases of C-cell hyperplasia, while one case of C-cell hyperplasia showed no staining. Expression of E-cadherin was particularly high in the thyroid follicles. Altogether staining in all areas of the tumor was observed in 15 cases of MTC, with 8 MTC cases showing partial expression and 3 MTC cases showing no expression at all. There were no significant differences in E-cadherin expression between MTC and C-cell hyperplasia. As expected form a membrane bound protein, E-cadherin expression was primarily observed in the plasma membrane of cells (Figure 2). Immunoreactivity scores in E-cadherin samples ranged from 1 to 9 (full range) with a mean score of 4.69 ± 2.4.

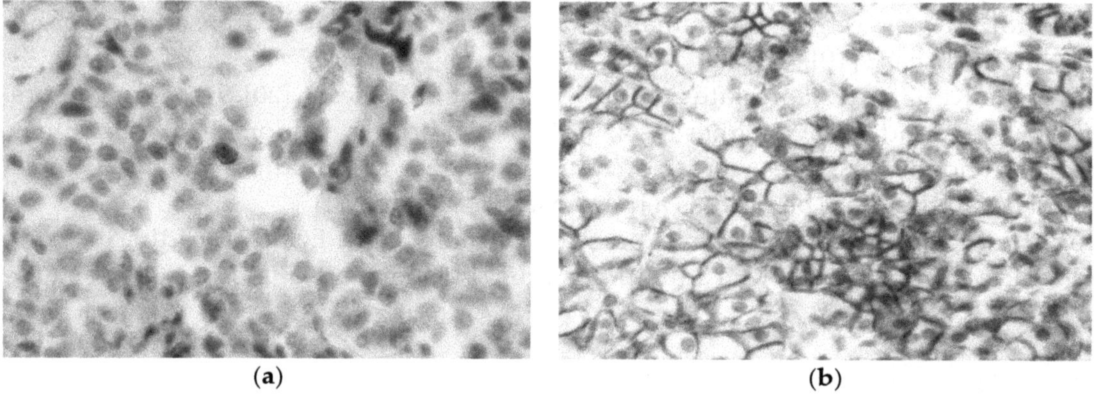

(a) (b)

Figure 2. (**a**) 40× magnification, depicting the staining results of Ki-67 (note the proliferating cell in the center); (**b**) 40× magnification, showing strong plasma-membrane expression of E-cadherin.

EGFR expression was very weak, with six positively stained cases consisting of four cases of MTC and two cases of C-cell hyperplasia. Staining was primarily found in the cytoplasm of cells and endothelial cells. The highest staining intensity was found in non-neoplastic follicular cells scattered amid the tumor mass (Figure 3). Inside the tumor area, staining was relatively weak. The mean immunoreactivity score was 1.58 ± 1.20.

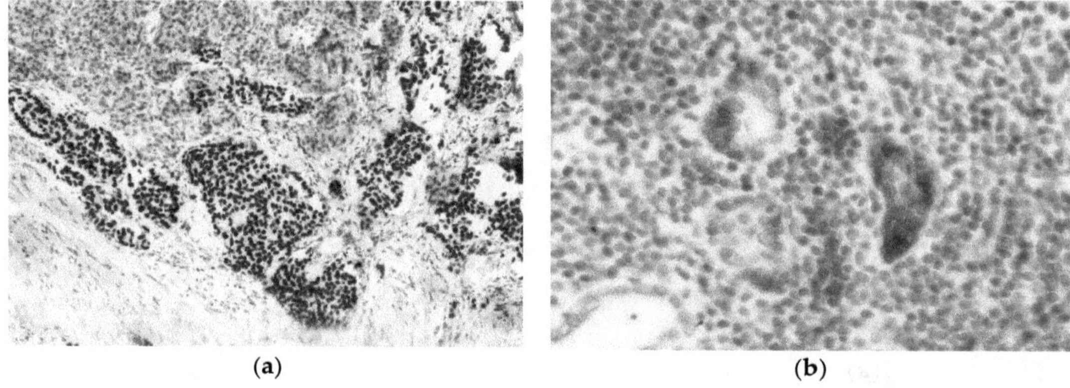

(a) (b)

Figure 3. (**a**) 10× magnification, showing thyroid transcription factor-1 (TTF-1) expression in a metastasis in a Meckel's diverticulum; (**b**) 40× magnification, illustrating epidermal growth factor receptor (EGFR) expression in follicular cells scattered between medullary thyroid carcinoma (MTC) cells.

With exception of the metastasis to the adrenal gland all tissue samples, including the metastasis in a Meckel's diverticulum showed TTF-1 expression (Figure 3). The entire tumor area and all of the follicles showed strong staining with the TTF-1 antibody. The samples only differed in the staining intensity, which was moderate to strong. The mean immunoreactivity score was 7.77 ± 1.89.

The staining results for the proliferation marker Ki-67 showed positive staining results in all 30 samples. As expected, protein expression was only seen in the nucleus (Figure 2). Immunoreactivity scores ranged from 1.5 to 6.75 after correction with the correlation coefficient. The mean score was 3.35 ± 1.57. The four cases of C-cell hyperplasia had the lowest Ki-67 expression ($p < 0.001$) with only 1–2 cells per high power field. Tenascin C expression correlated moderately to strongly with the level of the proliferation marker Ki-67 in the tumor tissue. A weak correlation could be observed with E-cadherin, whereas EGFR and TTF-1 showed no significant correlation (Table 1).

Table 1. Correlation of tenascin C, EGFR, E-cadherin, and TTF-1 expression with the proliferation marker Ki-67.

MTC	Tenascin C	EGFR	E-Cadherin	TTF-1
Overall MTC				
r-value	0.61	−0.04	−0.19	0.13
p-value	<0.005	ns	<0.05	ns
RET-mutated MTC				
r-value	0.81	0.14	−0.11	−0.12
p-value	<0.01	ns	ns	ns
Wild-type MTC				
r-value	0.08	–	−0.40	0.72
p-value	ns	–	ns	<0.001

EGFR: epidermal growth factor receptor; TTF-1: thyroid transcription factor-1; MTC: medullary thyroid carcinoma; RET: rearranged during transfection; *r*: Pearson correlation coefficient; *p*: probability of obtaining a positive test result; ns: not significant.

All 15 tumors that showed RET mutation were analyzed regarding their expression of tenascin C, EGFR, E-cadherin, and TTF-1. They were then correlated with the proliferation marker Ki-67. Tenascin C expression showed a very strong correlation with the proliferation of RET-mutated tumors, while EGFR, E-cadherin, and TTF-1 showed a very weak correlation (Table 1).

The group of RET-mutated tumors was then split in germ-line-mutated ($n = 7$) and somatic-mutated ($n = 8$) tumors. Expression profiles of both groups were then correlated with proliferation in those tumors. In the case of the germ-line-mutated tumors, tenascin C expression correlated highly ($r = 0.86$) with proliferation. A weak correlation could be observed with E-cadherin and TTF-1 ($r = -0.26$ and -0.33, respectively), whereas EGFR only showed a very weak correlation ($r = -0.11$). In the case of MTC with somatic RET mutation, tenascin C still showed a moderate-to-strong correlation with proliferation ($r = 0.67$). EGFR correlation with proliferation was moderate ($r = 0.51$), while E-cadherin and TTF-1 showed low ($r = 0.39$) and very low correlations ($r = 0.02$), respectively.

MTC with RET wild-type were also investigated. Tenascin C showed a very weak correlation, E-cadherin a weak to moderate correlation, and TTF-1 a strong correlation with tumor proliferation (Table 1). EGFR analysis was not performed in this group because none of the specimens showed positivity for EGFR. Only EGFR expression differed significantly between RET-mutated and RET wild-type tumors ($r = 0.51$, $p = 0.001$). Tenascin C, E-cadherin, and TTF-1 did not differ in their respective expression levels.

RET-mutated and wild-type tumors were compared to evaluate whether the mutation status of RET affects TTF-1 expression. No significant difference in TTF-1 expression was found between both groups. RET-mutated MTC showed no correlation with TTF-1 expression for germ-line- and somatic-mutated tumors ($r = -0.33$ and 0.02, respectively, p-value is not significant (p ns)). TTF-1 expression correlated with tenascin C, EGFR, and E-cadherin expression. Tenascin C correlation was very weak ($r = -0.10$, p ns), while the EGFR and E-cadherin correlation was weak ($r = 0.37$ and 0.21, respectively, p ns).

EGFR positively stained tumors (all RET wild-type) did not show a significantly higher Ki-67 index, as compared with EGFR negatively stained tumors.

A weak to moderate correlation ($r = 0.08$–0.40, p ns) between calcitonin levels and Ki-67 was found. Preoperative calcitonin levels only showed a weak correlation with tenascin C expression ($r = 0.18$, $p < 0.05$) and Ki-67 ($r = 0.10$, p ns). Post-operative calcitonin levels correlated moderately with tenascin C expression ($r = 0.53$, $p < 0.005$) and Ki-67 ($r = 0.40$, p ns). Except for the inverse correlation for EGFR ($r = -0.38$, $p < 0.05$), post-operative calcitonin levels showed weak to no correlation with E-cadherin, TTF-1, and EGFR expression ($r = 0.22$, 0.08 and 0.07, respectively, p ns).

Both pre-operative and post-operative calcitonin levels were not significantly different between RET-mutated and wild-type tumors.

3. Discussion

In this study, we found tenascin C expression in all MTC, but in none of the C-cell hyperplasia cases. Tenascin C was primarily located in the stromal areas of tumors, but could also be detected in the cytoplasm and plasma membrane. Our results are in agreement with the findings by Koperek et al. [7] of tenascin C expression in all cases of MTC and in only 52% of C-cell hyperplasia cases. The difference in tenascin C expression in C-cell hyperplasia is most likely due to the larger study group used by Koperek et al. Our study cohort included only 30 patients because of the rarity of the disease. Furthermore, we investigated only four C-cell hyperplasia and two MTC metastases. The relationship between tenascin C expression and tumor proliferation needs to be further investigated. It seems that RET mutation is associated with a higher level of tenascin C expression, even though we found no significant difference between RET-mutated and wild-type MTC. It might be that, with a larger study cohort, a significant difference between RET-mutated and wild-type MTC could be established. Furthermore, it seems that the bc-24 clone used for tenascin C staining does not uniquely bind to tenascin C, but to other tenascin subtypes over the EGF-like repeats. Therefore, the results might not solely represent tenascin C, but also the expression of other tenascin isoforms.

EGFR plays an important role in driving proliferation in a variety of tumors [8]. In the study of Rodriguez-Antona et al. [9], EGFR expression was shown in a subset of 18 tumors, and it was thus concluded that EGFR might be a target for drug therapy. We therefore evaluated if MTC expresses EGFR and, if so, to what degree. In our study, EGFR expression could be detected in six cases (15%), with few staining cells and scattered expression. Our results are consistent with the reported EGFR expression of 9% and 35% in primary MTC and metastasis, respectively. Additionally, it seems that EGFR expression is significantly higher in MTC carrying a RET mutation [9]. Due to these reports, we performed EGFR mutation analysis on three cases with the highest EGFR expression. However, no mutations could be detected using the Cobas® EGFR mutation analysis kit. Our results are consistent with the finding by Rodriguez-Antona et al. [9] of nucleotide changes of unknown significance in only one sample. It thus seems that, although some EGFR expression can be detected, the role of EGFR in MTC is of a minor nature. Therefore, the absence of activating mutations questions the use of EGFR inhibitor drugs. This suggestion is further backed by Vitagliano et al. [21], who found that EGFR downstream signaling is of minor significance in the presence of active RET.

We also looked at the expression of E-cadherin, a plasma membrane protein important for cell–cell adhesion [11,12]. In our findings, E-cadherin showed staining in 26 cases of MTC (87%). The remaining samples showed no staining including one case of C-cell hyperplasia. Naito et al. [13] reported that low E-cadherin expression was associated with a higher malignant potential as well as regional lymph node metastasis. We therefore compared the expression levels of E-cadherin in C-cell hyperplasia and MTC, which showed no statistical significance. This is probably due to the small number of cases with C-cell hyperplasia in our study cohort.

In our study, with the exception of a metastasis in the adrenal gland, TTF-1 staining was moderate to strong in all tissue samples. We also found TTF-1 expression in a metastasis in a Meckel's diverticulum. These data seem to indicate that TTF-1 can be used as a useful marker for detecting primary MTC or metastasis, as previously suggested by Katho et al. [17].

The expression of the proliferation marker Ki-67 was generally low in our study cohort. As expected, C-cell hyperplasia showed the lowest Ki-67 indices, which were significantly lower than those found in MTC. Ishihara et al. [22] reported that breast cancers staining positive for tenascin carried a less favorable prognosis. We therefore evaluated if the expression of tenascin C in MTC correlates with tumor proliferation. We found that the Ki-67 index correlated moderately to strong with tenascin C expression. It might therefore be that tenascin C expression can be used as a marker for the malignant potential of a MTC. On the other hand, we observed that E-cadherin shows weak inverse correlation to tumor proliferation. As previously found by Naito et al. [13], low E-cadherin expression correlates with higher malignant potential of the tumor. This might also be true for our study group, but the size of our cohort may be a limiting factor.

The RET proto-oncogene is an important molecule in the development of MTC. We investigated if RET mutation correlates with a higher expression of tenascin C, EGFR, E-cadherin, or TTF-1. Furthermore, we evaluated whether proliferation is higher in RET-mutated MTC. We found that tenascin C expression in RET-mutated tumors showed a high correlation to proliferation. However, except for a significantly higher degree of EGFR expression in RET wild-type tumors, no significant difference in the expression of E-cadherin or TTF-1 could be detected between RET-mutated and wild-type MTC. Rodriguez-Antona et al. [9] also found that EGFR expression was higher in RET-mutated tumors, depending on the localization of the mutation.

We thereafter investigated RET-mutated tumors where the mutation was germ-line-derived or a somatic mutation. The expression profiles of the tumors in each group were then correlated with the proliferation marker Ki-67. Tenascin C correlated highly to proliferation in the germ-line-mutated group, whereas EGFR, E-cadherin, and TTF-1 showed a weak correlation. In the somatic-mutated tumors, tenascin C correlation was lower but showed a higher correlation to EGFR.

Calcitonin has proven to be a useful marker in the diagnosis and prognosis of MTC [23]. We found that both basal and pentagastrin stimulated calcitonin levels did not differ significantly between RET-mutated and wild-type MTC. Furthermore, no correlation between basal calcitonin levels and the Ki-67 index, tenascin C, EGFR, E-cadherin, or TTF-1 was observed. A moderate correlation was found between post-operative calcitonin levels and both Ki-67 index and tenascin C expression. However, due to the low level of correlation, it is possible that these results are stochastic.

The role of TTF-1 in the development of Hirschsprung's disease by RET interaction has been recently outlined [19]. Furthermore, not only papillary thyroid carcinoma but also MTC show expression of TTF-1 [17]. Garcia-Barcelò et al. [24] found that mutations in single nucleotide polymorphisms (SNPs) of NKX2 (codes for TTF-1) and the RET promoter region correlated with the decreased TTF-1 binding and activation of RET, leading to Hirschsprung's disease. It is known that a loss of RET activation leads to Hirschsprung's disease [3], whereas a gain in function leads to MTC [2]. It is possible therefore that TTF-1 expression in RET-mutated MTCs might be higher, leading to consecutive RET activation. However, we found no significant difference in TTF-1 levels between RET-mutated (germ-line- and somatic-mutated) and RET wild-type tumors. Our data seem thus to indicate that TTF-1 does not play a role in the consecutive activation of RET. Moreover, we observed that TTF-1 has a weak correlation with EGFR and E-cadherin, but no correlation with tenascin-C or the Ki-67 index. However, the role of TTF-1 in MTC has yet to be established by a study with a larger cohort.

4. Materials and Methods

In the present study, 30 patients (16 females, 14 males; age: 2–81 years, mean age: 51 $\pm$ 18 years) with diagnosed MTC (n = 26) or C-cell hyperplasia (n = 4) at the Medical University of Salzburg were investigated. Eight patients showed MEN (MEN2A, 7 patients; MEN2B, 1 patient). All subjects gave their informed consent for inclusion before they participated in the study. The study was conducted in accordance with the Declaration of Helsinki, and the protocol (Approval: 14 February 2014) was approved by an institutional review board.

Routinely performed formalin-fixed paraffin embedded (FFPE) tissue was obtained from the primary thyroid site in 22 patients, lymph node metastasis in 6 patients, metastasis in a Meckel's diverticulum in 1 patient, and metastasis in the adrenal gland in 1 patient.

Genetic analysis of RET mutations was carried out in 21 patients, 6 of them with MEN2. RET gene mutations were detected in 15 patients (Table 2), while 6 patients showed RET wild-type.

Table 2. Rearranged during transfection (RET) mutations detected in the study group.

Mutation Detected	Sporadic MTC/MEN2
Codon 769 on Exon 13 (n = 5)	Sporadic
Codon 904 on Exon 15 (n = 3)	Sporadic
Codon L790F on Exon 13 + Codon 769 on Exon 13 (n = 3)	MEN2A (familial)
Codon L790F on Exon 13 + Codon 904 on Exon 15 (n = 1)	MEN2A
Codon 790 on Exon 13 (n = 1)	MEN2A
Codon 634 on Exon 11 (n = 1)	MEN2A
Codon 836 on Exon 14 (n = 1)	Sporadic

n, number of patients; MEN, multiple endocrine neoplasia.

Preoperative serum calcitonin levels (2.2–3293.4 ng/L, mean: 596.4 ng/L) were measured in 23 patients and pentagastrin tests (calcitonin: 17.7–2936.7 ng/L; mean: 708.3 ng/L) were performed in 11 patients. At time of the study, serum calcitonin levels (0.7–289,951.0 ng/L, mean: 11,056.6 ng/L) and pentagastrin test results (calcitonin: 2.6–971.7 ng/L; mean: 188.9 ng/L) were available in 29 patients and 16 patients, respectively. The normal calcitonin levels were <15 ng/L for males and <5 ng/L for females.

The expression of tenascin C, EGFR, E-cadherin, TTF-1, and Ki-67 was evaluated by immunohistochemistry. The primary antibodies used, with the working dilutions and pH of antigen retrieval buffers, are listed in Table 3.

Table 3. List of primary antibodies, working dilutions and pH of antigen retrieval buffers used.

Antibody	Source	Clone	Type	Species	pH-Retrieval	Working Dilution
Tenascin C	Sigma Aldrich™	bc-24	mc	Mouse	pH 6	1:4000
	Santa Cruz™	bc-24	mc	Mouse	pH 6	1:4000
EGFR	Dako™	E30	mc	Mouse	pH 6	1:20
E-Cadherin	Thermo Scientific™	SPM471	mc	Mouse	pH 9	1:100
TTF-1	Novocastra™	SPT24	mc	Mouse	pH 9	1:50
Ki-67	Dako™	MIB-1	mc	Mouse	pH 9	1:500

EGFR: epidermal growth factor receptor; TTF-1: thyroid transcription factor-1; mc: monoclonal antibody.

EGFR mutation analysis was performed using the Roche™ Cobas® EGFR mutation kit (Roche Molecular Systems, Inc., Branchburg, NJ, USA) on a Cobas® 4800 platform, v2.0 (Roche Molecular Systems, Inc.).

Statistical Analysis

Excel® software (Microsoft Corporation, Vienna, Austria) was used for the statistical evaluation of results.

Correlation analysis of tenascin C, EGFR, E-cadherin, and TTF-1 with the Ki-67 index was done by using the Pearson correlation coefficient test. For the assessment of statistical significance, the *t*-test for unpaired variance was used. Statistical significance was defined as $p < 0.05$.

5. Conclusions

MTC express tenascin C, E-cadherin, and TTF-1. Tenascin C expression correlates significantly with tumor proliferation, especially in RET-mutated tumors. EGFR expression is low in MTC and tumors showing EGFR expression do not exhibit higher proliferation. However, EGFR expression is significantly higher in MTC with RET mutation. No EGFR mutation was found in MTC. TTF-1 expression does not correlate with RET mutation status. TTF-1 expression has a weak correlation with tenascin C, E-cadherin, and EGFR expression.

Acknowledgments: The authors declare that no funds or grants were received.

Author Contributions: Cornelia Hauser-Kronberger and Christian Pirich conceived and designed the experiments; Florian Steiner and Gundula Rendl performed the experiments; Cornelia Hauser-Kronberger, Margarida Rodrigues, and Christian Pirich analyzed the data; Florian Steiner and Margarida Rodrigues wrote the paper.

References

1. Lairmore, T.C.; Wells, S.A.; Moley, J.F. Molecular biology of endocrine tumors. In *Cancer: Principles and Practice of Oncology*, 6th ed.; DeVita, V.T., Jr., Hellman, S., Rosenberg, S.A., Eds.; Lippincott: Philadelphia, PA, USA, 2001; pp. 1727–1740.
2. Edery, P.; Eng, C.; Munnich, A.; Lyonnet, S. RET in human development and oncogenesis. *Bioessays* **1997**, *19*, 389–395. [CrossRef] [PubMed]
3. Pasini, B.; Borrello, M.G.; Greco, A.; Bongarzone, I.; Luo, Y.; Mondellini, P.; Alberti, L.; Miranda, C.; Arighi, E.; Bocciardi, R.; et al. Loss of function effect of RET mutations causing Hirschsprung disease. *Nat. Genet.* **1995**, *10*, 35–40. [CrossRef] [PubMed]
4. Yoshida, T.; Matsumoto, E.; Hanamura, N.; Kalembeyi, I.; Katsuta, K.; Ishihara, A.; Sakakura, T. Co-expression of tenascin and fibronectin in epithelial and stromal cells of benign lesions and ductal carcinomas in the human breast. *J. Pathol.* **1997**, *182*, 421–428. [CrossRef]
5. Bourdon, M.A.; Wikstrand, C.J.; Furthmayr, H.; Matthews, T.J.; Bigner, D.D. Human glioma-mesenchymal extracellular matrix antigen defined by monoclonal antibody. *Cancer Res.* **1983**, *43*, 2796–2805. [PubMed]
6. Herold-Mende, C.; Mueller, M.M.; Bonsanto, M.M.; Schmitt, H.P.; Kunze, S.; Steiner, H.H. Clinical impact and functional aspects of tenascin-C expression during glioma progression. *Int. J. Cancer* **2002**, *98*, 362–369. [CrossRef] [PubMed]
7. Koperek, O.; Prinz, A.; Scheuba, C.; Niederle, B.; Kaserer, K. Tenascin C in medullary thyroid microcarcinoma and C-cell hyperplasia. *Virchows Arch.* **2009**, *455*, 43–48. [CrossRef] [PubMed]
8. Wikstrand, C.J.; Hale, L.P.; Batra, S.K.; Hill, M.L.; Humphrey, P.A.; Kurpad, S.N.; McLendon, R.E.; Moscatello, D.; Pegram, C.N.; Reist, C.J.; et al. Monoclonal antibodies against EGFRvIII are tumor specific and react with breast and lung carcinomas and malignant gliomas. *Cancer Res.* **1995**, *55*, 3140–3148. [PubMed]
9. Rodriguez-Antona, C.; Pallares, J.; Montero-Conde, C.; Inglada-Pérez, L.; Castelblanco, E.; Landa, I.; Leskelä, S.; Leandro-García, L.J.; López-Jiménez, E.; Letón, R.; et al. Overexpression and activation of EGFR and VEGFR2 in medullary thyroid carcinomas is related to metastasis. *Endocr. Relat. Cancer* **2010**, *17*, 7–16. [CrossRef] [PubMed]
10. Croyle, M.; Akeno, N.; Knauf, J.A.; Fabbro, D.; Chen, X.; Baumgartner, J.E.; Lane, H.A.; Fagin, J.A. RET/PTC-induced cell growth is mediated in part by epidermal growth factor receptor (EGFR) activation: Evidence for molecular and functional interactions between RET and EGFR. *Cancer Res.* **2008**, *68*, 4183–4191. [CrossRef] [PubMed]
11. Shimoyama, Y.; Hirohashi, S. Expression of E- and P-cadherin in gastric carcinomas. *Cancer Res.* **1991**, *51*, 2185–2192. [PubMed]

12. Vleminckx, K.; Vakaet, L.; Mareel, M.; Fiers, W.; van Roy, F. Genetic manipulation of E-cadherin expression by epithelial tumor cells reveals an invasion suppressor role. *Cell* **1991**, *66*, 107–119. [CrossRef]
13. Naito, A.; Iwase, H.; Kuzushima, T.; Nakamura, T.; Kobayashi, S. Clinical significance of E-cadherin expression in thyroid neoplasms. *J. Surg. Oncol.* **2001**, *76*, 176–180. [CrossRef] [PubMed]
14. Francis-Lang, H.; Price, M.; Polycarpou-Schwarz, M.; Di Lauro, R. Cell-type-specific expression of the rat thyroperoxidase promoter indicates common mechanisms for thyroid-specific gene expression. *Mol. Cell. Biol.* **1992**, *12*, 576–588. [CrossRef] [PubMed]
15. Civitareale, D.; Lonigro, R.; Sinclair, A.J.; di Lauro, R. A thyroid-specific nuclear protein essential for tissue-specific expression of the thyroglobulin promoter. *EMBO J.* **1989**, *8*, 2537–2542. [PubMed]
16. Fabbro, D.; di Loreto, C.; Beltrami, C.A.; Belfiore, A.; di Lauro, R.; Damante, G. Expression of thyroid-specific transcription factors TTF-1 and PAX-8 in human thyroid neoplasms. *Cancer Res.* **1994**, *54*, 4744–4749. [PubMed]
17. Katoh, R.; Miyagi, E.; Nakamura, N.; Li, X.; Suzuki, K.; Kakudo, K.; Kobayashi, M.; Kawaoi, A. Expression of thyroid transcription factor-1 (TTF-1) in human C cells and medullary thyroid carcinomas. *Hum. Pathol.* **2000**, *31*, 386–393. [CrossRef]
18. Suzuki, K.; Lavaroni, S.; Mori, A.; Okajima, F.; Kimura, S.; Katoh, R.; Kawaoi, A.; Kohn, L.D. Thyroid transcription factor 1 is calcium modulated and coordinately regulates genes involved in calcium homeostasis in C cells. *Mol. Cell. Biol.* **1998**, *18*, 7410–7422. [CrossRef] [PubMed]
19. Zhu, J.; Garcia-Barcelo, M.M.; Tam, P.K.H.; Lui, V.C.H. HOXB5 cooperates with NKX2–1 in the transcription of human RET. *PLoS ONE* **2011**, *6*, e20815. [CrossRef] [PubMed]
20. Tisell, L.E.; Oden, A.; Muth, A.; Altiparmak, G.; Mõlne, J.; Ahlman, H.; Nilsson, O. The Ki67 index a prognostic marker in medullary thyroid carcinoma. *Br. J. Cancer* **2003**, *89*, 2093–2097. [CrossRef] [PubMed]
21. Vitagliano, D.; de Falco, V.; Tamburrino, A.; Coluzzi, S.; Troncone, G.; Chiappetta, G.; Ciardiello, F.; Tortora, G.; Fagin, J.A.; Ryan, A.J.; et al. The tyrosine kinase inhibitor ZD6474 blocks proliferation of RET mutant medullary thyroid carcinoma cells. *Endocr. Relat. Cancer* **2011**, *18*, 1–11. [CrossRef] [PubMed]
22. Ishihara, A.; Yoshida, T.; Tamaki, H.; Sakakura, T. Tenascin expression in cancer cells and stroma of human breast cancer and its prognostic significance. *Clin. Cancer Res.* **1995**, *1*, 1035–1041. [PubMed]
23. Kloos, R.T.; Eng, C.; Evans, D.B.; Francis, G.L.; Gagel, R.F.; Gharib, H.; Moley, J.F.; Pacini, F.; Ringel, M.D.; Schlumberger, M.; et al. Medullary thyroid cancer: Management guidelines of the American Thyroid Association. *Thyroid* **2009**, *19*, 565–612. [CrossRef] [PubMed]
24. Garcia-Barcelo, M.; Ganster, R.W.; Lui, V.C.; Leon, T.Y.; So, M.T.; Lau, A.M.; Fu, M.; Sham, M.H.; Knight, J.; Zannini, M.S.; et al. TTF-1 and RET promoter SNPs: Regulation of RET transcription in Hirschsprung's disease. *Hum. Mol. Genet.* **2005**, *14*, 191–204. [CrossRef] [PubMed]

15

Association between Family Histories of Thyroid Cancer and Thyroid Cancer Incidence: A Cross-Sectional Study Using the Korean Genome and Epidemiology Study Data

Soo-Hwan Byun [1,2], Chanyang Min [3], Hyo-Geun Choi [2,3,4,*] and Seok-Jin Hong [2,5,*]

1 Department of Oral & Maxillofacial Surgery, Dentistry, Hallym University College of Medicine, Anyang 14068, Korea; purheit@daum.net
2 Research Center of Clinical Dentistry, Hallym University Clinical Dentistry Graduate School, Chuncheon 24252, Korea
3 Hallym Data Science Laboratory, Hallym University College of Medicine, Anyang 14068, Korea; joicemin@naver.com
4 Department of Otorhinolaryngology-Head & Neck Surgery, Hallym University College of Medicine, Anyang 14068, Korea
5 Department of Otorhinolaryngology-Head & Neck Surgery, Hallym University College of Medicine, Dongtan 18450, Korea
* Correspondence: pupen@naver.com (H.-G.C.); enthsj@hanmail.net (S.-J.H.)

Abstract: This study assessed the association between thyroid cancer and family history. This cross-sectional study used epidemiological data from the Korean Genome and Epidemiology Study from 2001 to 2013. Among 211,708 participants, 988 were in the thyroid cancer group and 199,588 were in the control group. Trained interviewers questioned the participants to obtain their thyroid cancer history and age at onset. The participants were examined according to their age, sex, monthly household income, obesity, smoking, alcohol consumption, and past medical history. The adjusted odds ratios (95% confidence intervals) for the family histories of fathers, mothers, and siblings were 6.59 (2.05–21.21), 4.76 (2.59–8.74), and 9.53 (6.92–13.11), respectively, and were significant. The results for the subgroup analyses according to sex were consistent. The rate of family histories of thyroid cancer for fathers and siblings were not different according to the thyroid cancer onset, while that of mothers were higher in participants with a younger age at onset (<50 years old group, 11/523 [2.1%], $p = 0.007$). This study demonstrated that thyroid cancer incidence was associated with thyroid cancer family history. This supports regular examination of individuals with a family history of thyroid cancer to prevent disease progression and ensure early management.

Keywords: epidemiology; thyroid cancer; family history; differentiated thyroid cancer; papillary thyroid cancer

---

1. Introduction

The incidence of thyroid cancer is increasing worldwide [1], and it has increased by approximately two folds over the past few decades [2]. The incidence of thyroid nodules diagnosed by palpation of the thyroid gland is approximately 5–10% in adults [3]. Because of the frequent use and accessibility of thyroid ultrasonography (US), there has been an increase in thyroid cancer detection [4]. The objective of the examination of patients with thyroid nodules is to identify thyroid cancer. As a result, its incidence in South Korea in 2011 was 15 times higher than in 1993 [5]. Korean women had the highest age-standardized incidence of thyroid cancer globally [6]. Differentiated thyroid carcinoma (DTC) comprises approximately 90% of all thyroid cancers and includes the papillary type and follicular type [7,8]. In Korea, the most common histological type (94.9%) of DTC is papillary thyroid cancer (PTC) [9]. Total thyroidectomy is usually recommended for treatment of thyroid cancer, followed by radioiodine therapy in some cases. Inoperable or radiotherapy refractory differentiated thyroid cancers are commonly the main causes of thyroid cancer-related deaths and do not have effective treatments [10]. Cytotoxic chemotherapy with innovative medicines should be studied because they appear to be effective in some patients [11,12].

The etiology of DTC is still unknown. However, environmental and genetic predisposing factors including ionizing radiation might affect the development of thyroid cancer [13]. Air pollution and iodine intake are considered risk factors for thyroid cancer [14–17]. Obesity, smoking, and alcohol consumption are also associated with thyroid cancer [18]. A family history of thyroid cancer is also a suggested risk factor in 5–15% of cases. There are several genetic mutations identified to have a role in the development of DTC [7]. Rearranged during transfection (RET) chromosomal rearrangement genes, and mutation of RAS or BRAF proto-oncogenes can trigger the activation of the mitogen-activated protein kinase cascade in PTC. Mutations of the BRAF, RAS, or RET genes are found in nearly 70% of PTC cases [19,20]. A previous study mentioned that BRAF mutation is associated with aggressiveness of PTC and the loss of radiotherapy effectiveness in recurrent disease. Surgical resection of mutation-positive cancer is recommended [10]. For instance, lobectomy is recommended by the American Thyroid Association for treatment of PTCs < 1 cm [21]. However, because of the definite association of BRAF mutation with aggressiveness of PTC, total thyroidectomy might be a better treatment option if BRAF mutation is positive in preoperative testing [21].

The familial risk of thyroid cancer is known to be highest in all cancer sites, for which the increased risk extends beyond the nuclear family [22–24]. Family history is a possible risk factor which could be associated with medical and psychosocial benefits. To provide definite information, the clinicians and entire medical system need to recognize the familial risks that are not included in the conventional familial risk guidelines.

Nevertheless, only few studies have studied the risk factors of familial history for thyroid cancer in Asian adults. Most of the studies were focused on familial non-medullary thyroid cancer, or the study sample sizes were relatively small [25]. Myung et al. reported that a family history of cancer and alcohol consumption were associated with a decreased risk of thyroid cancer, whereas a higher body mass index (BMI) and family history of thyroid cancer were associated with an increased risk of thyroid cancer in 34,211 patients [26]. The study was a case-control study. A total of 802 thyroid cancer cases out of 34,211 patients was included. A total of 802 control cases was also selected from the same cohort group and matched using the ratio 1:1 by age and area of residence. Multivariate conditional logistic regression analysis was used. The results show that females and those with a family history of thyroid cancer had an increased risk of thyroid cancer, and a family history of cancer and alcohol consumption were associated with a decreased risk of thyroid cancer, whereas a higher BMI and family history of thyroid cancer were associated with an increased risk of thyroid cancer. The study suggested that females and those with a family history of thyroid cancer have an increased risk of thyroid cancer. Hwang et al. showed that multicollinearity existed between US assessment and patient age, and first-degree family history of thyroid cancer and serum thyroid hormone values in 1254 patients [25]. A retrospective study investigated 1310 thyroid nodules of 1254 euthyroid asymptomatic patients who underwent US-guided fine needle aspiration. The study evaluated nodule size, first-degree family history of thyroid cancer, gender, age, and thyroid-stimulating hormone (TSH) levels with US examination to distinguish between benign and malignant nodules. Multiple logistic regression analysis was conducted to evaluate the risk of thyroid malignancy according to clinical and US features. A first-degree family history of thyroid cancer, age, and high TSH levels did not independently significantly increase the risk of thyroid cancer. The study concluded that a first-degree family history as a risk factor for thyroid malignancy should be further investigated in asymptomatic patients.

Similar to those studies, previous studies of familial risk were performed without a control group or with a small control group. Moreover, those studies did not include many confounding factors that could influence the study results. To the best of our knowledge, there has been no study on the association between family history and thyroid cancer using large Korean population data.

A clear picture of the association between thyroid cancer and family history will help both patients and clinicians. This could serve as a basis for guidelines governing clinical risk factor assessment and the management of thyroid nodules. Therefore, this study assessed the association between thyroid cancer and family history.

2. Materials and Methods

2.1. Study Population and Data Collection

Authorization was obtained from the ethics committee of the Hallym University (2019-02-020). The requirement for written informed consent was waived by the Institutional Review Board. This cross-sectional study relied on the data from the Korean Genome and Epidemiology Study (KoGES) from 2001 to 2013.

The Korean Genome and Epidemiology Study Health Examinee (KoGES HEXA) is a large cohort project initiated to reveal gene-environmental factors and their interactions in diseases [27,28]. Among this, we have selected the questionnaires. Therefore, this study had a cross-sectional design. KoGES was designed to identify gene-environment factors and their interactions in common chronic diseases, such as hypertension, cardiovascular disease, type 2 diabetes, obesity, and metabolic syndrome, in Korea. KoGES collected epidemiological data and biospecimens, such as urine, blood, and genome, from many patients aged 40–69 years by performing a medical examination and health survey. Familial data were well-organized and systemized, and the data were collected using a questionnaire, which was confirmed by expert clinicians. The KoGES data were collected from both urban and rural areas. Therefore, the study sample size was relatively larger than that reported in previous studies.

2.2. Participant Selection

Among 211,708 participants, we excluded the participants with no family history of thyroid cancer (n = 10,030) and no BMI data (n = 1102) (Figure 1). In total, 200,576 participants (69,693 men, 130,883 women) were evaluated. According to their cancer thyroid histories, they were divided into two groups: the thyroid cancer group and control group.

2.3. Survey

Trained interviewers asked the participants questions to obtain relevant data including previous thyroid cancer history, age at onset, household monthly income, past metabolic disease history (hypertension, diabetes mellitus, and hyperlipidemia), smoking history, and alcohol consumption history. Anthropometric and clinical measurements were obtained [27,28]. This study categorized the family histories of thyroid cancer into groups: fathers, mothers, and siblings (brothers or sisters). Income was categorized into four groups according to the household monthly income: no information, low (<\$1500), middle (≥\$1500–<\$3000), and high (≥\$3000). BMI was used to measure obesity (kg/m^2), wherein height and weight were considered as continuous variables [27,29]. Total smoking histories were calculated in pack-year, and alcohol consumption was measured as the mean daily alcohol consumption (g/day) using the frequency and alcohol types [30,31].

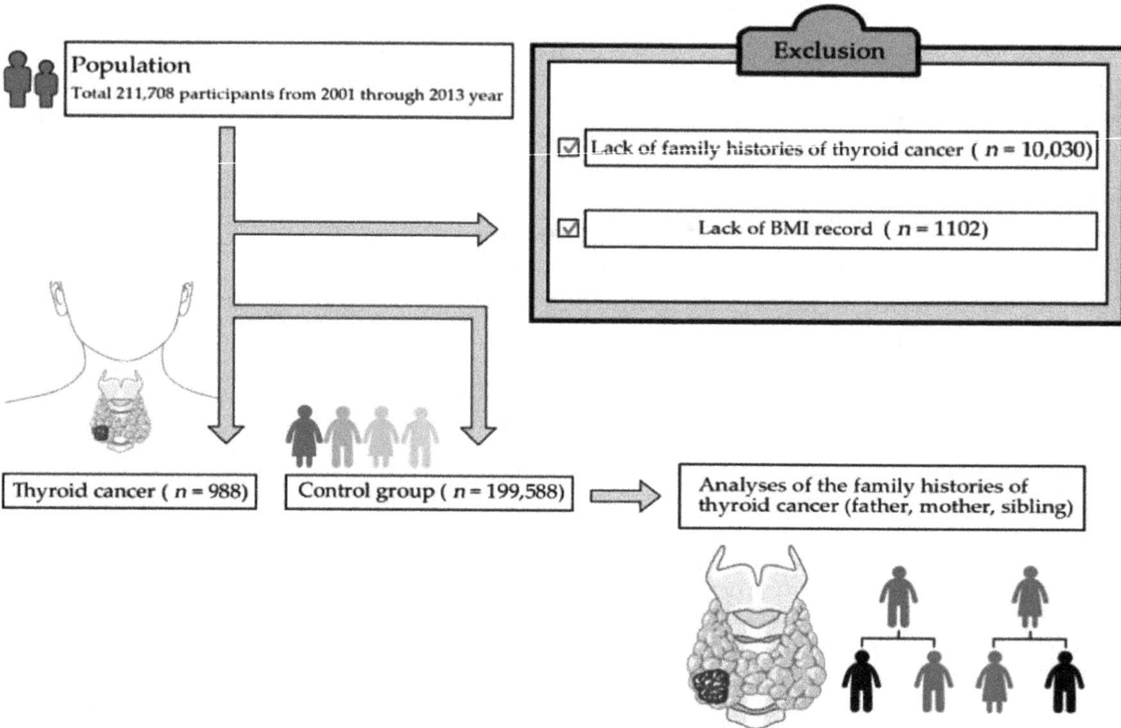

Figure 1. Participant selection.

2.4. Statistical Analyses

The chi-square test or Fisher's exact test was used to compare the differences between sex, income, metabolic disease history, and thyroid cancer family history between both groups. The independent *t*-test was used to compare the age, BMI, smoking pack year, and alcohol consumption.

To analyze the odds ratio (OR) of thyroid cancer history for the thyroid cancer group, a logistic regression model was used. In the crude model, this study only inserted each family history of thyroid cancer as an independent variable. In Model 1, this study inserted each family history of thyroid cancer and age, sex, income, BMI, smoking, alcohol intake, and past medical histories of hypertension, diabetes mellitus, and dyslipidemia as independent variables. In Model 2, this study inserted thyroid cancer history of the father, mother, and siblings as independent variables. In Model 3, this study inserted the variables of Models 2 and 3. To analyze the interaction between the different family histories of thyroid cancer, we designed Model 4. In this model, the variables included: thyroid cancer history of father, mother, siblings, father × siblings, and mother × siblings.

The 95% confidence intervals (CIs) were calculated. For the subgroup analysis, this study stratified the participants according to sex: male and female.

Two-tailed analyses were conducted, and p values < 0.05 were considered as statistically significant. The results were analyzed using SPSS v. 22.0 (IBM, Armonk, NY, USA).

3. Results

The participant age ranged from 40 to 91 years. In total, 988 participants were in the thyroid cancer group, while 199,588 were in the control group. The differences between the mean age, BMI, smoking duration, and daily alcohol consumption of both groups were significant (Table 1). The rates of sex, income, past medical history of diabetes mellitus, and dyslipidemia were also different between both groups.

Table 1. General characteristics of participants.

Characteristics	Total Participants		
	Thyroid Cancer (*n*, %)	Control (*n*, %)	*p*-Value
Total number (*n*, %)	988 (100.0)	199,588 (100.0)	
Age (years, mean, SD)	53.2 (7.6)	53.9 (8.7)	0.007 [1]
Sex (*n*, %)			<0.001 [1]
Male	79 (8.0)	69,614 (34.9)	
Female	909 (92.0)	129,974 (65.1)	
Income (*n*, %)			<0.001 [1]
No information	95 (9.6)	40,590 (20.3)	
Low	166 (16.8)	41,060 (20.6)	
Middle	292 (29.6)	51,899 (26.0)	
High	435 (44.0)	66,039 (33.1)	
Hypertension (*n*, %)	220 (22.3)	40,930 (20.5)	0.172
Diabetes (*n*, %)	50 (5.1)	14,584 (7.3)	0.007 [1]
Dyslipidemia (*n*, %)	117 (11.8)	17,834 (8.9)	0.001 [1]
Obesity (BMI, kg/m^2, mean, SD)	23.8 (2.9)	24.0 (3.0)	<0.001 [1]
Tobacco index (pack-year, mean, SD)	1.63 (6.5)	6.62 (12.5)	<0.001 [1]
alcohol consumption (g/day, mean, SD)	2.0 (10.1)	7.2 (22.1)	<0.001 [1]
Family history of father (*n*, %)	3 (0.3)	86 (0.0)	0.010 [1]
Family history of mother (*n*, %)	12 (1.2)	307 (0.2)	<0.001 [1]
Family history of siblings (*n*, %)	44 (4.5)	653 (0.3)	<0.001 [1]

BMI, body mass index, kg/m^2; SD, Standard deviation. [1] Independent *t*-test, Chi-square test, or Fisher's exact test. Significance at $p < 0.05$.

In Model 1, adjusted for general characteristics, the adjusted ORs for the family histories of fathers, mothers, and siblings were 6.72 (95% CI = 2.10–21.50), 6.33 (95% CI = 3.52–11.36), and 10.16 (95% CI = 7.42–13.93), respectively.

In Model 2, adjusted for only family histories of thyroid cancer, the adjusted ORs for family histories of fathers, mothers, and siblings were 6.75 (95% CI = 2.10–21.67), 5.55 (95% CI = 3.02–10.19), and 13.09 (95% CI = 9.53–17.99), respectively.

In Model 3, adjusted for both general characteristics and family histories of thyroid cancer, the adjusted OR was slightly lower than in Models 1 and 2. The adjusted ORs for the family histories of fathers, mothers, and siblings were 6.59 (95% CI = 2.05–21.21), 4.76 (95% CI = 2.59–8.74), and 9.53 (95% CI = 6.92–13.11), respectively, and were significant (Table 2).

Table 2. Association between thyroid cancer history and their family thyroid cancer histories.

Family History	ORs of Thyroid Cancer for the Thyroid Cancer Family Histories							
	Crude	*p*-Value	Model 1	*p*-Value	Model 2	*p*-Value	Model 3	*p*-Value
ORs of the thyroid cancer history of father								
Thyroid cancer	7.07 (2.23–22.38)	0.001 [1]	6.72 (2.10–21.50)	0.001 [1]	6.75 (2.10–21.67)	0.001 [1]	6.59 (2.05–21.21)	0.002 [1]
Control	1.00		1.00		1.00		1.00	
ORs of the thyroid cancer history of mother								
Thyroid cancer	7.98 (4.47–14.26)	<0.001 [1]	6.33 (3.52–11.36)	<0.001 [1]	5.55 (3.02–10.19)	<0.001 [1]	4.76 (2.59–8.74)	<0.001 [1]
Control	1.00		1.00		1.00		1.00	
ORs of the thyroid cancer history of siblings								
Thyroid cancer	14.20 (10.40–19.40)	<0.001 [1]	10.16 (7.42–13.93)	<0.001 [1]	13.09 (9.53–17.99)	<0.001 [1]	9.53 (6.92–13.11)	<0.001 [1]
Control	1.00		1.00		1.00		1.00	

ORs, odds ratios. Model 1: adjusted for age, sex, income, body mass index, smoking, alcohol intake, and past medical histories of hypertension, diabetes mellitus, and dyslipidemia. Model 2: adjusted for thyroid cancer history of father, mother, and siblings. Model 3: adjusted for Models 1 and 2. [1] Logistic regression analyses, Statistical significance at $p < 0.05$.

In the subgroup analyses according to sex, the results were consistent with the results of the total participants (Table 3). In men, the adjusted ORs for the family histories of fathers and siblings were 29.09 (95% CI = 3.84–220.29) and 14.15 (95% CI = 3.39–58.95), respectively, in Model 3, while that of mother did not converge. In women, the adjusted ORs for the family histories of fathers, mothers, and siblings were 4.71 (95% CI = 1.13–19.52), 5.06 (95% CI = 2.75–9.31) and 9.37 (95% CI = 6.75–13.00), respectively.

Table 3. Subgroup analyses of association between thyroid cancer history and their family thyroid cancer histories according to sex.

Family History	ORs of Thyroid Cancer for the Thyroid Cancer Histories of Families							
	Crude	***p*-Value**	**Model 1**	***p*-Value**	**Model 2**	***p*-Value**	**Model 3**	***p*-Value**
Men (*n* = 69,693)								
ORs of the thyroid cancer history of father								
Thyroid cancer	27.88 (3.76–206.55)	0.001 [1]	28.21 (3.73–213.69)	0.001 [1]	28.53 (3.85–211.44)	0.001 [1]	29.09 (3.84–220.29)	0.001 [1]
Control	1.00		1.00		1.00		1.00	
ORs of the thyroid cancer history of mother								
Thyroid cancer	No convergence	0.997	No convergence	0.997	No convergence	0.997	No convergence	0.997
Control	1.00		1.00		1.00		1.00	
ORs of the thyroid cancer history of siblings								
Thyroid cancer	15.43 (3.75–63.54)	<0.001 [1]	13.90 (3.34–57.94)	<0.001 [1]	16.02 (3.89–66.00)	<0.001 [1]	14.15 (3.39–58.95)	<0.001 [1]
Control	1.00		1.00		1.00		1.00	
Women (*n* = 130,883)								
ORs of the thyroid cancer history of father								
Thyroid cancer	5.31 (1.29–21.79)	0.021 [1]	4.84 (1.18–19.94)	0.029 [1]	4.92 (1.18–20.61)	0.029 [1]	4.71 (1.13–19.52)	0.033 [1]
Control	1.00		1.00		1.00		1.00	
ORs of the thyroid cancer history of mother								
Thyroid cancer	7.89 (4.40–14.16)	<0.001 [1]	6.75 (3.75–12.14)	<0.001 [1]	5.70 (3.09–10.51)	<0.001 [1]	5.06 (2.75–9.31)	<0.001 [1]
Control	1.00		1.00		1.00		1.00	
ORs of the thyroid cancer history of siblings								
Thyroid cancer	11.70 (8.49–16.13)	<0.001 [1]	10.04 (7.27–13.87)	<0.001 [1]	10.81 (7.80–14.98)	<0.001 [1]	9.37 (6.75–13.00)	<0.001 [1]
Control	1.00		1.00		1.00		1.00	

Model 1: adjusted for age, sex, income, body mass index, smoking, alcohol intake, and past medical histories of hypertension, diabetes mellitus, and dyslipidemia. Model 2: adjusted for thyroid cancer history of father, thyroid cancer history of mother, and thyroid cancer history of siblings. Model 3: adjusted for Models 1 and 2. [1] Logistic regression analyses, Statistical significance at $p < 0.05$.

Because no father had a thyroid cancer history when mother had thyroid cancer, we did not make the interaction model for father × mother. In the interaction model, we did not find any interaction in father × siblings and mother × siblings (Table 4).

Table 4. Interaction model of each family history of thyroid cancer.

Variable	ORs for Thyroid Cancer	
	Model 4	***p*-Value**
Father	No convergence	1.00
Mother	12.84 (2.02–81.86)	0.007
Siblings	26.87 (5.69–126.91)	<0.001
Father × siblings	No convergence	1.000
Mother × siblings	0.51 (0.12–2.17)	0.362

Model 4: adjusted for thyroid cancer history of father, mother, siblings, father × siblings, and mother × siblings.

The rate of family histories of thyroid cancer of father and siblings were not different according to thyroid cancer onset (Table 5), while that of mother was higher in patients with a younger age at onset (<50 years group, 11/523 [2.1%]) compared with those with an older age at onset (≥50 years group, 1/456 [0.2%], $p = 0.007$).

Table 5. Ratio of family histories of thyroid cancer according to thyroid cancer onset among the thyroid cancer participants.

Histories	Onset of Thyroid Cancer		
	<50 Years Old	≥50 Years Old	*p*-Value
Thyroid cancer histories of father (*n*, %)			
Yes	3 (0.6)	0 (0.0)	0.253
No	520 (99.4)	456 (100.0)	
Thyroid cancer histories of mother (*n*, %)			
Yes	11 (2.1)	1 (0.2)	0.007 [1]
No	512 (97.9)	455 (99.8)	
Thyroid cancer histories of siblings (*n*, %)			
Yes	23 (4.4)	21 (4.6)	0.876
No	500 (95.6)	435 (95.4)	

[1] Fisher's exact test. Significance at $p < 0.05$.

4. Discussion

The definite association between family history and thyroid cancer incidence is not yet completely known. Although most cases of PTC occur sporadically, it seems that there are family components in some cases of PTC. Familial non-medullary thyroid cancer (FNMTC) is defined as a condition in which two or more first-degree relatives are affected by thyroid cancer in the absence of a known familial syndrome [32,33]. FNMTC shows a tendency to be more aggressive than sporadic cases with higher rates of extra-thyroid extension, lymph node metastases, larger tumor size in younger patients, and worse prognosis [32,33]. This study focused on the family history of PTC in a large population and not FNMTC. The most common histological type (94.9%) of DTC in Korea was PTC [9]. Most participants with thyroid cancer in the KoGES data would have PTC based on the results of previous studies [9,34–36]. There are few studies on the family history of PTC in a large population. Therefore, this study investigated the association between thyroid cancer and family history using data from a large Korean study.

This study showed that the adjusted OR for family history was higher in all thyroid cancer patients than in the control group (Table 2). Family history was significantly associated with the incidence of thyroid cancer after adjustment for age, sex, income, hypertension, diabetes, dyslipidemia, obesity, smoking, and alcohol consumption (Table 1). A meta-analysis of seven cohort studies by Zhao et al. showed that obesity increased the risk of thyroid cancer [37]. The meta-analysis evaluated the association between body weight or BMI and risk of thyroid cancer. A total of 5154 thyroid cancer cases was included. The pooled relative risk (RR) of thyroid cancer was 1.13 (95% CI 1.04–1.22) for overweight. Obesity was related with increased thyroid cancer risk in both genders, the strength of the association increasing with increasing BMI. The combined RR of thyroid cancer was 1.18 (95% CI 1.11–1.25) for excess body weight. Being overweight was associated with a significant increase in the thyroid cancer risk among non-Asians, but not among Asians. Overweight, obesity, and excess body weight were linked to PTC risk. Han et al. reported that obesity was associated with a higher prevalence of thyroid cancer in women [38]. The study collected data from 15,068 subjects who received a health examination from 2007 to 2008 at the Health Screening and Promotion Center of Asan Medical Center in Korea. Thyroid US was conducted in the examination, and suspected nodules were additionally examined by US-guided aspiration. Those with a history of thyroid disease or family history of thyroid cancer were excluded from the study. In total, 15,068 participants were screened by thyroid US. The prevalence of thyroid cancer in females was related with a high BMI (per 5 kg/m^2 increase) (OR = 1.63, 95% CI 1.24–2.10, $p < 0.001$) after adjustment for age, smoking status, and TSH levels. There was no significant correlation between the prevalence of thyroid cancer in males and a high BMI (OR = 1.16, 95% CI 0.85–1.57, $p = 0.336$). There was no association between age, fasting serum insulin, or basal TSH levels and thyroid cancer in either gender. In a meta-analysis of observational studies, Cho et al. showed that the risk of thyroid cancer was decreased by 21% in smokers compared to non-smokers [39]. The study investigated 31 studies to analyze the relationship between thyroid cancer occurrence and smoking. These studies consisted of 6260 thyroid cancer cases and 32,935 controls. The cohort studies included 2715 thyroid cancer patients. Summary RRs and 95% CIs were calculated using a random effects model. The risk of thyroid cancer was decreased in participants with a past smoking history (RR = 0.79; 95% CI 0.70–0.88) compared with those without. However, strong evidence of heterogeneity was found among the investigated studies; therefore, subgroup analyses were performed according to study location, study type, source of controls, smoking status, sex, and histological type of thyroid cancer. When the data were stratified by smoking status, an inverse association was observed only among current smokers (RR = 0.74; 95% CI 0.64–0.86), not former smokers (RR = 1.01; 95% CI 0.92–1.10). Previous studies demonstrated that alcohol consumption was found to be significantly associated with a decreased risk of thyroid cancer when the analysis was performed using the control group [40–42]. Kitahara et al. evaluated data from five prospective United States studies (384,433 males and 361,664 females) [40]. Hazard ratios and 95% CIs for thyroid cancer were calculated from adjusted models of smoking and alcohol consumption with additional adjustment of age, sex, race, education, and BMI. In total, 1003 thyroid cancer cases (335 males and 668 females) were identified. Alcohol intake was also inversely associated with thyroid cancer risk (≥7 drinks/week versus 0, HR = 0.72, 95% CI 0.58–0.90). Inverse associations with alcohol consumption were more pronounced for papillary versus follicular tumors. Hong et al. investigated 33 observational studies with two cross-sectional studies, 20 case-control studies, and 11 cohort studies [42]. The studies involved 7725 thyroid cancer participants and 3,113,679 participants without thyroid cancer. In the fixed-effect model meta-analysis of all 33 studies, alcohol intake was related with a reduced risk of thyroid cancer (OR = 0.74; 95% CI 0.67–0.83). In the subgroup meta-analysis, alcohol consumption also reduced the risk of thyroid cancer in both case-control studies (OR = 0.77; 95% CI 0.65–0.92) and cohort studies (RR = 0.70; 95% CI 0.60–0.82). Subgroup meta-analyses showed that alcohol consumption was significantly related with a reduced risk of thyroid cancer.

The present study adjusted for various confounding factors to reduce the surveillance bias. The adjusted ORs in this study were similar to those in previous studies performed in other countries [7,8,23]. Kust et al. reported that family history plays a significant role in the development of thyroid cancer. Having first-degree relatives with thyroid cancer is a risk factor in both medullary and papillary thyroid cancer. The first-degree relatives could predict the risk of thyroid cancer [7]. A total of 10,709 participants was included in the study. Correlation of cytological findings and family history was evaluated using Fisher's exact test. There were 2580 (24.09%) patients with non-malignant thyroid diseases in the family and 198 (1.85%) patients with a history of thyroid cancer in the family. A total of 2778 (25.94%) patients had a positive family history of thyroid diseases, and 7931 (74.06%) patients had a negative family history. In patients with a family history of papillary thyroid carcinoma, the difference between those with benign and malignant thyroid tumors was found to be significant (p = 0.0432). Thyroid cancer may be more aggressive in younger patients and may have a higher rate of lymph node metastasis [7]. The rates for family histories of fathers and siblings were not different according to the age at onset of thyroid cancer, while those of mothers were higher in patients with a younger age at onset of thyroid cancer (Table 5). In addition, this study analyzed the interaction among familial histories by using the interaction model. There was no significant interactional effect in father with siblings and mother with siblings (Table 4).

Despite our large sample size, this study has few limitations. First, it was impossible to consider all the confounding factors for the association. KoGES did not cover all of the potentially influencing factors such as history of radiation therapy and CT, iodine intake, and history of thyroiditis. Second, KoGES HEXA was started based on a questionnaire survey [27]. The patient's thyroid cancer history was asked. However, in the cases of positivity, no biopsy or ultrasonography was performed for a definitive diagnosis. This study included all participants who had thyroid cancer as PTC given that about 95% of DTC cases in Korea were PTC [9]. Third, this study included only the participants who were survivors after being diagnosed with thyroid cancer. The survey could not be performed with the dead participants. However, this was not a huge problem because the survival rate of thyroid cancer in Korea is high. Thyroid cancer has an excellent prognosis and a five-year relative survival rate of 100.1% in Korea [43]. Lastly, this study did not include the family history of grandparents or distant relatives. Last, the reliability of the questionnaires on the smoking, alcohol consumption, and nutritional intake frequencies were unclear [27]. To collect accurate data, the reliability and validity of the questionnaire survey should be examined in future studies.

In contrast, this study has several advantages. To the best of our knowledge, this study is the first population-based study examining the association between thyroid cancer family history and the incidence of thyroid cancer in Asia. Second, this study is a large population-based study compared with studies in other countries. This study investigated detailed associations in subgroups in a large population. In addition, the risk of family history on incidence was evaluated using a large control group. This study provides more precise information than most previous individual studies. Third, this study considered many more influential factors than in previous studies. Obesity, smoking, and alcohol consumption were further adjusted in this study. These confounding factors would be important adjustments for the analysis of family history as a risk factor.

5. Conclusions

This study demonstrated that the incidence of thyroid cancer was associated with thyroid cancer family history. This finding supports regular examination of individuals with a family history of thyroid cancer to prevent the progression of thyroid cancer. The identification of family history would provide opportunities for early detection and prevention. Further studies including those on gene mutations associated with family history are recommended to demonstrate the pathophysiology and prevalence of thyroid cancer.

Author Contributions: Conceptualization, H.-G.C.; Data curation, C.M. and H.-G.C.; Formal analysis, C.M. and H.-G.C.; Funding acquisition, H.-G.C.; Investigation, S.-H.B. and H.-G.C.; Methodology, H.-G.C.; Project administration, S.-H.B. and H.-G.C.; Resources, S.-H.B.; Software, S.-J.H.; Supervision, S.-H.B. and S.-J.H.; Validation, S.-H.B.; Visualization, S.-J.H.; Writing—original draft, S.-H.B. and S.-J.H.; and Writing—review and editing, S.-H.B. and S.-J.H. All authors have read and agreed to the published version of the manuscript.

References

1. Vigneri, R.; Malandrino, P.; Vigneri, P. The changing epidemiology of thyroid cancer: Why is incidence increasing? *Curr. Opin. Oncol.* **2015**, *27*, 1–7. [CrossRef] [PubMed]
2. Morris, L.G.; Sikora, A.G.; Tosteson, T.D.; Davies, L. The increasing incidence of thyroid cancer: The influence of access to care. *Thyroid* **2013**, *23*, 885–891. [CrossRef] [PubMed]
3. Mazzaferri, E.L. Management of a solitary thyroid nodule. *N. Engl. J. Med.* **1993**, *328*, 553–559. [CrossRef] [PubMed]
4. Wartofsky, L. Increasing world incidence of thyroid cancer: Increased detection or higher radiation exposure? *Hormones* **2010**, *9*, 103–108. [CrossRef]
5. Ahn, H.S.; Kim, H.J.; Welch, H.G. Korea's thyroid-cancer "epidemic"—Screening and overdiagnosis. *N. Engl. J. Med.* **2014**, *371*, 1765–1767. [CrossRef]
6. Ferlay, J.; Colombet, M.; Soerjomataram, I.; Mathers, C.; Parkin, D.M.; Pineros, M.; Znaor, A.; Bray, F. Estimating the global cancer incidence and mortality in 2018: GLOBOCAN sources and methods. *Int. J. Cancer* **2019**, *144*, 1941–1953. [CrossRef]

7. Kust, D.; Stanicic, J.; Matesa, N. Bethesda thyroid categories and family history of thyroid disease. *Clin. Endocrinol.* **2018**, *88*, 468–472. [CrossRef]
8. Schmidbauer, B.; Menhart, K.; Hellwig, D.; Grosse, J. Differentiated Thyroid Cancer-Treatment: State of the Art. *Int. J. Mol. Sci.* **2017**, *18*, 1292. [CrossRef]
9. Park, S.; Oh, C.M.; Cho, H.; Lee, J.Y.; Jung, K.W.; Jun, J.K.; Won, Y.J.; Kong, H.J.; Choi, K.S.; Lee, Y.J.; et al. Association between screening and the thyroid cancer "epidemic" in South Korea: Evidence from a nationwide study. *BMJ* **2016**, *355*, i5745. [CrossRef]
10. Xing, M.; Haugen, B.R.; Schlumberger, M. Progress in molecular-based management of differentiated thyroid cancer. *Lancet* **2013**, *381*, 1058–1069. [CrossRef]
11. Spano, J.P.; Vano, Y.; Vignot, S.; De La Motte Rouge, T.; Hassani, L.; Mouawad, R.; Menegaux, F.; Khayat, D.; Leenhardt, L. GEMOX regimen in the treatment of metastatic differentiated refractory thyroid carcinoma. *Med. Oncol.* **2012**, *29*, 1421–1428. [CrossRef]
12. Crouzeix, G.; Michels, J.J.; Sevin, E.; Aide, N.; Vaur, D.; Bardet, S.; French, T.N. Unusual short-term complete response to two regimens of cytotoxic chemotherapy in a patient with poorly differentiated thyroid carcinoma. *J. Clin. Endocrinol. Metab.* **2012**, *97*, 3046–3050. [CrossRef]
13. Xu, L.; Li, G.; Wei, Q.; El-Naggar, A.K.; Sturgis, E.M. Family history of cancer and risk of sporadic differentiated thyroid carcinoma. *Cancer* **2012**, *118*, 1228–1235. [CrossRef]
14. Albi, E.; Cataldi, S.; Lazzarini, A.; Codini, M.; Beccari, T.; Ambesi-Impiombato, F.S.; Curcio, F. Radiation and Thyroid Cancer. *Int. J. Mol. Sci.* **2017**, *18*, 911. [CrossRef]
15. Pacini, F.; Castagna, M.G.; Brilli, L.; Pentheroudakis, G.; Group, E.G.W. Thyroid cancer: ESMO Clinical Practice Guidelines for diagnosis, treatment and follow-up. *Ann. Oncol.* **2012**, *23* (Suppl. 7), vii110–vii119. [CrossRef]
16. Cong, X. Air pollution from industrial waste gas emissions is associated with cancer incidences in Shanghai, China. *Environ. Sci. Pollut. Res. Int.* **2018**, *25*, 13067–13078. [CrossRef]
17. Fiore, M.; Oliveri Conti, G.; Caltabiano, R.; Buffone, A.; Zuccarello, P.; Cormaci, L.; Cannizzaro, M.A.; Ferrante, M. Role of Emerging Environmental Risk Factors in Thyroid Cancer: A Brief Review. *Int. J. Environ. Res. Public Health* **2019**, *16*, 1185. [CrossRef]
18. Mack, W.J.; Preston-Martin, S.; Dal Maso, L.; Galanti, R.; Xiang, M.; Franceschi, S.; Hallquist, A.; Jin, F.; Kolonel, L.; La Vecchia, C.; et al. A pooled analysis of case-control studies of thyroid cancer: Cigarette smoking and consumption of alcohol, coffee, and tea. *Cancer Causes Control.* **2003**, *14*, 773–785. [CrossRef]
19. Nikiforova, M.N.; Tseng, G.C.; Steward, D.; Diorio, D.; Nikiforov, Y.E. MicroRNA expression profiling of thyroid tumors: Biological significance and diagnostic utility. *J. Clin. Endocrinol. Metab.* **2008**, *93*, 1600–1608. [CrossRef]
20. Abdullah, M.I.; Junit, S.M.; Ng, K.L.; Jayapalan, J.J.; Karikalan, B.; Hashim, O.H. Papillary Thyroid Cancer: Genetic Alterations and Molecular Biomarker Investigations. *Int. J. Med. Sci.* **2019**, *16*, 450–460. [CrossRef]
21. Cooper, D.S.; Doherty, G.M.; Haugen, B.R.; Kloos, R.T.; Lee, S.L.; Mandel, S.J.; Mazzaferri, E.L.; McIver, B.; Pacini, F.; Schlumberger, M.; et al. Revised American Thyroid Association management guidelines for patients with thyroid nodules and differentiated thyroid cancer. *Thyroid* **2009**, *19*, 1167–1214. [CrossRef]
22. Fallah, M.; Sundquist, K.; Hemminki, K. Risk of thyroid cancer in relatives of patients with medullary thyroid carcinoma by age at diagnosis. *Endocr. Relat. Cancer* **2013**, *20*, 717–724. [CrossRef]
23. Goldgar, D.E.; Easton, D.F.; Cannon-Albright, L.A.; Skolnick, M.H. Systematic population-based assessment of cancer risk in first-degree relatives of cancer probands. *J. Natl. Cancer Inst.* **1994**, *86*, 1600–1608. [CrossRef]
24. Amundadottir, L.T.; Thorvaldsson, S.; Gudbjartsson, D.F.; Sulem, P.; Kristjansson, K.; Arnason, S.; Gulcher, J.R.; Bjornsson, J.; Kong, A.; Thorsteinsdottir, U.; et al. Cancer as a complex phenotype: Pattern of cancer distribution within and beyond the nuclear family. *PLoS Med.* **2004**, *1*, e65. [CrossRef]
25. Hwang, S.H.; Kim, E.K.; Moon, H.J.; Yoon, J.H.; Kwak, J.Y. Risk of Thyroid Cancer in Euthyroid Asymptomatic Patients with Thyroid Nodules with an Emphasis on Family History of Thyroid Cancer. *Korean J. Radiol.* **2016**, *17*, 255–263. [CrossRef]
26. Myung, S.K.; Lee, C.W.; Lee, J.; Kim, J.; Kim, H.S. Risk Factors for Thyroid Cancer: A Hospital-Based Case-Control Study in Korean Adults. *Cancer Res. Treat.* **2017**, *49*, 70–78. [CrossRef]
27. Byun, S.H.; Min, C.; Hong, S.J.; Choi, H.G.; Koh, D.H. Analysis of the Relation between Periodontitis and Chronic Gastritis/Peptic Ulcer: A Cross-Sectional Study Using KoGES HEXA Data. *Int. J. Environ. Res. Public Health* **2020**, *17*, 4387. [CrossRef]

28. Kim, Y.; Han, B.G.; KoGES Group. Cohort Profile: The Korean Genome and Epidemiology Study (KoGES) Consortium. *Int. J. Epidemiol.* **2017**, *46*, 1350. [CrossRef]
29. Byun, S.H.; Min, C.; Kim, Y.B.; Kim, H.; Kang, S.H.; Park, B.J.; Wee, J.H.; Choi, H.G.; Hong, S.J. Analysis of Chronic Periodontitis in Tonsillectomy Patients: A Longitudinal Follow-Up Study Using a National Health Screening Cohort. *Appl. Sci.* **2020**, *10*, 3663. [CrossRef]
30. Byun, S.H.; Min, C.; Park, I.S.; Kim, H.; Kim, S.K.; Park, B.J.; Choi, H.G.; Hong, S.J. Increased Risk of Chronic Periodontitis in Chronic Rhinosinusitis Patients: A Longitudinal Follow-Up Study Using a National Health-Screening Cohort. *J. Clin. Med.* **2020**, *9*, 1170. [CrossRef]
31. Byun, S.H.; Lee, S.; Kang, S.H.; Choi, H.G.; Hong, S.J. Cross-Sectional Analysis of the Association between Periodontitis and Cardiovascular Disease Using the Korean Genome and Epidemiology Study Data. *Int. J. Environ. Res. Public Health* **2020**, *17*, 5237. [CrossRef]
32. Tavarelli, M.; Russo, M.; Terranova, R.; Scollo, C.; Spadaro, A.; Sapuppo, G.; Malandrino, P.; Masucci, R.; Squatrito, S.; Pellegriti, G. Familial Non-Medullary Thyroid Cancer Represents an Independent Risk Factor for Increased Cancer Aggressiveness: A Retrospective Analysis of 74 Families. *Front. Endocrinol.* **2015**, *6*, 117. [CrossRef]
33. Oakley, G.M.; Curtin, K.; Pimentel, R.; Buchmann, L.; Hunt, J. Establishing a familial basis for papillary thyroid carcinoma using the Utah Population Database. *JAMA Otolaryngol. Head Neck Surg.* **2013**, *139*, 1171–1174. [CrossRef]
34. Ahn, H.S.; Kim, H.J.; Kim, K.H.; Lee, Y.S.; Han, S.J.; Kim, Y.; Ko, M.J.; Brito, J.P. Thyroid Cancer Screening in South Korea Increases Detection of Papillary Cancers with No Impact on Other Subtypes or Thyroid Cancer Mortality. *Thyroid* **2016**, *26*, 1535–1540. [CrossRef]
35. Brito, J.P.; Kim, H.J.; Han, S.J.; Lee, Y.S.; Ahn, H.S. Geographic Distribution and Evolution of Thyroid Cancer Epidemic in South Korea. *Thyroid* **2016**, *26*, 864–865. [CrossRef]
36. Oh, C.M.; Kong, H.J.; Kim, E.; Kim, H.; Jung, K.W.; Park, S.; Won, Y.J. National Epidemiologic Survey of Thyroid cancer (NEST) in Korea. *Epidemiol. Health* **2018**, *40*, e2018052. [CrossRef]
37. Zhao, Z.G.; Guo, X.G.; Ba, C.X.; Wang, W.; Yang, Y.Y.; Wang, J.; Cao, H.Y. Overweight, obesity and thyroid cancer risk: A meta-analysis of cohort studies. *J. Int. Med. Res.* **2012**, *40*, 2041–2050. [CrossRef]
38. Han, J.M.; Kim, T.Y.; Jeon, M.J.; Yim, J.H.; Kim, W.G.; Song, D.E.; Hong, S.J.; Bae, S.J.; Kim, H.K.; Shin, M.H.; et al. Obesity is a risk factor for thyroid cancer in a large, ultrasonographically screened population. *Eur. J. Endocrinol.* **2013**, *168*, 879–886. [CrossRef]
39. Cho, Y.A.; Kim, J. Thyroid cancer risk and smoking status: A meta-analysis. *Cancer Causes Control.* **2014**, *25*, 1187–1195. [CrossRef]
40. Kitahara, C.M.; Linet, M.S.; Beane Freeman, L.E.; Check, D.P.; Church, T.R.; Park, Y.; Purdue, M.P.; Schairer, C.; Berrington de Gonzalez, A. Cigarette smoking, alcohol intake, and thyroid cancer risk: A pooled analysis of five prospective studies in the United States. *Cancer Causes Control.* **2012**, *23*, 1615–1624. [CrossRef]
41. Balhara, Y.P.; Deb, K.S. Impact of alcohol use on thyroid function. *Indian J. Endocrinol. Metab.* **2013**, *17*, 580–587. [CrossRef]
42. Hong, S.H.; Myung, S.K.; Kim, H.S.; Korean Meta-Analysis Study, G. Alcohol Intake and Risk of Thyroid Cancer: A Meta-Analysis of Observational Studies. *Cancer Res. Treat.* **2017**, *49*, 534–547. [CrossRef]
43. Hong, S.; Won, Y.J.; Park, Y.R.; Jung, K.W.; Kong, H.J.; Lee, E.S.; The Community of Population-Based Regional Cancer Registries. Cancer Statistics in Korea: Incidence, Mortality, Survival, and Prevalence in 2017. *Cancer Res. Treat.* **2020**, *52*, 335–350. [CrossRef]

16

Genetic Heterogeneity of *HER2* Amplification and Telomere Shortening in Papillary Thyroid Carcinoma

Paola Caria [1], Silvia Cantara [2], Daniela Virginia Frau [1], Furio Pacini [2,†], Roberta Vanni [1,*,†] and Tinuccia Dettori [1]

1 Department of Biomedical Sciences, University of Cagliari, Cittadella Universitaria, Monserrato 09042, Italy; paola.caria@unica.it (P.C.); dvfrau@unica.it (D.V.F.); dettorit@unica.it (T.D.)
2 Department of Medical, Surgical and Neurological Sciences, University of Siena, Siena 53100, Italy; cantara@unisi.it (S.C.); pacini8@unisi.it (F.P.)
* Correspondence: vanni@unica.it
† These authors contributed equally to this work.

Academic Editor: Daniela Gabriele Grimm

Abstract: Extensive research is dedicated to understanding if sporadic and familial papillary thyroid carcinoma are distinct biological entities. We have previously demonstrated that familial papillary thyroid cancer (fPTC) cells exhibit short relative telomere length (RTL) in both blood and tissues and that these features may be associated with chromosome instability. Here, we investigated the frequency of *HER2* (*Human Epidermal Growth Factor Receptor 2*) amplification, and other recently reported genetic alterations in sporadic PTC (sPTC) and fPTC, and assessed correlations with RTL and *BRAF* mutational status. We analyzed *HER2* gene amplification and the integrity of *ALK, ETV6, RET*, and *BRAF* genes by fluorescence in situ hybridization in isolated nuclei and paraffin-embedded formalin-fixed sections of 13 fPTC and 18 sPTC patients. We analyzed $BRAF^{V600E}$ mutation and RTL by qRT-PCR. Significant *HER2* amplification ($p = 0.0076$), which was restricted to scattered groups of cells, was found in fPTC samples. *HER2* amplification in fPTCs was invariably associated with $BRAF^{V600E}$ mutation. RTL was shorter in fPTCs than sPTCs ($p < 0.001$). No rearrangements of other tested genes were observed. These findings suggest that the association of *HER2* amplification with $BRAF^{V600E}$ mutation and telomere shortening may represent a marker of tumor aggressiveness, and, in refractory thyroid cancer, may warrant exploration as a site for targeted therapy.

Keywords: papillary thyroid carcinoma; *HER2* (*Human Epidermal Growth Factor Receptor 2*); Telomere; FISH (fluorescence in situ hybridization)

---

1. Introduction

The most common histological subtype of non-medullary thyroid carcinoma (NMTC) is papillary thyroid carcinoma (PTC), which represents 75%–85% of all thyroid cancer. Although mostly sporadic (sPTC), there is some evidence for a familial form of PTC (fPTC) not associated with known Mendelian syndromes. Familial PTC is observed in approximately 5%–10% of NMTC cases [1] and, despite the extensive research dedicated to understand if it is a distinct biological entity than sPTC [2], this distinction remains controversial. Indeed, the most common somatic alterations, such as mutations in *RAS* and *BRAF* and rearrangements of *RET/PTC* and *NTRK1*, exhibit similar prevalence and distribution in both sPTC and fPTC [3]. No oncogenic germline mutations of these genes have been detected in fPTC cases [4]. However, there is an ongoing debate on the possible association of *HAPB2* germline mutation to the predisposition to familial forms of NMTC [5–8]. Generally speaking, most PTC can be treated effectively with surgery and radioactive iodine therapy. However, for cases in which these treatments are not effective, targeted drugs might be considered. Kinase inhibitors, such as sorafenib and lenvatinib, are now used as targeted drugs [9,10]. Less frequent genetic alterations, such as rearrangements of *ALK* [11] and *ETV6* [12], identified in sPTC, but not yet investigated in fPTC, also represent new therapeutic targets. In addition, the amplification of the *HER2* gene, reported in highly-malignant PTC nodules [13], might be added to the list of drug-targetable genes. The *HER2* amplification in PTC was observed by fluorescence in situ hybridization (FISH), and average telomere length in *HER2*-positive (*HER2*+) PTC was significantly shorter than *HER2*-negative (*HER2*−) PTC [13]. Of possible significance, shorter average telomere length has also been reported in fPTC compared to sPTC [14]. These observations prompted us to verify *HER2* amplification and telomere length status in 13 fPTC and 18 sPTC. Tumors were also investigated for integrity of the *RET* gene, which is rearranged in 10%–40% of PTC, and *ALK*, *ETV6*, and *BRAF* genes, which are rearranged in a minority of PTC. $BRAF^{V600E}$ mutation, which is associated with an aggressive biological behavior [15], was also evaluated. Our results indicate an increased prevalence of occasional *HER2* gene intermediate amplification in fPTC compared to sPTC, and shorter telomeres in all fPTC, including those with *HER2* amplification, compared to sPTC. In addition, all *HER2*+ samples invariably possessed the $BRAF^{V600E}$ mutation, but not vice versa. The association might represent a marker of tumor aggressiveness and, in refractory thyroid cancer, may indicate possible exploration for targeted therapy. Additionally, the simultaneous occurrence of these three specific molecular alterations may be suggestive of the existence of a specific fPTC subgroup.

2. Results

2.1. Human Epidermal Growth Factor Receptor 2 (HER2) Amplification in Familial Papillary Thyroid Carcinoma (fPTC) and Sporadic Papillary Thyroid Carcinoma (sPTC)

HER2 amplification was evaluated in 13 fPTC (seven females, mean age at diagnosis of 53.7 ± 14.2; six males, mean age at diagnosis 49.0 ± 21.5) and 18 sPTC (15 females, mean age at diagnosis 46.6 ± 7.8; three males, mean age at diagnosis 43.6 ± 13.6). We found that isolated fPTC and sPTC nuclei were *HER2*− according to the Wolff criteria (originally developed for breast cancer formalin-fixed paraffin-embedded (FFPE) examination) [16], although a number of cases showed scattered *HER2*+ cells, ranging from 1.4% to 9% in fPTC and from 1% to 2.4% in sPTC (Figure 1A,B). Based on these observations, and on the lack of specific criteria for the evaluation of *HER2* amplification in thyroid tumors, we analyzed the distribution of HER2+ cells in these cases to determine if they met the criteria for the presence of genetic heterogeneity (>5% and <50%) according to Vance [17]. We found significant genetic heterogeneity in the distribution of *HER2* amplification in fPTC compared to sPTC ($p = 0.0076$) (Figure 1C–E). We found that 5/13 (38.5%) fPTC cases showed 5.1% to 10% HER2+ cells. FISH on FFPE from sPTC confirmed the findings obtained from isolated nuclei that no sPTC case exceeded the cut-off value. When fPTCs were analyzed by immunohistochemistry using an anti-c-erbB2 antibody [18] to detect HER2 protein expression, inconsistent results compared to the FISH analysis were obtained. However, this result was possibly biased by the age of the available histological sections (7–20 years).

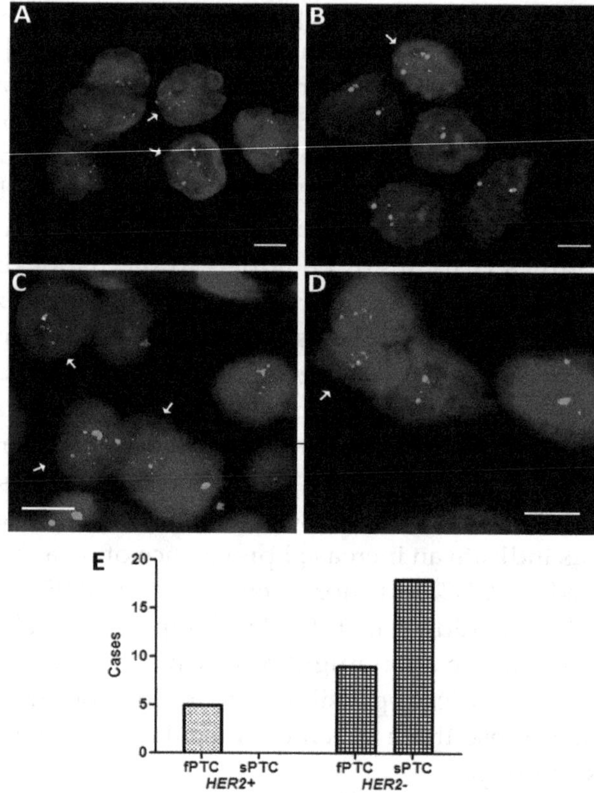

Figure 1. Distribution of *HER2* (*human epidermal growth factor receptor 2*) amplification in familial papillary thyroid carcinoma (fPTC) and sporadic papillary thyroid carcinoma (sPTC) nuclei. Arrows point to isolated nuclei with extra copies of the *HER2* gene (**red spots**) in the presence of disomy 17 (chromosome 17 centromere-specific alphoid repetitive DNA, **green spots**) in fPTC (**A**); and sPTC (**B**); and in nuclei in formalin-fixed paraffin-embedded (FFPE) sections of fPTC (**C**); and sPTC (**D**). The distribution of the amplification in FFPE sections of fPTC versus sPTC was significant ($p = 0.0076$) (Fisher exact test) and indicative of genetic heterogeneity heterogeneity according to Vance criteria [17] (**E**). Scare bar = 10 μm.

2.2. Rearrangements of ALK, BRAF, ETV6, and RET Genes

We found no rearrangements of *ALK*, *BRAF*, and *ETV6* genes by fluorescence in situ hybridization. We found one case of sPTC with a *RET* rearrangement, the remaining cases exhibited neither disruptions nor numerical changes in *RET* gene (see examples in Figure 2A,B).

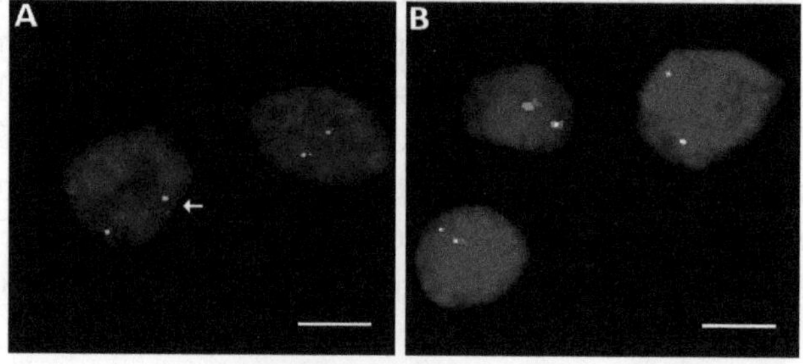

Figure 2. Examples of fluorescence in situ hybridization (FISH) in isolated nuclei for the identification of genes specifically rearranged in papillary thyroid carcinoma (PTC). Arrows point to the split of the red/green signal of a *RET* break-apart [19] probe in the case of sPTC, indicating broken *RET* (**A**); and to un-split red/green signals of an *ALK* break-apart probe in the case of fPTC, indicating unbroken *ALK* (**B**). **Red spot**: 300 kb probe DNA fragment; **Green spot**: 442 kb probe DNA fragment; Scare bar = 10 μm.

2.3. Telomere Length and BRAF^{V600E} Mutation in fPTC and sPTC Patients

Relative telomere length was significantly shorter in fPTC samples than in sPTC samples: median = 0.93 (25th–75th percentile: 0.6–1.2) vs. 1.9 (25th–75th percentile: 1.8–2.3) for fPTC vs. sPTC, respectively ($p < 0.001$) (Figure 3). This result was not due to a difference in the patient's age and sex, as sporadic cases were selected to be age/sex-matched with familial patients (Table 1).

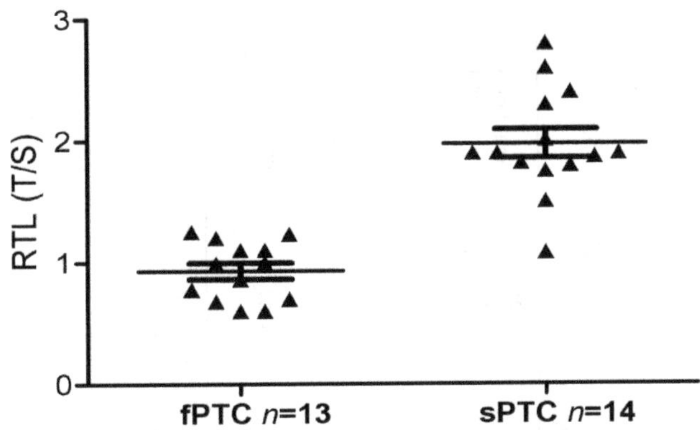

Figure 3. fPTC and sPTC relative telomere length (RTL). RTL was measured by q-PCR, and was expressed as the ratio (T/S) of the telomere (T) repeat copy number to a single-copy gene (S). The difference in RLT between fPTC and sPTC samples was significant ($p < 0.001$) (Mann-Whitney *U*-test). Triangles represent the RTL of each case; the upper and lower lines represent the interquartile range of the distribution (25th–75th percentile); the middle line represents the median.

BRAF^{V600E} mutation was detected in 9/13 (69.0%) fPTC and 14/18 (78%) sPTC ($p = 0.68$), which was not statistically significant. All *HER2*+ fPTC were *BRAF*^{V600E}-positive (*BRAF*+), although not all *BRAF*+ fPTC were *HER2*+ (Figure 4).

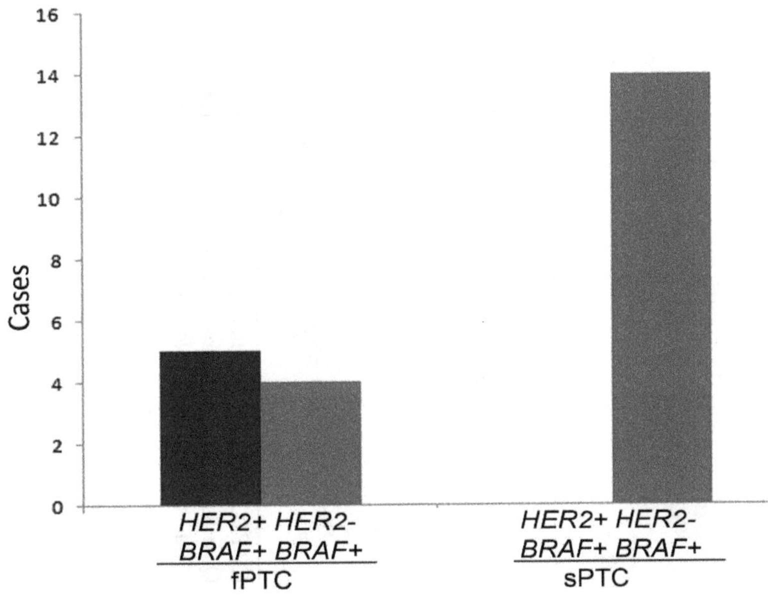

Figure 4. Distribution of *HER2* amplification and *BRAF*^{V600E} mutation in fPTC and sPTC tumors.

Table 1. Characteristics of patients.

Tumor	Age at Diagnosis (Mean ± SD)	Sex (Males %)	PTC Size (Median/IQR)	TNM	Extrathyroidal Invasion *N* (%)	Multifocality *N* (%)	Lymphonode Metastases at Diagnosis *N* (%)	Final Outcome * *N* (%)	Follow-up (Mean Years)	Histology
fPTC (*n* = *13*)	51.5 ± 17.0	6 (46.1%)	11/11.5	*pT1* 8 (61.5%) *pT2* 2 (11.7%) *pT3* 3 (23.0%)	5 (38.5%)	7 (53.8%)	3 (23%)	*Remission* 9 (69.2%) *Persistent disease* 4 (30.8%)	7.59 ± 3.9	9 CV-PTC 4 FV-PTC
sPTC (*n* = *18*)	46.1 ± 8.5	3 (16.6%)	9.5/8.5	*pT1* 8 (44.4%) *pT2* 1 (5.5%) *pT3* 9 (50.%)	9 (50%)	6 (33.3%)	5 (27.7%)	*Remission* 11 (61.1%) *Persistent disease* 2 (11.1%)	5.5 ± 2.8	14 CV-PTC 2 FV-PTC 1 SV-PTC 1 TR-PTC

CV-PTC—classical variant of papillary thyroid carcinoma; fPTC—familial papillary thyroid carcinoma; FV-PTC—follicular variant of papillary thyroid carcinoma; IQR—Inter Quartile Range; *N*—number of cases; PTC—papillary thyroid carcinoma; sPTC—sporadic papillary thyroid carcinoma; SV-PTC—sclerosing variant of papillary thyroid carcinoma; TNM—(Tumor (limph) Node Metastasis) classification [20]; TR-PTC: trabecular variant of papillary thyroid carcinoma; *—six patients were lost to follow-up.

3. Discussion

Amplification of the *HER2* gene in thyroid cancer was first uncovered by FISH analysis of follicular cells from highly malignant PTC nodules [13]. They observed that *HER2+* PTC exhibited shorter telomeres than *HER2−* PTC. PTC is an entity mostly recognized as sporadic, although the familial form may account for approximately 5% of cases [1,2]. Familial PTC may occur in combination with other Mendelian cancer syndromes (familial adenomatous polyposis, Gardner's syndrome, Peutz-Jeghers syndrome, and Cowden's syndrome) or may be unassociated with other neoplasms in familial aggregates. However, although the risk of developing extra-thyroidal malignancy in non-Cowden's syndrome is documented [21,22], the clinical correlation between sporadic breast cancer (20% of which are *HER2+*) [23] and PTC is still controversial [24,25], and the co-occurrence of both disorders in the same individual is a subject of extensive debate [26,27]. None of our fPTC patients had clinical or pathological evidence of hereditary syndromes associated with NMTC, breast cancer, or other types of sporadic tumors, except for one male patient who had a previous squamous cell carcinoma of the auricle. The thyroid cancer of this patient was not associated with any genetic alterations of the genes examined here. As more than 5%, but fewer than 50%, of nuclei were found to be amplified in our FFPE sections, we use the Vance criteria [17] in the interpretation of our results. Our data indicated a significant difference in *HER2* amplification ($p = 0.019$) in fPTC compared to sPTC. This finding indicates a degree of genetic heterogeneity in the fPTC group and suggests that *HER2+* cells in fPTC possibly undergo apoptosis to a lesser extent than in sPTC. The observation adds thyroid carcinoma to the list of tumors that exhibit *HER2+*. *HER2+* is indeed observed in a growing number of other tumors, including advanced gastric and esophageal cancer [28], ovarian [29], colon [30], bladder, lung, uterine, cervix, head and neck, and endometrial cancer [31]. The extracellular domain of the HER2 receptor has an essential role in cell proliferation and anti-apoptotic processes, making *HER2+* breast and gastric/gastroesophageal cancers more likely to respond to targeted therapies in combination with chemotherapy than *HER2−* tumors. A wide range of solid tumors showing deregulation of *HER2* expression are regarded as biologically aggressive. Familial PTC is often associated with a more severe phenotype than its sporadic counterpart [32], and often harbor $BRAF^{V600E}$ mutation. $BRAF^{V600E}$ is considered to have a prognostic value in PTC [33], and usually identifies differentiated thyroid tumors with advanced clinicopathological features. $BRAF^{V600E}$ is also strongly associated with PTC patient mortality [15]. In contrast to lung adenocarcinoma, in which *HER2* amplification and $BRAF^{V600E}$ mutation appear to be mutually exclusive events [34], here we found that all *HER2+* fPTC bore the $BRAF^{V600E}$ mutation, although not all $BRAF^{V600E}$-positive nodules had *HER2* amplification. Of significance, none of the $BRAF^{V600E}$-positive sPTC were *HER2+*, despite the high frequency of $BRAF^{V600}$ mutations in this cohort. It is not entirely clear how this discrepancy should be interpreted, considering the limited size of our cohorts. In addition, we do not know whether *HER2* amplification and $BRAF^{V600E}$ mutation coexist in the same cells within a tumor or if they are segregated in different clones. We do not know, either, if the condition is different in our *HER2+* fPTC versus sPTC with *HER2+* cells <5%.

The other evaluated genes, *ALK*, *BRAF*, *ETV6*, and *RET*, exhibited extensive integrity. The only case bearing a *RET* disruption was $BRAF^{V600E}$-negative. Moreover, we found a significant difference ($p < 0.001$) of RTL in fPTC nodules compared to sPTC nodules, in agreement with our previous investigations [14,35]. Telomere length regulation plays a crucial role in genome instability and tumorigenesis [36]. Dysfunctional telomeres can increase chromosome instability by causing either fusion of chromosomes or fusion of sister chromatids, bringing the formation of anaphase bridges and the beginning of the so-called breakage-bridge-fusion cycles [37]. Although biased by the small number of patients investigated in our two cohorts (forced by the low frequency of fPTC), our data stigmatize significantly shorter RTL in fPTC cells versus sPTC cells. This result is in line with the reported predisposition of fPTC patients toward spontaneous chromosome fragility [35]. This observation poses the basis for further investigation exploring the existence of a possible specific three-dimensional (3D) altered telomere organization in fPTC. Telomere remodeling is a feature of cancer cells [38] and may identify tumor subgroups [39,40]. On the other hand, alterations in the telomere 3D profile have been reported in a murine model of thyroid tumors [41]. Recurrent somatic mutations in the promoter of TERT, the catalytic subunit of the enzyme telomerase, has been reported in PTC [42], often in concomitance with mutated *BRAF* [43]. A subclonal distribution in the rare PTC that harbor the alteration, in contrast to a clonal distribution in the poorly-differentiated and anaplastic tumors has been observed [44]. Unfortunately, the scanty material available from our cases prevented the possibility to establish a putative association of TERT promoter mutations with telomere length in our PTCs.

Our finding on RTL are, substantially, in keeping with the Sugishita data [13]. However, in contrast, 38.5% of our fPTC, but none of our sPTC, showed *HER2* amplification, indicating an apparently preferential association with fPTC. In this regard, the small number of patients investigated in our two cohorts might constitute a bias. Nevertheless, as a whole, the finding of $BRAF^{V600E}$ mutation in association with *HER2*+ genetic heterogeneity, short telomere length, and prevalence of multifocal tumors seems to not be a rare molecular event in fPTC and may characterize a subgroup of fPTC. The response of refractory fPTC patients of this subgroup to target therapy of trastuzumab and lapatinib should be explored.

4. Materials and Methods

4.1. Sample Collection

The PTCs (13 fPTC and 18 sPTC) considered in the present study were selected from the pathological files of the University of Siena. Familial recurrence of the disease was defined as the presence of at least one first-degree relative with differentiated thyroid carcinoma in the absence of any other familial syndrome. None of the fPTC patients presented with any other sporadic tumor, including breast cancer, except for one male patient with a previous squamous cell carcinoma of the auricle. The histology of all tumor samples was classified according to the World Health Organization guidelines [20]. The fPTC cases were selected from 13 families, randomly choosing one affected subject from each family (the oldest affected subject): seven females (mean age at diagnosis of 53.7 ± 14.2, with an age range of 29–69 years) and six males (mean age at diagnosis of 49.0 ± 21.5, range 24–81). Four fPTC tumors were classified as follicular variants and nine were classical PTC. Seven out of the 13 families (53.8%) had three or more affected members, two out of 13 (15.3%) had two members with PTC and at least three members operated for multi-nodular goiter, and four out of 13 had only two members affected by thyroid cancer. In these cases, the phenomenon of genetic anticipation was observed with the second generation acquiring the disease at an earlier age and having more advanced disease at presentation.

The sPTC cases were from 15 females (mean age at diagnosis of 46.6 ± 7.8, range 31–64) and three males (mean age at diagnosis 43.6 ± 13.6, range 31–58). Fourteen were classified as classical PTC, two as follicular variants, one as a diffuse sclerosing variant, and one as a trabecular variant (Table 1). Informed consent was obtained from each patient after a full explanation of the purpose and nature of all of the procedures to be used. All data from the patients were handled in accordance with local ethical committee-approved protocols and in compliance with the Helsinki declaration

4.2. Fluorescence In Situ Hybridization

Thick sections (30 μm) were obtained from formalin-fixed paraffin-embedded (FFPE) tissue blocks of the thyroid nodules or, to assess probe cut-off, from the apparently tumor-free tissue of the contralateral lobe. Nuclei were isolated as reported [45], and were investigated by FISH, using specific probes and a standard protocol [46].

4.3. Detection of HER2 Gene Copy Number Alterations or Amplification

HER2 amplification was determined by counting the total numbers of *HER2* and CEP17 (chromosome 17 centromere-specific alphoid repetitive DNA, Abbott Molecular, Abbott Park, IL, USA) signals per nucleus with a mean of 89.5 (range 34–175) nuclei. The ratio of *HER2* signals to CEP17 (centromeric probe for chromosome 17) signals was calculated according to ASCO/CAP (American Society of Clinical Oncology/College of American Pathologists Guideline) criteria refined for breast cancer [16].

Nodules with, or suspected to have, *HER2* amplification were then re-evaluated by FISH on 4 μm histological sections to assess the distribution of possible clones. The tumor area, marked by the pathologist [47], was entirely scored. As more than 5%, but fewer than 50%, of nuclei were found to be amplified, the Vance criteria were used to define the distribution of abnormal cells [17].

Consecutive histologic sections were used to assess *HER2* expression by immunohistochemistry. The expression of HER2 protein was determined using anti-c-erbB2 antibody (Dako, Glostrup, Denmark) in accordance with the manufacturer's instructions.

Detection of *ALK*, *BRAF*, *ETV6*, and *RET* rearrangements. Commercially available break-apart or single gene probes for *ALK*, *BRAF* (Abbott Molecular, Abbott Park, IL, USA), and *ETV6* (Kreatech Diagnostic, Amsterdam, The Netherlands) were used to verify gene integrity in nuclei isolated from FFPE tissue blocks. An arbitrary cut-off of 3% was employed, as control cells showed no split signal in 200 scored nuclei per sample. For the *RET* gene, a homebrew probe and a previously described cut-off value were used [19]. Microscopic analysis was performed with an Olympus BX41 epifluorescence microscope and a charge-coupled device camera (Cohu, San Diego, CA, USA) interfaced with the CytoVision system (software version 3.9; Applied Imaging, Pittsburg, PA, USA).

4.4. Telomere Length and $BRAF^{V600E}$ Mutation

DNA was extracted from fresh or FFPE tissues, using the QIAamp® DNA Mini Kit (Qiagen, Milano, Italy) following the manufacturer's instructions. RTL of sPTC was determined by quantitative PCR, carried out on 30 ng/μL genomic DNA using an MJ Mini Personal Thermal cycler (Bio-Rad, Milano, Italy) as described [14]. RTL values of the fPTC examined in the present study were reported previously [14]. Relative telomere length was calculated as the ratio of telomere repeats to a single-copy gene in experimental samples using standard curves. This ratio is proportional to the average telomere length. The *36B4* gene, which encodes acidic ribosomal phosphoprotein P0, was used as the single-copy gene [14]. For analysis of the $BRAF^{V600E}$ mutation, DNA was amplified in a final volume of 50 μL of 2× PCR Master Mix (AmpliTaq Gold® PCR Master Mix, Applied Biosystems, Milano, Italy) and a final primer concentration of 200 nM. Primer sequences, PCR conditions, and interpretation of results were as previously described [48].

4.5. Statistical Analyses

Mann-Whitney *U*-test (IBM SPSS Statistic version 2.1 software, Armonk, NY, USA) was used for statistical analysis of differences in RTL. Fisher exact test was used to compare *HER2* gene amplification. All p-values were two-sided and p less than 0.05 was considered significant.

Epidemiological data are presented as the mean ± SD and median when necessary. The t-test for independent data was performed for normal variables. To evaluate significant differences in data frequency we analyzed 2 × 2 contingency tables by the Fisher exact test. Tables with sizes larger than 2 × 2 were examined by the Chi-squared test.

Acknowledgments: We thank Sandra Orrù from the Pathology Service Businco Hospital (Cagliari, Italy), Azienda Ospedaliera Brotzu for analysis of specimens by immunohistochemistry. This work was partially supported by the program "Projects of national interest (PRIN)" of the Italian Ministry of Education, University and Research (MIUR) (grant No 20122ZF7HE-002).

Author Contributions: Paola Caria, Daniela Virginia Frau, and Tinuccia Dettori carried out the FISH studies and drafted the manuscript. Silvia Cantara carried out the qPCR studies and the *BRAF*^{V600E} mutational analysis. Silvia Cantara and Furio Pacini participated in the design of the study and took care of the clinical approach to patients. Roberta Vanni and Tinuccia Dettori conceived of the study, participated in its design and coordination, and drafted the manuscript. All authors read and approved the final version.

References

1. Thyroid Disease Manager. Available online: http://www.thyroidmanager.org/ (accessed on 31 July 2016).
2. Bonora, E.; Tallini, G.; Romeo, G. Genetic predisposition to familial nonmedullary thyroid cancer: An update of molecular findings and state-of-the-art studies. *J. Oncol.* **2010**, 385206. [CrossRef] [PubMed]
3. Moses, W.; Weng, J.; Kebebew, E. Prevalence, clinicopathologic features, and somatic genetic mutation profile in familial versus sporadic nonmedullary thyroid cancer. *Thyroid* **2011**, *21*, 367–371. [CrossRef] [PubMed]
4. Hou, P.; Xing, M. Absence of germline mutations in genes within the MAP kinase pathway in familial non medullary thyroid cancer. *Cell Cycle* **2006**, *5*, 2036–2039. [CrossRef] [PubMed]
5. Gara, S.K.; Jia, L.; Merino, M.J.; Agarwa, S.K.; Zhang, L.; Cam, M.; Patel, D.; Kebebew, E. Germline *HABP2* mutation causing familial non medullary thyroid cancer. *N. Engl. J. Med.* **2015**, *373*, 448–455. [CrossRef] [PubMed]
6. Carvajal-Carmona, L.G.; Tomlinson, I.; Sahasrabudhe, R. Re: HABP2 G534E mutation in familial nonmedullary thyroid cancer. *J. Natl. Cancer Inst.* **2016**, *108*, djw108. [CrossRef] [PubMed]
7. Weeks, A.L.; Wilson, S.G.; Ward, L.; Goldblatt, J.; Hui, J.; Walsh, J.P. HABP2 germline variants are uncommon in familial nonmedullary thyroid cancer. *BMC Med. Genet.* **2016**, *17*, 60. [CrossRef] [PubMed]
8. Tomsic, J.; Fultz, R.; Liyanarachchi, S.; He, H.; Senter, L.; de la Chapelle, A. HABP2 G534E variant in papillary thyroid carcinoma. *PLoS ONE* **2016**, *11*, e0146315. [CrossRef] [PubMed]
9. Fallahi, P.; Mazzi, V.; Vita, R.; Ferrari, S.M.; Materazzi, G.; Galleri, D.; Benvenga, S.; Miccoli, P.; Antonelli, A. New therapies for dedifferentiated papillary thyroid cancer. *Int. J. Mol. Sci.* **2015**, *16*, 6153–6182. [CrossRef] [PubMed]
10. Bikas, A.; Vachhani, S.; Jensen, K.; Vasko, V.; Burman, K.D. Targeted therapies in thyroid cancer: An extensive review of the literature. *Expert Rev. Clin. Pharmacol.* **2016**, *15*, 1–15. [CrossRef] [PubMed]
11. Nikiforov, Y.E. Thyroid cancer in 2015: Molecular landscape of thyroid cancer continues to be deciphered. *Nat. Rev. Endocrinol.* **2016**, *12*, 67–68. [CrossRef] [PubMed]
12. Ricarte-Filho, J.C.; Li, S.; Garcia-Rendueles, M.E.; Montero-Conde, C.; Voza, F.; Knauf, J.A.; Heguy, A.; Viale, A.; Bogdanova, T.; Thomas, G.A.; Mason, C.E.; et al. Identification of kinase fusion oncogenes in post-Chernobyl radiation-induced thyroid cancers. *J. Clin. Investig.* **2013**, *123*, 4935–4944. [CrossRef] [PubMed]
13. Sugishita, Y.; Kammori, M.; Yamada, O.; Poon, S.S.; Kobayashi, M.; Onoda, N.; Yamazaki, K.; Fukumori, T.; Yoshikawa, K.; Onose, H.; et al. Amplification of the human epidermal growth factor receptor 2 gene in differentiated thyroid cancer correlates with telomere shortening. *Int. J. Oncol.* **2013**, *42*, 1589–1596. [PubMed]
14. Capezzone, M.; Cantara, S.; Marchisotta, S.; Busonero, G.; Formichi, C.; Benigni, M.; Capuano, S.; Toti, P.; Pazaitou-Panayiotou, K.; Caruso, G.; et al. Telomere length in neoplastic and nonneoplastic tissues of patients with familial and sporadic papillary thyroid cancer. *J. Clin. Endocrinol. Metab.* **2011**, *96*, E1852–E1856. [CrossRef] [PubMed]
15. Xing, M.; Haugen, B.R.; Schlumberger, M. Progress in molecular-based management of differentiated thyroid cancer. *Lancet* **2013**, *381*, 1058–1069. [CrossRef]
16. Wolff, A.C.; Hammond, M.E.H.; Hicks, D.G.; Dowsett, M.; McShane, L.M.; Allison, K.H.; Allred, D.C.; Bartlett, J.M.S.; Bilous, M.; Fitzgibbons, P.; et al. Recommendations for human epidermal growth factor receptor 2 testing in breast cancer: American Society of Clinical Oncology/College of American Pathologists clinical practice guideline update. *J. Clin. Oncol.* **2013**, *31*, 3997–4013. [CrossRef] [PubMed]
17. Vance, G.H.; Barry, T.S.; Bloom, K.J.; Fitzgibbons, P.L.; Hicks, D.G.; Jenkins, R.B.; Persons, D.L.; Tubbs, R.R.; Hammond, M.E.H. Genetic heterogeneity in HER2 testing in breast cancer panel summary and guidelines. *Arch. Pathol. Lab. Med.* **2009**, *133*, 611–612. [PubMed]

18. Wright, C.; Angus, B.; Nicholson, S.; Sainsbury, J.R.; Cairns, J.; Gullick, W.J.; Kelly, P.; Harris, A.L.; Horne, C.H. Expression of c-erbB-2 oncoprotein: A prognostic indicator in human breast cancer. *Cancer Res.* **1989**, *49*, 2087–2090. [PubMed]
19. Caria, P.; Dettori, T.; Frau, D.V.; Borghero, A.; Cappai, A.; Riola, A.; Lai, M.L.; Boi, F.; Calò, P.; Nicolosi, A.; et al. Assessing RET/PTC in thyroid nodule fine-needle aspirates: The FISH point of view. *Endocr. Relat. Cancer* **2013**, *20*, 527–536. [CrossRef] [PubMed]
20. De Lellis, R.A. *WHO Classification of Tumours, Pathology and Genetics of Tumours of Endocrine Organs*, 3rd ed.; Ronald, A., de Lellis, R.A., Riccardo, V.L., Philipp, U.H., Charis, E., Eds.; IARC Press: Lyon, France, 2004; Volume 8, p. 230.
21. Ronckers, C.M.; McCarron, P.; Ron, E. Thyroid cancer and multiple primary tumors in the SEER cancer registries. *Int. J. Cancer* **2005**, *117*, 281–288. [CrossRef] [PubMed]
22. Omür, O.; Ozcan, Z.; Yazici, B.; Akgün, A.; Oral, A.; Ozkiliç, H. Multiple primary tumors in differentiated thyroid carcinoma and relationship to thyroid cancer outcome. *Endocr. J.* **2008**, *55*, 365–372. [CrossRef] [PubMed]
23. Burstein, H.J. The distinctive nature of HER2-positive breast cancers. *N. Engl. J. Med.* **2005**, *353*, 1652–1654. [CrossRef] [PubMed]
24. Joseph, K.R.; Edirimanne, S.; Eslick, G.D. The association between breast cancer and thyroid cancer: A meta-analysis. *Breast Cancer Res. Treat.* **2015**, *152*, 173–181. [CrossRef] [PubMed]
25. Sogaard, M.; Farkas, D.K.; Ehrenstein, V.; Jørgensen, J.O.; Dekkers, O.M.; Sorensen, H.T. Hypothyroidism and hyperthyroidism and breast cancer risk: A nationwide cohort study. *Eur. J. Endocrinol.* **2016**, *174*, 409–414. [CrossRef] [PubMed]
26. Brown, A.P.; Chen, J.; Hitchcock, Y.J.; Szabo, A.; Shrieve, D.C.; Tward, J.D. The risk of second primary malignancies up to three decades after the treatment of differentiated thyroid cancer. *J. Clin. Endocrinol. Metab.* **2008**, *93*, 504–515. [CrossRef] [PubMed]
27. Verkooijen, R.B.; Smit, J.W.; Romijn, J.A.; Stokkel, M.P. The incidence of second primary tumors in thyroid cancer patients is increased, but not related to treatment of thyroid cancer. *Eur. J. Endocrinol.* **2006**, *155*, 801–806. [CrossRef] [PubMed]
28. Nagaraja, V.; Eslick, G.D. HER2 expression in gastric and oesophageal cancer: A metaanalytic review. *J. Gastrointest. Cancer* **2015**, *6*, 143–154.
29. Verri, E.; Guglielmini, P.; Puntoni, M.; Perdelli, L.; Papadia, A.; Lorenzi, P.; Rubagotti, A.; Ragni, N.; Boccardo, F. HER2/neuoncoprotein overexpression in epithelial ovarian cancer: Evaluation of its prevalence and prognostic significance. *Oncology* **2005**, *68*, 154–161. [CrossRef] [PubMed]
30. Seo, A.N.; Kwak, Y.; Kim, D.W.; Kang, S.B.; Choe, G.; Kim, W.H.; Lee, H.S. HER2 status in colorectal cancer: Its clinical significance and the relationship between *HER2* gene amplification and expression. *PLoS ONE* **2014**, *9*, e98528. [CrossRef] [PubMed]
31. Iqbal, N.; Iqbal, N. Human epidermal growth factor receptor 2 (HER2) in cancers: Overexpression and therapeutic implications. *Mol. Biol. Int.* **2014**, *2014*, 1–9. [CrossRef] [PubMed]
32. Capezzone, M.; Marchisotta, S.; Cantara, S.; Busonero, G.; Brilli, L.; Pazaitou-Panayiotou, K.; Carli, A.F.; Caruso, G.; Toti, P.; Capitani, S.; et al. Familial non-medullary thyroid carcinoma displays the features of clinical anticipation suggestive of a distinct biological entity. *Endocr. Relat. Cancer* **2008**, *15*, 1075–1081. [CrossRef] [PubMed]
33. Xing, M.; Alzahrani, A.S.; Carson, K.A.; Shong, Y.K.; Kim, T.Y.; Viola, D.; Elisei, R.; Bendlová, B.; Yip, L.; Mian, C.; et al. Association between BRAF V600E mutation and recurrence of papillary thyroid cancer. *J. Clin. Oncol.* **2015**, *33*, 42–50. [CrossRef] [PubMed]
34. Shan, L.; Qiu, T.; Ling, Y.; Guo, L.; Zheng, B.; Wang, B.; Li, W.; Li, L.; Ying, J. Prevalence and clinicopathological characteristics of HER2 and BRAF mutation in Chinese patients with lung adenocarcinoma. *PLoS ONE* **2015**, *10*, e0130447. [CrossRef] [PubMed]
35. Cantara, S.; Pisu, M.; Frau, D.V.; Caria, P.; Dettori, T.; Capezzone, M.; Capuano, S.; Vanni, R.; Pacini, F. Telomere abnormalities and chromosome fragility in patients affected by familial papillary thyroid cancer. *J. Clin. Endocrinol. Metab.* **2012**, *97*, E1327–E1331. [CrossRef] [PubMed]
36. Meeker, A.K.; Hicks, J.L.; Iacobuzio-Donahue, C.A.; Montgomery, E.A.; Westra, W.H.; Chan, T.Y.; Ronnett, B.M.; De Marzo, A.M. Telomere length abnormalities occur early in the initiation of epithelial carcinogenesis. *Clin. Cancer Res.* **2004**, *10*, 3317–3326. [CrossRef] [PubMed]

37. Gisselsson, D.; Jonson, T.; Petersen, A.; Strombeck, B.; Dal Cin, P.; Hoglund, M.; Mitelman, F.; Mertens, F.; Mandahl, N. Telomere dysfunction triggers extensive DNA fragmentation and evolution of complex chromosome abnormalities in human malignant tumors. *Proc. Natl. Acad. Sci. USA* **2001**, *98*, 12683–12688. [CrossRef] [PubMed]
38. Gadji, M.; Vallente, R.; Klewes, L.; Righolt, C.; Wark, L.; Kongruttanachok, N.; Knecht, H.; Mai, S. *Nuclear Remodeling as a Mechanism for Genomic Instability in Cancer*; Gisselsson, D., Ed.; Academic Press: New York, NY, USA, 2011; Volume 112, pp. 77–126.
39. Gadji, M.; Adebayo Awe, J.; Rodrigues, P.; Kumar, R.; Houston, D.S.; Klewes, L.; Dièye, T.N.; Rego, E.M.; Passetto, R.F.; de Oliveira, F.M.; et al. Profiling three-dimensional nuclear telomeric architecture of myelodysplastic syndromes and acute myeloid leukemia defines patient subgroups. *Clin. Cancer Res.* **2012**, *18*, 3293–3304. [CrossRef] [PubMed]
40. Kuzyk, A.; Gartner, J.; Mai, S. Identification of neuroblastoma subgroups based on three-dimensional telomere organization. *Transl. Oncol.* **2016**, *9*, 348–356. [CrossRef] [PubMed]
41. Wark, L.; Danescu, A.; Natarajan, S.; Zhu, X.; Cheng, S.Y.; Hombach-Klonisch, S.; Mai, S.; Klonisch, T. Three-dimensional telomere dynamics in follicular thyroid cancer. *Thyroid* **2014**, *24*, 296–304. [CrossRef] [PubMed]
42. Liu, R.; Xing, M. TERT promoter mutations in thyroid cancer. *Endocr. Relat. Cancer* **2016**, *23*, R143–R155. [PubMed]
43. Liu, R.; Bishop, J.; Zhu, G.; Zhang, T.; Ladenson, P.W.; Xing, M. Mortality risk stratification by combining BRAF V600E and TERT promoter mutations in papillary thyroid cancer: Genetic duet of BRAF and TERT promoter mutations in thyroid cancer mortality. *JAMA Oncol.* **2016**. [CrossRef] [PubMed]
44. Landa, I.; Ibrahimpasic, T.; Boucai, L.; Sinha, R.; Knauf, J.A.; Shah, R.H.; Dogan, S.; Ricarte-Filho, J.C.; Krishnamoorthy, G.P.; Xu, B.; et al. Genomic and transcriptomic hallmarks of poorly differentiated and anaplastic thyroid cancers. *J. Clin. Investig.* **2016**, *126*, 1052–1066. [CrossRef] [PubMed]
45. Petersen, B.L.; Sorensen, M.C.; Pedersen, S.; Rasmussen, M. Fluorescence in situ hybridization on formalin-fixed and paraffin-embedded tissue: Optimizing the method. *Appl. Immunohistochem. Mol. Morphol.* **2004**, *12*, 259–265. [CrossRef] [PubMed]
46. Caria, P.; Frau, D.V.; Dettori, T.; Boi, F.; Lai, M.L.; Mariotti, S.; Vanni, R. Optimizing detection of RET and PPARg rearrangements in thyroid neoplastic cells using a home-brew tetracolor probe. *Cancer Cytopathol.* **2014**, *122*, 377–385. [CrossRef] [PubMed]
47. Hastings, R.; Bown, N.; Tibiletti, M.G.; Debiec-Rychter, M.; Vanni, R.; Espinet, B.; van Roy, N.; Roberts, P.; van den Berg-de-Ruiter, E.; Bernheim, A.; et al. Guidelines for cytogenetic investigations in tumours. *Eur. J. Hum. Genet.* **2015**, *24*, 1–8. [CrossRef] [PubMed]
48. Cantara, S.; Capezzone, M.; Marchisotta, S.; Capuano, S.; Busonero, G.; Toti, P.; di Santo, A.; Caruso, G.; Carli, A.F.; Brilli, L.; et al. Impact of proto-oncogene mutation detection in cytological specimens from thyroid nodules improves the diagnostic accuracy of cytology. *J. Clin. Endocrinol. Metab.* **2010**, *95*, 1365–1369. [CrossRef] [PubMed]

Permissions

All chapters in this book were first published by MDPI; hereby published with permission under the Creative Commons Attribution License or equivalent. Every chapter published in this book has been scrutinized by our experts. Their significance has been extensively debated. The topics covered herein carry significant findings which will fuel the growth of the discipline. They may even be implemented as practical applications or may be referred to as a beginning point for another development.

The contributors of this book come from diverse backgrounds, making this book a truly international effort. This book will bring forth new frontiers with its revolutionizing research information and detailed analysis of the nascent developments around the world.

We would like to thank all the contributing authors for lending their expertise to make the book truly unique. They have played a crucial role in the development of this book. Without their invaluable contributions this book wouldn't have been possible. They have made vital efforts to compile up to date information on the varied aspects of this subject to make this book a valuable addition to the collection of many professionals and students.

This book was conceptualized with the vision of imparting up-to-date information and advanced data in this field. To ensure the same, a matchless editorial board was set up. Every individual on the board went through rigorous rounds of assessment to prove their worth. After which they invested a large part of their time researching and compiling the most relevant data for our readers.

The editorial board has been involved in producing this book since its inception. They have spent rigorous hours researching and exploring the diverse topics which have resulted in the successful publishing of this book. They have passed on their knowledge of decades through this book. To expedite this challenging task, the publisher supported the team at every step. A small team of assistant editors was also appointed to further simplify the editing procedure and attain best results for the readers.

Apart from the editorial board, the designing team has also invested a significant amount of their time in understanding the subject and creating the most relevant covers. They scrutinized every image to scout for the most suitable representation of the subject and create an appropriate cover for the book.

The publishing team has been an ardent support to the editorial, designing and production team. Their endless efforts to recruit the best for this project, has resulted in the accomplishment of this book. They are a veteran in the field of academics and their pool of knowledge is as vast as their experience in printing. Their expertise and guidance has proved useful at every step. Their uncompromising quality standards have made this book an exceptional effort. Their encouragement from time to time has been an inspiration for everyone.

The publisher and the editorial board hope that this book will prove to be a valuable piece of knowledge for researchers, students, practitioners and scholars across the globe.

List of Contributors

Benedikt Schmidbauer, Karin Menhart, Dirk Hellwig and Jirka Grosse
Department of Nuclear Medicine, University of Regensburg, 93053 Regensburg, Germany

Fabíola Yukiko Miasaki and Gisah Amaral de Carvalho
Department of Endocrinology and Metabolism (SEMPR), Hospital de Clínicas, Federal University of Paraná, Curitiba 80030-110, Brazil

Cesar Seigi Fuziwara and Edna Teruko Kimura
Department of Cell and Developmental Biology, Institute of Biomedical Sciences, University of São Paulo, São Paulo 05508-000, Brazil

Rosaria M. Ruggeri and Francesco Trimarchi
Department of Clinical and Experimental Medicine, Unit of Endocrinology, University of Messina, AOU Policlinico G. Martino, 98125 Messina, Italy

Alfredo Campennì and Massimiliano Siracusa
Department of Biomedical Sciences and Morphological and Functional Images, Unit of Nuclear Medicine, University of Messina, AOU Policlinico G. Martino, 98125 Messina, Italy

Giuseppe Giuffrè, Angela Simone, Giovanni Branca, Rosa Scarfì, Antonio Ieni and Giovanni Tuccari
Department of Human Pathology in Adult and Developmental Age "Gaetano Barresi", Unit of Pathological Anatomy, University of Messina, AOU Policlinico G. Martino, 98125 Messina, Italy

Luca Giovanella
Department of Nuclear Medicine, Thyroid and PET/CT Center, Oncology Institute of Southern Switzerland, 6500 Bellinzona, Switzerland

Paul J. Davis
Department of Medicine, Albany Medical College, Albany, NY 12208, USA
Pharmaceutical Research Institute, Albany College of Pharmacy and Health Sciences, Rensselaer, NY 12144, USA

Shaker A. Mousa
Pharmaceutical Research Institute, Albany College of Pharmacy and Health Sciences, Rensselaer, NY 12144, USA

Hung-Yun Lin
Ph.D. Program for Cancer Molecular Biology and Drug Discovery, College of Medical Science and Technology, Taipei Medical University, Taipei 11031, Taiwan
Cancer Center, Wan Fang Hospital, Taipei Medical University, Taipei 11031, Taiwan
Traditional Herbal Medicine Research Center of Taipei Medical University Hospital, Taipei Medical University, Taipei 11031, Taiwan

Aleck Hercbergs
Department of Radiation Oncology, The Cleveland Clinic, Cleveland, OH 44195, USA

Silvia Cantara, Carlotta Marzocchi, Tania Pilli, Sandro Cardinale, Raffaella Forleo, Maria Grazia Castagna and Furio Pacini
Department of Medical, Surgical and Neurological Sciences, University of Siena, 53100 Siena, Italy

Leonardo P. Stuchi, Márcia Maria U. Castanhole-Nunes, Patrícia M. Biselli-Chicote, Erika C. Pavarino and Eny Maria Goloni-Bertollo
Research Unit in Genetics and Molecular Biology—UPGEM, Faculty of Medicine of São José do Rio Preto—FAMERP, São José do Rio Preto 15090-000, Brazil

Nathália Maniezzo-Stuchi and Ana Paula Girol
Padre Albino University Center—UNIFIPA, Catanduva, São Paulo 15809-144, Brazil

Tiago Henrique
Laboratory of Molecular Markers and Bioinformatics, Department of Molecular Biology, Faculty of Medicine of São José do Rio Preto —FAMERP, São José do Rio Preto 15090-000, Brazil

João Armando Padovani Neto
Department of Otolaryngology and Head and Neck Surgery, Faculty of Medicine of São José do Rio Preto —FAMERP, São José do Rio Preto 15090-000, Brazil

Dalisio de-Santi Neto
Pathological Anatomy Service, Hospital de Base, Foundation Regional Faculty of Medicine of São José do Rio Preto—FUNFARME, São José do Rio Preto 15090-000, Brazil

Ole Vincent Ancker
Department of Biomedicine, Aarhus University, Wilhelm Meyers Allé 4, 8000 Aarhus C, Denmark

Daniela Grimm
Department of Biomedicine, Aarhus University, Wilhelm Meyers Allé 4, 8000 Aarhus C, Denmark
Clinic and Policlinic for Plastic, Aesthetic and Hand Surgery, Otto von Guericke University, Leipziger Str. 44, 39120 Magdeburg, Germany

Markus Wehland and Manfred Infanger
Clinic and Policlinic for Plastic, Aesthetic and Hand Surgery, Otto von Guericke University, Leipziger Str. 44, 39120 Magdeburg, Germany

Johann Bauer
Max-Planck-Institute for Biochemistry, Am Klopferspitz 18, 82152 Martinsried, Germany

Dumitru A. Iacobas
Personalized Genomics Laboratory, CRI Center for Computational Systems Biology, Roy G Perry College of Engineering, Prairie View A&M University, Prairie View, TX 77446, USA

Stefan Schob and Karl-Titus Hoffmann
Department for Neuroradiology, University Hospital Leipzig, Leipzig 04103, Germany

Hans Jonas Meyer, Nikita Garnov and Alexey Surov
Department for Diagnostic and Interventional Radiology, University Hospital Leipzig, Leipzig 04103, Germany

Julia Dieckow
Department for Ophthalmology, University Hospital Leipzig, Leipzig 04103, Germany

Bhogal Pervinder and Diana Horvath-Rizea
Department for Diagnostic and Interventional Neuroradiology, Katharinenhospital Stuttgart, Stuttgart 70174, Germany

Nikolaos Pazaitis
Institute for Pathology, University Hospital Halle-Wittenberg, Martin-Luther-University Halle-Wittenberg, Halle 06112, Germany

Anne Kathrin Höhn
Institute for Pathology, University Hospital Leipzig, Leipzig 04103, Germany

Luís S. Santos
Centre for Toxicogenomics and Human Health (ToxOmics), Genetics, Oncology and Human Toxicology, NOVA Medical School; Faculdade de Ciências Médicas, Universidade Nova de Lisboa, 1169-056 Lisboa, Portugal
Institute of Health Sciences (ICS), Center for Interdisciplinary Research in Health (CIIS), Universidade Católica Portuguesa, 3504-505 Viseu, Portugal

Octávia M. Gil
Centro de Ciências e Tecnologias Nucleares, Instituto Superior Técnico, Universidade de Lisboa, 2695-066 Bobadela, Loures, Portugal

Teresa C. Ferreira
Serviço de Medicina Nuclear, Instituto Português de Oncologia de Lisboa (IPOLFG), 1099-023 Lisboa, Portugal

Edward Limbert
Serviço de Endocrinologia, Instituto Português de Oncologia de Lisboa (IPOLFG), 1099-023 Lisboa, Portugal

Susana N. Silva, Bruno C. Gomes and José Rueff
Centre for Toxicogenomics and Human Health (ToxOmics), Genetics, Oncology and Human Toxicology, NOVA Medical School; Faculdade de Ciências Médicas, Universidade Nova de Lisboa, 1169-056 Lisboa, Portugal

Bartosz Wojtas
Department of Nuclear Medicine and Endocrine Oncology, Maria Sklodowska-Curie Institute—Oncology Center, Gliwice Branch, Wybrzeze Armii Krajowej 15, 44-101 Gliwice, Poland
Laboratory of Molecular Neurobiology, Neurobiology Center, Nencki Institute of Experimental Biology, Pasteura 3, 02-093 Warsaw, Poland

Aleksandra Pfeifer
Department of Nuclear Medicine and Endocrine Oncology, Maria Sklodowska-Curie Institute—Oncology Center, Gliwice Branch, Wybrzeze Armii Krajowej 15, 44-101 Gliwice, Poland
Faculty of Automatic Control, Electronics and Computer Science, Silesian University of Technology, Akademicka 2A, 44-100 Gliwice, Poland

Agnieszka Czarniecka
The Oncologic and Reconstructive Surgery Clinic, Maria Sklodowska-Curie Institute—Oncology Center, Gliwice Branch, Wybrzeze Armii Krajowej 15, 44-101 Gliwice, Poland

Markus Eszlinger
Department of Oncology & Arnie Charbonneau Cancer Institute, Cumming School of Medicine, University of Calgary, Calgary, AB T2N 4N1, Canada

Thomas Musholt
Department of General, Visceral and Transplantation Surgery, University Medical Center of the Johannes Gutenberg University, D55099 Mainz, Germany

Tomasz Stokowy
Department of Nuclear Medicine and Endocrine Oncology, Maria Sklodowska-Curie Institute – Oncology Center, Gliwice Branch, Wybrzeze Armii Krajowej 15, 44-101 Gliwice, Poland
Faculty of Automatic Control, Electronics and Computer Science, Silesian University of Technology, Akademicka 2A, 44-100 Gliwice, Poland
Department of Clinical Science, University of Bergen, 5020 Bergen, Norway

Michal Swierniak
Department of Nuclear Medicine and EndocrineOncology, Maria Sklodowska-Curie Institute – Oncology Center, Gliwice Branch, Wybrzeze Armii Krajowej 15, 44-101 Gliwice, Poland
Genomic Medicine, Department of General, Transplant and Liver Surgery, Medical University of Warsaw, Zwirki iWigury 61, 02-093 Warsaw, Poland

Ewa Stobiecka, Ewa Chmielik and Dariusz Lange
Tumor Pathology Department, Maria Sklodowska-Curie Institute – Oncology Center, Gliwice Branch, Wybrzeze Armii Krajowej 15, 44-101 Gliwice, Poland

Steffen Hauptmann
Department of Pathology, Martin Luther University Halle-Wittenberg, 06108 Halle (Saale), Germany

Michal Jarzab
III Department of Radiotherapy and Chemotherapy, Maria Sklodowska-Curie Institute – Oncology Center, Gliwice Branch, Wybrzeze Armii Krajowej 15, 44-101 Gliwice, Poland

Ralf Paschke
Division of Endocrinology, Departments of Medicine, Pathology, Biochemistry & Molecular Biology and Oncology and Arnie Charbonneau Cancer Institute, Cumming School of Medicine, University of Calgary, Calgary, Alberta T2N 4N1, Canada

Malgorzata Oczko-Wojciechowska, Jolanta Krajewska, Aleksandra Kukulska, Dagmara Rusinek, Tomasz Tyszkiewicz, Monika Halczok and Barbara Jarzab
Department of Nuclear Medicine and Endocrine Oncology, Maria Sklodowska-Curie Institute – Oncology Center, Gliwice Branch, Wybrzeze Armii Krajowej 15, 44-101 Gliwice, Poland

Xingyun Su, Weibin Wang and Lisong Teng
Department of Surgical Oncology, First Affiliated Hospital, School of Medicine, Zhejiang University, Hangzhou 310003, China

Guodong Ruan
Department of Oncology, the Second Hospital of Shaoxing, Shaoxing 312000, China

Min Liang, Jing Zheng, Ye Chen and Minxin Guan
Institute of Genetics, School of Medicine, Zhejiang University, Hangzhou 310058, China

Huiling Wu
Department of Plastic Surgery, First Affiliated Hospital, School of Medicine, Zhejiang University, Hangzhou 310003, China

Thomas J. Fahey III
Department of Surgery, New York Presbyterian Hospital and Weill Medical College of Cornell University, New York, NY 10021, USA

Young Sin Ko
Diagnostic Pathology Center, Seegene Medical Foundation, Seoul KS013, Korea
Molecular Genetics and Pathology, Department of Medicine, Graduate School of Konkuk University, Seoul KS013, Korea

Tae Sook Hwang, Hye Seung Han and Wan Seop Kim
Molecular Genetics and Pathology, Department of Medicine, Graduate School of Konkuk University, Seoul KS013, Korea
Department of Pathology, Konkuk University School of Medicine, Seoul KS013, Korea

Ja Yeon Kim
Department of Pathology, Konkuk University School of Medicine, Seoul KS013, Korea

Yoon-La Choi
Department of Pathology and Translational Genomics, Samsung Medical Center, Sungkyunkwan University School of Medicine, Seoul KS013, Korea

Seung Eun Lee
Department of Pathology, Konkuk University Medical Center, Seoul KS013, Korea

Suk Kyeong Kim
Department of Internal Medicine, Konkuk University School of Medicine, Seoul KS013, Korea

Kyoung Sik Park
Department of Surgery, Konkuk University School of Medicine, Seoul KS013, Korea

Florian Steiner and Cornelia Hauser-Kronberger
Department of Pathology, Paracelsus Medical University Salzburg, Müllner Hauptstrasse 48, A-5020 Salzburg, Austria

Gundula Rendl, Margarida Rodrigues and Christian Pirich
Department of Nuclear Medicine and Endocrinology, Paracelsus Medical University Salzburg, Müllner Hauptstrasse 48, A-5020 Salzburg, Austria

Soo-Hwan Byun
Department of Oral & Maxillofacial Surgery, Dentistry, Hallym University College of Medicine, Anyang 14068, Korea
Research Center of Clinical Dentistry, Hallym University Clinical Dentistry Graduate School, Chuncheon 24252, Korea

Chanyang Min
Hallym Data Science Laboratory, Hallym University College of Medicine, Anyang 14068, Korea

Hyo-Geun Choi
Research Center of Clinical Dentistry, Hallym University Clinical Dentistry Graduate School, Chuncheon 24252, Korea
Hallym Data Science Laboratory, Hallym University College of Medicine, Anyang 14068, Korea
Department of Otorhinolaryngology-Head & Neck Surgery, Hallym University College of Medicine, Anyang 14068, Korea

Seok-Jin Hong
Research Center of Clinical Dentistry, Hallym University Clinical Dentistry Graduate School, Chuncheon 24252, Korea
Department of Otorhinolaryngology-Head & Neck Surgery, Hallym University College of Medicine, Dongtan 18450, Korea

Paola Caria, Daniela Virginia Frau, Roberta Vanni and Tinuccia Dettori
Department of Biomedical Sciences, University of Cagliari, Cittadella Universitaria, Monserrato 09042, Italy

Index

Printed in the USA
CPSIA information can be obtained
at www.ICGtesting.com
JSHW051408091023
49903JS00006B/333